TWELFTH EDITION

FIT&WELL

BRIEF EDITION

Core Concepts and Labs in Physical Fitness and Wellness

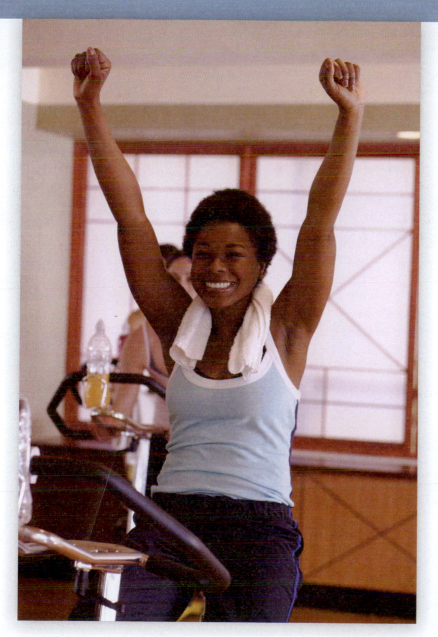

Thomas D. Fahey
California State University, Chico

Paul M. Insel
Stanford University

Walton T. Roth
Stanford University

Claire E. A. Insel
California Institute of Human Nutrition

McGraw
Hill
Education

FIT & WELL: CORE CONCEPTS AND LABS IN PHYSICAL FITNESS AND WELLNESS, BRIEF EDITION, TWELFTH EDITION

Published by McGraw-Hill Education, 2 Penn Plaza, New York, NY 10121. Copyright © 2017 by McGraw-Hill Education. All rights reserved. Printed in the United States of America. Previous editions © 2015, 2013, and 2011. No part of this publication may be reproduced or distributed in any form or by any means, or stored in a database or retrieval system, without the prior written consent of McGraw-Hill Education, including, but not limited to, in any network or other electronic storage or transmission, or broadcast for distance learning.

Some ancillaries, including electronic and print components, may not be available to customers outside the United States.

This book is printed on acid-free paper.

1 2 3 4 5 6 7 8 9 0 DOW/DOW 1 0 9 8 7 6

ISBN 978-1-25-975126-4
MHID 1-25-975126-0

Senior Vice President, Products & Markets: *Kurt L. Strand*
Vice President, General Manager, Products & Markets: *Michael Ryan*
Vice President, Content Design & Delivery: *Kimberly Meriwether David*
Managing Director: *Gina Boedeker*
Director, Product Development: *Meghan Campbell*
Product Developer: *Kirstan Price*
Marketing Manager: *Philip Weaver*
Lead Product Developer: *Rhona Robbin*
Digital Product Developer: *Jessica Portz*
Director, Content Design & Delivery: *Terri Schiesl*
Program Manager: *Marianne Musni*
Content Project Managers: *Rick Hecker/Katie Klochan*
Buyer: *Jennifer Pickel*
Design: *iSrdj Savanovic*
Content Licensing Specialists: *Shawntel Schmitt/Jacob Sullivan*
Cover Image: © *Erik Isakson/Getty Images*
Compositor: *SPi Global*
Printer: *R. R. Donnelley*
All credits appearing on page or at the end of the book are considered to be an extension of the copyright page.

The Internet addresses listed in the text were accurate at the time of publication. The inclusion of a website does not indicate an endorsement by the authors or McGraw-Hill Education, and McGraw-Hill Education does not guarantee the accuracy of the information presented at these sites.

BRIEF CONTENTS

CONTENTS

BOXES

LABORATORY ACTIVITIES

The laboratory activities are also found in an interactive format in Connect (connect.mheducation.com).

LEARN WITHOUT LIMITS

McGraw-Hill Connect®

McGraw-Hill Connect® is a digital teaching and learning environment that improves performance over a variety of critical outcomes; it is easy to use; and it is proven effective. Connect® empowers students by continually adapting to deliver precisely what they need, when they need it, and how they need it, so your class time is more engaging and effective. Connect for *Fit & Well* offers a wealth of interactive online content, including fitness labs and self-assessments, video activities on timely health topics and exercise technique, a behavior-change workbook, and practice quizzes with immediate feedback.

Connect INSIGHT™

Connect Insight® is Connect's new one-of-a-kind visual analytics dashboard—now available for both instructors and students—that provides at-a-glance information regarding student performance, which is immediately actionable. By presenting assignment, assessment, and topical performance results together with a time metric that is easily visible for aggregate or individual results, Connect Insight gives the user the capability to take a just-in-time approach to teaching and learning, which was never before available. Connect Insight presents data that empowers students and helps instructors improve class performance in a way that is efficient and effective.

SMARTBOOK®

Available within Connect, **SmartBook**® makes study time as productive and efficient as possible by identifying and closing knowledge gaps. SmartBook is powered by the proven **LearnSmart**® engine, which identifies what an individual student knows and doesn't know based on the student's confidence level, responses to questions, and other factors. LearnSmart builds an optimal, personalized learning path for each student, so students spend less time on concepts they already understand and more time on those they don't. As a student engages with SmartBook, the reading experience continuously adapts by highlighting the most impactful content a student needs to learn at that moment in time. This ensures that every minute spent with SmartBook is returned to the student as the most value-added minute possible. The result? More confidence, better grades, and greater success.

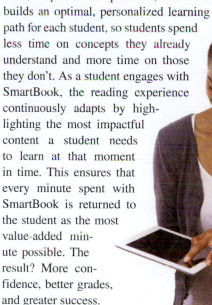

PROVEN, SCIENCE-BASED CONTENT

The digital teaching and learning tools within Connect are built on the solid foundation of *Fit & Well*'s authoritative, science-based content. *Fit & Well* is written by experts who work and teach in the fields of exercise science, physical education, and health education. *Fit & Well* provides accurate, reliable current information on key health and fitness topics while also addressing issues related to mind-body health, diversity, gender, research, and consumer health.

Wellness in the Digital Age sections focus on the many fitness- and wellness-related devices and applications that are appearing every day.

Diversity Matters features address the ways that our biological and cultural differences influence our health strengths, risks, and behaviors.

Evidence for Exercise sections demonstrate that physical activity and exercise recommendations are based on solid scientific evidence.

Fitness Tips and **Wellness Tips** catch students' attention and get them thinking about—and acting to improve—their fitness and wellness.

Critical Consumer boxes help students navigate the numerous and diverse set of health-related products currently available.

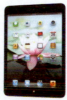
Hands-on lab activities give students the opportunity to assess their current level of fitness and wellness and to create their own individualized programs for improvement.

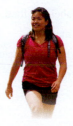
Take Charge features provide a wealth of practical advice for students on how to apply concepts from the text to their own lives.

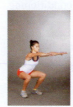
Exercise photos and online videos demonstrate exactly how to correctly perform exercises described in the text.

CHAPTER-BY-CHAPTER CHANGES

Changes to the twelfth edition reflect new research findings, updated statistics, and current hot topics that impact students' fitness and wellness behaviors. Revisions were also guided by student performance data anonymously collected from the tens of thousands of students who have used LearnSmart with *Fit & Well*. Because virtually every text paragraph is tied to several questions that students answer while using LearnSmart, the specific concepts that students are having the most difficulty with can be pinpointed through empirical data.

Chapter 1: Introduction to Wellness, Fitness, and Lifestyle Management

- Discussions of dimensions of wellness expanded to include cultural and occupational wellness
- All statistics updated to reflect the latest information on causes of death, life expectancy, and measures of quality of life
- New section on the Affordable Care Act

Chapter 2: Principles of Physical Fitness
- New Take Charge feature on reducing sedentary behaviors
- Updated information on medical clearance and risks from exercise

Chapter 3: Cardiorespiratory Endurance
- New Take Charge feature on high-intensity conditioning programs
- Updated coverage of warm-up and cool-down, high-intensity interval training, and cross-training

Chapter 4: Muscular Strength and Endurance
- New table summarizing pros and cons of stability balls
- Updated coverage of core training

Chapter 5: Flexibility and Low-Back Health
- Updated coverage of static and dynamic stretching and exercise safety for back pain
- New illustration of core musculature

Chapter 6: Body Composition
- Updated statistics on overweight and obesity in U.S. adults
- Updated and expanded coverage of diabetes

Chapter 7: Putting Together a Complete Fitness Program
- New Evidence for Exercise feature on the importance of reducing sedentary time
- Updated coverage of apps for tracking and motivation during a fitness program

Chapter 8: Nutrition
- Incorporation of information from the Scientific Report of the 2015 Dietary Guidelines Advisory Committee
- New tables summarizing recommended healthy dietary patterns, including vegetarian and Mediterranean patterns
- New Take Charge feature on making positive dietary changes
- Discussion of new FDA requirements for labels on food packaging, in restaurants, and for vending machines
- Expanded coverage of added sugars and updated discussion of dietary fats, including the FDA ban on trans fats

YOUR COURSE, YOUR WAY

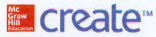

McGraw-Hill Create® is a self-service website that allows you to create customized course materials using McGraw-Hill Education's comprehensive, cross-disciplinary content and digital products. You can even access third party content such as readings, articles, cases, videos, and more.

- Select and arrange content to fit your course scope and sequence
- Upload your own course materials
- Select the best format for your students—print or eBook
- Select and personalize your cover
- Edit and update your materials as often as you'd like

Experience how McGraw-Hill Education's Create empowers you to teach your students your way: http://www.mcgrawhillcreate.com.

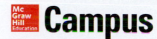

McGraw-Hill Campus® is a groundbreaking service that puts world-class digital learning resources just a click away for all faculty and students. All faculty—whether or not they use a McGraw-Hill title—can instantly browse, search, and access the entire library of McGraw-Hill instructional resources and services, including eBooks, test banks, PowerPoint slides, animations and learning objects—from any Learning Management System (LMS), at no additional cost to an institution. Users also have single sign-on access to McGraw-Hill digital platforms, including Connect, Create, and Tegrity, a fully automated lecture caption solution.

INSTRUCTOR RESOURCES

Instructor resources available through Connect for *Fit & Well* include a Course Integrator Guide, Test Bank, and PowerPoint presentations for each chapter.

ACKNOWLEDGMENTS

Fit & Well has benefited from the thoughtful commentary, expert knowledge, and helpful suggestions of many people. We are deeply grateful for their participation in the project.

Academic Advisors and Reviewers
Grady Armstrong, *Salisbury University*
David Campbell, *Concord University*
Renee Frimming, *University of Southern Indiana*

Christopher M. Keshock, *University of Southern Alabama*
Justin Kraft, *Missouri Western State University*
Lynn Hunt Long, *University of North Carolina at Wilmington*
Bradford Moore, *Pacific Lutheran University*
Joseph Mundt, *Kansas City Kansas Community College*
Susan Peterson, *Linn-Benton Community College*
Beverly D. Pittman, *Northern Virginia Community College*
Sheila Stepp, *SUNY Orange*

FIT&WELL

Core Concepts and Labs in Physical Fitness and Wellness

Introduction to Wellness, Fitness, and Lifestyle Management

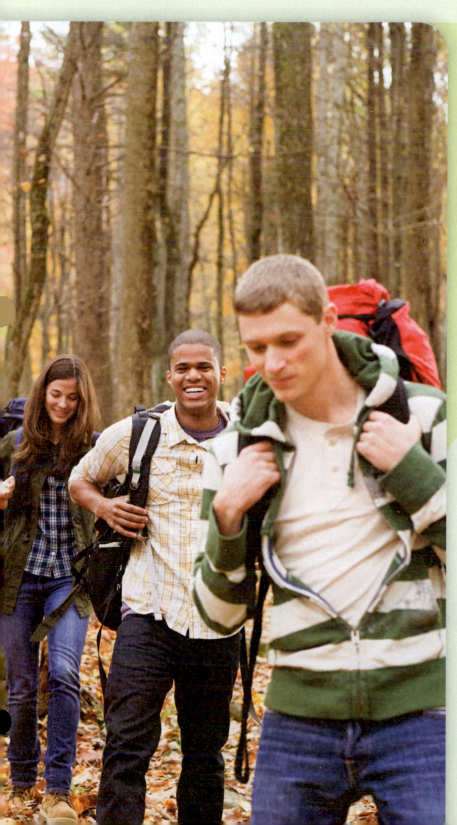

LOOKING AHEAD...

After reading this chapter, you should be able to

- Describe the dimensions of wellness.

- Identify the major health problems in the United States today and discuss their causes.

- Describe the behaviors that are part of a wellness lifestyle.

- Explain the steps in creating a behavior management plan to change a wellness-related behavior.

- List some of the available sources of wellness information and explain how to think critically about them.

TEST YOUR KNOWLEDGE

1. Which of the following lifestyle factors is the leading preventable cause of death for Americans?
   a. excess alcohol consumption
   b. cigarette smoking
   c. obesity

2. The terms *health* and *wellness* mean the same thing. True or false?

3. A person's genetic makeup determines whether he or she will develop certain diseases (such as breast cancer), regardless of that person's health habits. True or false?

See answers on the next page.

A college sophomore sets the following goals for herself:

- Join new social circles and make new friends whenever possible.
- Exercise every day.
- Clean up trash and plant trees in blighted neighborhoods in her community.

These goals may differ, but they have one thing in common. Each contributes, in its own way, to this student's health and well-being. Not satisfied merely to be free of illness, she wants more. She has decided to live actively and fully—not just to be healthy, but to pursue a state of overall wellness.

WELLNESS: NEW HEALTH GOALS

Generations of people have viewed health simply as the absence of disease, and that view largely prevails today. The word **health** typically refers to the overall condition of a person's body or mind and to the presence or absence of illness or injury. **Wellness** expands this idea of health to include our ability to achieve optimal health. Beyond the simple presence or absence of disease, wellness refers to optimal health and vitality—to living life to its fullest. Although we use the terms

health and *wellness* interchangeably, there are two important differences between them:

- Health—or some aspects of it—can be determined or influenced by factors beyond your control, such as your genes, age, and family history. For example, a man with a strong family history of prostate cancer will have a higher-than-average risk for developing prostate cancer himself.
- Wellness is largely determined by the decisions you make about how you live. That same man can reduce his risk of cancer by eating sensibly, exercising, and having regular screening tests. Even if he develops the disease, he may still rise above its effects to live a rich, meaningful life. This means not only caring for himself physically, but also maintaining a positive outlook, keeping up his relationships with others, challenging himself intellectually, and nurturing other aspects of his life.

Enhanced wellness, therefore, involves making conscious decisions to control **risk factors** that contribute to disease or injury. Age and family history are risk factors you cannot control. Behaviors such as choosing not to smoke, exercising, and eating a healthy diet are well within your control.

The Dimensions of Wellness

Here are nine dimensions of wellness:

- Physical
- Emotional
- Intellectual
- Interpersonal
- Cultural
- Spiritual
- Environmental
- Financial
- Occupational

Each dimension of wellness affects the others. Further, the process of achieving wellness is constant and dynamic (Figure 1.1), involving change and growth. Ignoring any dimension of wellness can have harmful effects on your life.

FIGURE 1.1 The wellness continuum.
The concept of wellness includes vitality in nine interrelated dimensions, all of which contribute to overall wellness.

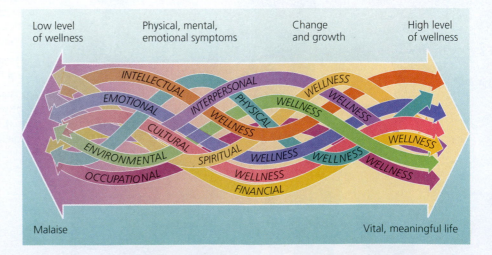

PHYSICAL WELLNESS	EMOTIONAL WELLNESS	INTELLECTUAL WELLNESS
• Eating well • Exercising • Avoiding harmful habits • Practicing safer sex • Recognizing symptoms of disease • Getting regular checkups • Avoiding injuries	• Optimism • Trust • Self-esteem • Self-acceptance • Self-confidence • Ability to understand and accept one's feelings • Ability to share feelings with others	• Openness to new ideas • Capacity to question • Ability to think critically • Motivation to master new skills • Sense of humor • Creativity • Curiosity • Lifelong learning
INTERPERSONAL WELLNESS	CULTURAL WELLNESS	SPIRITUAL WELLNESS
• Communication skills • Capacity for intimacy • Ability to establish and maintain satisfying relationships • Ability to cultivate a support system of friends and family	• Creating relationships with those who are different from you • Maintaining and valuing your own cultural identity • Avoiding stereotyping based on ethnicity, gender, religion, or sexual orientation	• Capacity for love • Compassion • Forgiveness • Altruism • Joy and fulfillment • Caring for others • Sense of meaning and purpose • Sense of belonging to something greater than oneself
ENVIRONMENTAL WELLNESS	FINANCIAL WELLNESS	OCCUPATIONAL WELLNESS
• Having abundant, clean natural resources • Maintaining sustainable development • Recycling whenever possible • Reducing pollution and waste	• Having a basic understanding of how money works • Living within one's means • Avoiding debt, especially for unnecessary items • Saving for the future and for emergencies	• Enjoying what you do • Feeling valued by your manager • Building satisfying relationships with co-workers • Taking advantage of opportunities to learn and be challenged

FIGURE 1.2 **Qualities and behaviors associated with the dimensions of wellness.**

The following sections briefly introduce the dimensions of wellness. Figure 1.2 lists some of the specific qualities and behaviors associated with each dimension. Lab 1.1 will help you learn what wellness means to you and where you fall on the wellness continuum.

Physical Wellness Your physical wellness includes not just your body's overall condition and the absence of disease, but your fitness level and your ability to care for yourself. The higher your fitness level (which is discussed throughout this book), the higher your level of physical wellness will be. Similarly, as you take better care of your own physical needs, you ensure greater physical wellness. To achieve optimum physical wellness, you need to make choices that help you avoid illnesses and injuries. The decisions you make now—and the habits you develop over your lifetime—will largely determine the length and quality of your life.

Emotional Wellness Your emotional wellness reflects your ability to understand and deal with your feelings. Emotional wellness involves attending to your own thoughts and feelings, monitoring your reactions, and identifying obstacles to emotional stability. *Self-acceptance* is your personal satisfaction with yourself, which might exclude society's expectations, whereas *self-esteem* relates to the way you think others perceive you. *Self-confidence* can be a part of both acceptance and esteem. Achieving this type of wellness means finding solutions to emotional problems, with professional help if necessary.

Intellectual Wellness Those who enjoy intellectual wellness constantly challenge their minds. An active mind is essential to wellness because it detects problems, finds solutions, and directs behavior. People who enjoy intellectual wellness never stop learning. They seek out and relish new experiences and challenges.

Interpersonal Wellness Satisfying and supportive relationships are important to physical and emotional wellness. Learning good communication skills, developing the capacity for intimacy, and cultivating a supportive network are all important to interpersonal (or social) wellness. Social wellness requires participating in and contributing to your community and to society.

Cultural Wellness Cultural wellness refers to the way you interact with others who are different from you in terms of ethnicity, religion, gender, sexual orientation, age, and customs (practices). It involves creating relationships with others and suspending judgment on others' behavior until you have lived

health The overall condition of body or mind and the presence or absence of illness or injury.

wellness Optimal health and vitality, encompassing all dimensions of well-being.

risk factor A condition that increases one's chances of disease or injury.

TERMS

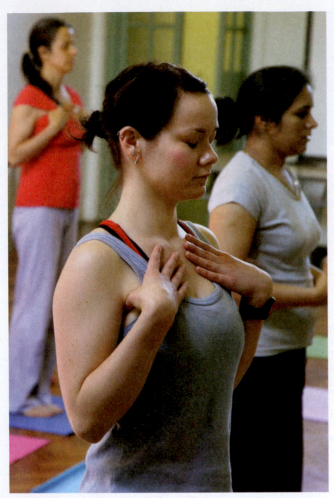

Wellness Tip Enhancing one dimension of wellness can have positive effects on others. For example, joining a meditation group can help you enhance your spiritual well-being, but it can also affect the emotional and interpersonal dimensions of wellness by enabling you to meet new people and develop new friendships.

with them or "walked in their shoes." It also includes accepting, valuing, and even celebrating the different cultural ways people interact in the world. The extent to which you maintain and value cultural identities is one measure of cultural wellness.

Spiritual Wellness To enjoy spiritual wellness is to possess a set of guiding beliefs, principles, or values that give meaning and purpose to your life, especially in difficult times. The well person uses spirituality to focus on positive aspects of life and to fend off negative feelings such as cynicism, anger, and pessimism. Organized religions help many people develop spiritual health. Religion, however, is not the only source or form of spiritual wellness. Many people find meaning and purpose in their lives on their own—through nature, art, meditation, or good works—or with their loved ones.

> **infectious disease** A disease that can spread from person to person; caused by microorganisms such as bacteria and viruses. **TERMS**

Environmental Wellness Your environmental wellness is defined by the livability of your surroundings. Personal health depends on the health of the planet—from the safety of the food supply to the degree of violence in society. To improve your environmental wellness, you can learn about and protect yourself against hazards in your surroundings and work to make your world a cleaner and safer place.

Financial Wellness Financial wellness refers to your ability to live within your means and manage your money in a way that gives you peace of mind. It includes balancing your income and expenses, staying out of debt, saving for the future, and understanding your emotions about money. For more on this topic, see the box "Financial Wellness".

Occupational Wellness Occupational wellness refers to the level of happiness and fulfillment you gain through your work. Although high salaries and prestigious titles are gratifying, they alone generally do not bring about occupational wellness. An occupationally well person truly likes his or her work, feels a connection with others in the workplace, and takes advantage of opportunities to learn and be challenged. Another important aspect of occupational wellness is recognition from managers and colleagues. An ideal job draws on your interests and passions, as well as your vocational skills, and allows you to feel that you are making a contribution in your everyday work.

New Opportunities for Taking Charge

A century ago, Americans considered themselves lucky just to survive to adulthood (Figure 1.3). A child born in 1900, for example, could expect to live only about 47 years. Many people died from common **infectious diseases** (such as pneumonia, tuberculosis, or diarrhea) and poor environmental conditions (such as water pollution and poor sanitation).

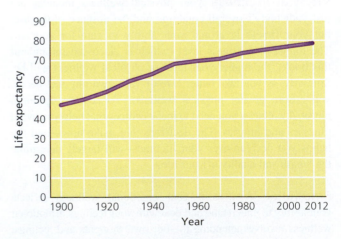

FIGURE 1.3 Life expectancy of Americans from birth, 1900–2011.
SOURCE: http://www.cdc.gov/nchs/data/nvsr/nvsr63/nvsr63_09.pdf, Table 10: Number of deaths from 113 selected causes, Enterocolitis due to Clostridium difficile, drug-induced causes, alcohol-induced causes, and injury by firearms, by age: United States, 2012.
[National Center for Health Statistics. Deaths: Final Data for 2013. *NVSR* Volume 64, Number 2 will be the final source, but it is forthcoming at time of editing]

With the news full of stories of home foreclosures, credit card debt, and personal bankruptcies, it has become painfully clear that many Americans do not know how to manage their finances. You can avoid such stress—and gain financial peace of mind—by developing skills that contribute to financial wellness.

Financial wellness means having a healthy relationship with money. It involves knowing how to manage your money, using self-discipline to live within your means, using credit cards wisely, staying out of debt, meeting your financial obligations, having a long-range financial plan, and saving.

Learn to Budget

Although the word *budget* may conjure up thoughts of deprivation, a budget is just a way of tracking where your money goes and making sure you're spending it on the things that are most important to you. To start one, list your monthly income and your expenditures. If you aren't sure where you spend your money, track your expenses for a few weeks or a month. Then organize them into categories, such as housing, food, transportation, entertainment, services, personal care, clothes, books and school supplies, health care, credit card and loan payments, and miscellaneous. Use categories that reflect the way you actually spend your money. Knowing where your money goes is the first step in gaining control of it.

Now total your income and expenditures. Are you taking in more than you spend, or vice versa? Are you surprised by your spending patterns? Use this information to set guidelines and goals for yourself. If your expenses exceed your income, identify ways to make some cuts. For example, instead of paying for cable TV, you can stream news and entertainment shows from the Internet through your television or Blu-ray player. Or you can view programs online on Hulu.com and Netflix.com. If you spend money going out at night, consider less expensive options like having a weekly game night with friends or organizing an occasional potluck.

Use Credit Cards Wisely

College students are prime targets for credit card companies: Some students tend to be overconfident in their financial decisions and have easy access to credit but little training in finance. The consequences of enhanced lifestyles and peer competition raise the risk of serious financial problems. Thus, the government passed the Credit Card Accountability, Responsibility, and Disclosure Act of 2009 to require people age 21 and younger to have a guarantor cosign their credit card applications to ensure they can make their payments. Students who learn about finance from parents are more likely to pay off their credit card balance in full and regularly.

It is important to understand terms like *APR* (annual percentage rate—the interest you're charged on your balance), *credit limit* (the maximum amount you can borrow at any one time), *minimum monthly payment* (the smallest payment your creditor will accept each month), *grace period* (the number of days you have to pay your bill before interest or penalties are charged), and *over-the-limit* and *late fees* (the amount you'll be charged if your payment is late or you go over your credit limit).

Get Out of Debt

A 2011 study indicated that graduating college students often had debts of $25,250 and that this number would likely increase by several thousand dollars over the next several years. If you have credit card debt, stop using your cards and start paying them off. If you can't pay the whole balance, at least try to pay more than the minimum payment each month. It can take a very long time to pay off a loan by making only the minimum payments. For example, to pay off a credit card balance of $2,000 at 10% interest with monthly payments of $20 would take 203 months—17 years. Check out an online credit card calculator like http://www.bankrate.com/calculators/credit-cards/balance-debt-payoff-calculator.aspx. Note that by carrying a balance and incurring finance charges, you are also paying back much more than your initial loan.

Start Saving

The same miracle of compound interest that locks you into years of credit card debt can work to your benefit if you start saving early (for an online compound interest calculator, visit http://www.moneychimp.com/calculator/compound_interest_calculator.htm). Experts recommend "paying yourself first" every month—that is, putting some money into savings before you start paying your bills, depending on what your budget allows. You may want to save for a large purchase, or you may even be looking ahead to retirement. If you work for a company with a 401(k) retirement plan, contribute as much as you can every pay period.

Become Financially Literate

How well do you manage your money? Most Americans have not received basic financial training. For this reason, the U.S. government has established the Financial Literacy and Education Commission (MyMoney.gov) to help Americans learn how to save, invest, and manage money better, a skill called *financial literacy*. Developing lifelong financial skills should begin in early adulthood, during the college years, if not earlier.

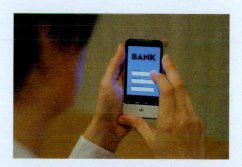

SOURCES: Smith, C., and G. A. Barboza. 2013. The role of trans-generational financial knowledge and self-reported financial literacy on borrowing practices and debt accumulation of college students. Social Science Electronic Publishing, Inc. (http://ssrn.com/abstract=2342168; Plymouth State University. 2013. Student Monetary Awareness and Responsibility Today! (http://www.plymouth.edu/office/financial-aid/smart/); U.S. Financial Literacy and Education Commission. 2013. MyMoney.gov (http://www.mymoney.gov).

connect

Since 1900, however, life expectancy has nearly doubled, and as of 2012, the average American's life expectancy was 78.8 years. This increase in life span is due largely to the development of vaccines and antibiotics to fight infections, and to public health measures to improve living conditions. But even though life expectancy has increased, poor health limits most Americans' activities during the last 15% of their lives, resulting in some sort of impaired life (Figure 1.4).

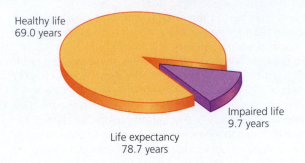

Healthy life
69.0 years

Impaired life
9.7 years

Life expectancy
78.7 years

FIGURE 1.4 Quantity of life versus quality of life. Years of healthy life as a proportion of life expectancy in the U.S. population.

SOURCE: National Center for Health Statistics. 2012. *Healthy People 2010 Final Review.* Hyattsville, MD.

Today, a different set of diseases has emerged as our major health threat: heart disease, cancer, and chronic lower respiratory diseases are now the three leading causes of death for Americans (Table 1.1). Treating such **chronic diseases** is costly and difficult.

The good news is that people have some control over whether they develop chronic diseases. People make choices every day that increase or decrease their risks for such diseases. These **lifestyle choices** include behaviors such as smoking, diet, exercise, and alcohol use. As Table 1.2 makes clear, lifestyle factors contribute to many deaths in the United States, and people can influence their own health risks. The need to make good choices is especially true for teens and young adults. For Americans age 15–24, for example, the top three causes of death are accidents, suicide, and homicide (Table 1.3).

National Health

Wellness is a personal concern, but the U.S. government has financial and humanitarian interests in it, too. A healthy population is the nation's source of vitality, creativity, and wealth. Poor health drains the nation's resources and raises health care costs for all.

Table 1.1	Leading Causes of Death in the United States, 2012

RANK	CAUSE OF DEATH	NUMBER OF DEATHS	PERCENTAGE OF TOTAL DEATHS	LIFESTYLE FACTORS
1	Heart disease	611,105	23.5	D I S A
2	Cancer	584,881	22.5	D I S A
3	Chronic lower respiratory diseases	149,205	5.7	■ ■ S ■
4	Unintentional injuries (accidents)	130,557	5.0	■ I S A
5	Stroke	128,978	5.0	D I S A
6	Alzheimer's disease	84,767	3.3	
7	Diabetes	75,578	2.9	D I S ■
8	Influenza and pneumonia	56,979	2.2	D I S A
9	Kidney disease	47,112	1.8	■ ■ S ■
10	Intentional self-harm (suicide)	41,149	1.6	■ ■ S A
11	Septicemia	38,156	1.5	■ ■ S A
12	Chronic liver disease and cirrhosis	36,427	1.4	■ ■ S A
13	Hypertension (high blood pressure)	30,770	1.2	D I S A
14	Parkinson's disease	25,196	1.0	
15	Lung inflammation due to inhaling solids and liquids	18,579	0.7	■ ■ S A
	All other causes	537,554		
	All causes	2,596,993	100.0	

Key					
	D	Diet plays a part		S	Smoking plays a part
	I	Inactive lifestyle plays a part		A	Excessive alcohol use plays a part

NOTE: Although not among the overall top 15 causes of death, HIV/AIDS is a major killer, responsible for 6,955 deaths in 2013. HIV/AIDS was the 13th leading cause of death for Americans aged 15–24 years and the 8th leading cause of death for those aged 25–44 years.

SOURCE: National Center for Health Statistics. 2015. Deaths: Final data for 2013. *National Vital Statistics Report 64*(2), http://www.cdc.gov/nchs/data/nvsr/nvsr64/nvsr64_02.pdf.

Table 1.2 — Key Contributors to Death among Americans

	NUMBER OF DEATHS PER YEAR	PERCENTAGE OF TOTAL DEATHS PER YEAR
Tobacco	481,000	18.5
Obesity-related deaths*	216,000	8.3
Alcohol	87,798	3.4
Microbial agents**	56,979	2.2
Illicit drug use	43,819	1.7
Unintentional poisonings	38,851	1.5
Motor vehicles	34,935	1.4
Firearms	33,636	1.3
Sexual behavior***	32,296	1.3

*The number of deaths due to obesity is an area of ongoing controversy and research. Recent estimates have ranged from 112,000 to 365,000.

**Microbial agents include bacterial and viral infections, such as influenza and pneumonia.

***The number of deaths due to sexual behavior includes deaths from HIV/AIDS, cervical cancer, and hepatitis B and C infections.

SOURCES: National Center for Health Statistics. 2014. Deaths: final data for 2013 (data release). *National Vital Statistics Report* 64(2); Stahre, M., et al. 2014. Contribution of excessive alcohol consumption to deaths and years of potential life lost in the United States. *Preventing Chronic Disease: Research, Practice, and Policy* 11:130293; U.S. Department of Health and Human Services. 2014. The health consequences of smoking—50 years of progress: a report of the surgeon general. Atlanta: U.S. Department of Health and Human Services, Centers for Disease Control and Prevention; American Cancer Society. 2015. Cervical cancer. Atlanta, GA: ACS; CDC. 2015. Disease burden from viral hepatitis A, B, and C in the United States. Atlanta, GA: Centers for Disease Control and Prevention

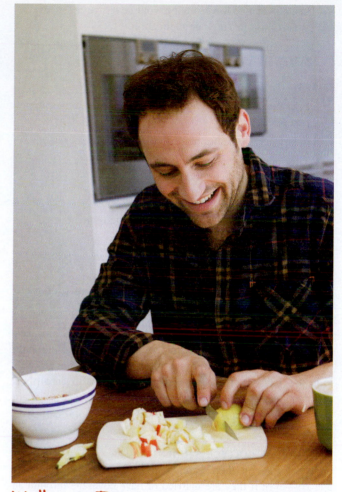

Wellness Tip In Table 1.1, notice how many causes of death are related to lifestyle. This is an excellent motivator for adopting healthy habits and staying in good condition. Maintaining physical fitness and a healthy diet can lead to a longer life. It's a fact!

Table 1.3 — Leading Causes of Death among Americans Age 15–24, 2012

RANK	CAUSE OF DEATH	NUMBER OF DEATHS	PERCENTAGE OF TOTAL DEATHS
1	Accidents	11,619	40.8
	Motor vehicle	6,692	23.5
	All other accidents	4,927	17.3
2	Suicide	4,874	17.1
3	Homicide	4,329	15.2
4	Cancer	1,496	5.3
5	Heart disease	941	3.3
	All causes	28,486	100.0

SOURCE: National Center for Health Statistics. 2015. Deaths: Final Data for 2013. *National Vital Statistics Report* 64(2), http://www.cdc.gov/nchs/data/nvsr/nvsr64/nvsr64_02.pdf.

The Affordable Care Act The Affordable Care Act (ACA), also called "Obamacare," was signed into law on March 23, 2010, and upheld by the Supreme Court in 2012 and 2015. The new law requires most people to obtain health insurance or pay a federal penalty. Here is a brief summary of the new law.

COVERAGE

- Health plans can no longer deny or limit benefits due to a pre-existing condition.
- If you are under 26, you may be eligible to be covered under your parent's health plan.

TERMS

chronic disease A disease that develops and continues over a long period of time, such as heart disease or cancer.

lifestyle choice A conscious behavior that can increase or decrease a person's risk of disease or injury; such behaviors include smoking, exercising, and eating a healthy diet.

- Insurers can no longer cancel your coverage because of honest mistakes in your application.
- If your plan denies payment, you are guaranteed the right to appeal.

COSTS

- Lifetime dollar limits on most benefits you receive are not permitted.
- Insurance companies must now publicly justify rate hikes.
- Your premium dollars must be spent primarily on health care—not administrative costs.

CARE

- Recommended preventive health services are covered with no copayment.
- From your plan's network, you can choose the primary care doctor you want.
- You can seek emergency care at a hospital outside your health plan's network.

FINDING A PLAN Under the ACA, a health insurance marketplace, also called health exchanges, facilitates the purchase of health insurance in every state. The health exchanges provide a selection of government-regulated health care plans that students and others may choose from. Those who are below income requirements are eligible for federal help with the premiums.

BENEFITS TO COLLEGE STUDENTS The ACA permits students to stay on their parents' health insurance plan until age 26—even if they are married or have coverage through an employer. Students not on their parents' plan who do not want to purchase insurance through their school can do so through the health insurance marketplace.

If you're under 30, you have the option of buying a "catastrophic" health plan. Such plans tend to have low premiums but require you to pay all medical costs up to a certain amount, usually several thousand dollars. The insurance company would pay for essential health benefits over that amount.

Students whose income is below a certain level may qualify for Medicaid. Check with your state. Individuals with non-immigrant status, which includes worker visas and student visas, qualify for insurance coverage through the exchanges.

You can browse plans and apply for coverage at HealthCare.gov.

The Healthy People Initiative The national Healthy People initiative aims to prevent disease and improve Americans' quality of life. Healthy People reports, published each decade since 1980, set national health goals based on 10-year agendas. The initiative's most recent iteration, *Healthy People 2020,* was developed in 2008–2009 and released to the public in 2010. *Healthy People 2020* envisions "a society in which all people live long, healthy lives" and proposes the eventual achievement of the following broad national health objectives:

- *Eliminate preventable disease, disability, injury, and premature death.* This objective involves taking more concrete steps to prevent diseases and injuries, promoting healthy lifestyle choices, improving the nation's preparedness for emergencies, and strengthening the public health infrastructure.
- *Achieve health equity, eliminate disparities, and improve the health of all groups.* This objective involves identifying, measuring, and addressing health differences between individuals or groups that result from social or economic disadvantage. (See the box "Wellness Issues for Diverse Populations.")
- *Create social and physical environments that promote good health for all.* This objective involves the use of health interventions at many levels (such as anti-smoking campaigns by schools, workplaces, and local agencies), providing a broader array of educational and job opportunities for undereducated and poor Americans, and actively developing healthier living and natural environments for everyone.
- *Promote healthy development and healthy behaviors across every stage of life.* This goal involves taking a cradle-to-grave approach to health promotion by encouraging disease prevention and healthy behaviors in Americans of all ages.

In a shift from the past, *Healthy People 2020* emphasizes the importance of health determinants—factors that affect the health of individuals, demographic groups, or entire populations. Health determinants are social (including factors such as ethnicity, education level, and economic status) and environmental (including natural and human-made environments). Thus, one goal is to improve living conditions in ways that reduce the impact of negative health determinants.

Table 1.4 shows examples of individual health promotion goals from *Healthy People 2020,* as well as estimates of how well Americans are achieving those goals.

Behaviors That Contribute to Wellness

A lifestyle based on good choices and healthy behaviors maximizes quality of life. It helps people avoid disease, remain strong and fit, and maintain their physical and mental health as long as they live.

Be Physically Active The human body is designed to be active. It readily adapts to nearly any level of activity and exertion. **Physical fitness** is a set of physical attributes that allows the body to respond or adapt to the demands and stress of physical effort. The more we ask of our bodies, the stronger and

physical fitness A set of physical attributes that allows the body to respond or adapt to the demands and stress of physical effort.

TERMS

DIVERSITY MATTERS
Wellness Issues for Diverse Populations

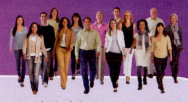

We all need to exercise, eat well, manage stress, and cultivate positive relationships. We all need to know how to protect ourselves from disease and injuries. But some of our differences—both as individuals and as members of groups—have important implications for wellness. These differences can be biological (determined genetically) or cultural (acquired as patterns of behavior through daily interactions with family, community, and society); many health conditions are a function of biology and culture combined. You share patterns of influences with others; and information about groups can be useful in identifying areas that may be of concern to you and your family. Wellness-related differences among groups can be described in terms of different characteristics, including the following:

Sex and Gender. *Sex* represents the biological and physiological characteristics that define men, women, and intersex people. *Gender* refers to the roles, behaviors, activities, and attributes that a given society considers appropriate for men and women. A person's gender is rooted in biology and physiology, but it is shaped by experience and environment—how society responds to individuals based on their sex. Examples of gender-related characteristics that affect wellness include higher rates of smoking and drinking among men and lower earnings among women compared with men doing similar work. Although men are more biologically likely than women to suffer from certain diseases (a sex issue), men are less likely to visit their physicians for regular exams (a gender issue). Men have higher rates of death from injuries, suicide, and homicide, whereas women are at greater risk for Alzheimer's disease and depression. Men and women also differ in body composition and certain aspects of physical performance.

Ethnicity. Compared with the U.S. population as a whole, American ethnic minorities have higher rates of death and disability from many causes. These disparities result from a complex mix of genetic variations, environmental factors, and health behaviors. Some diseases are concentrated in certain gene pools, the result of each ethnic group's relatively distinct history. Diabetes is more prevalent among individuals of Native American or Latino heritage, for example, and African Americans have higher rates of hypertension. Ethnic groups may vary in their traditional diets; their family and interpersonal relationships; their attitudes toward tobacco, alcohol, and other drugs; and their health beliefs and practices.

Income and Education. Of all the variables contributing to health status, inequalities in income and education are the most important. Income and education are closely related, and groups with the highest poverty rates and least education have the worst health status. These Americans have higher rates of infant mortality, traumatic injury, violent death, and many diseases. They are more likely to eat poorly, be overweight, smoke, drink, and use drugs. They are exposed to more day-to-day stressors and have less access to health care services.

Table 1.4	Selected *Healthy People 2020* Objectives			
OBJECTIVE	BASELINE (% MEETING GOAL IN 2008)	MOST RECENT PROGRESS (% MEETING GOAL IN 2012)	TARGET (% BY 2020)	PROGRESS
Increase proportion of people with health insurance	83.2	83.1	100.0	o
Help adults with hypertension get blood pressure under control	43.7	48.9	61.2	+
Reduce proportion of obese adults	33.9	35.3	30.5	−
Reduce proportion of adults who drank excessively in past 30 days	27.1	27.1	24.4	o
Increase proportion of adults who meet federal guidelines for aerobic physical activity and muscle strengthening	18.2	20.6	20.1	✓
Reduce proportion of adults who use cigarettes	20.6	18.2	12.0	+

✓ Target met   + Improving   o Insignificant or no change   − Getting worse

SOURCE: *Healthy People 2020 Leading Health Indicators: Progress Update, March 2014* (http://www.healthypeople.gov/sites/default/files/LHI-ProgressReport-ExecSum_0.pdf.)

more fit they become. When our bodies are not kept active, they deteriorate: Bones lose density, joints stiffen, muscles become weak, and cellular energy systems degenerate. To be truly well, human beings must be active.

Unfortunately, a **sedentary** lifestyle is common among Americans. According to a 2013 survey, only about half of adult Americans met the federal physical activity guidelines in 2013 (150 minutes or more per week of moderate aerobic exercise or 75 minutes per week of vigorous aerobic exercise). The older the adults, the less likely they met the guidelines.

The benefits of physical activity are both physical and mental, immediate and long term (Figure 1.5). In the short term, being physically fit makes it easier to do everyday tasks, such as lifting; it provides reserve strength for emergencies; and it helps people look and feel good. In the long term, being physically fit confers protection against chronic diseases and lowers the risk of dying prematurely. (See the box "Does Being Physically Active Make a Difference in How Long You Live?") Physically active people are less likely to develop or die from heart disease, respiratory disease, high blood pressure, cancer, osteoporosis, and type 2 diabetes (the most common form of diabetes). As they get older, they may be able to avoid weight gain, muscle and bone loss, fatigue, and other problems associated with aging.

Choose a Healthy Diet
In addition to being sedentary, many Americans have a diet that is too high in calories, unhealthy fats, and added sugars, as well as too low in fiber, complex carbohydrates, fruits, and vegetables. Like physical inactivity, this diet is linked to a number of chronic diseases. A healthy diet provides necessary nutrients and sufficient energy without also providing too much of the dietary substances linked to diseases.

- Increased endurance, strength, and flexibility
- Healthier muscles, bones, and joints
- Increased energy (calorie) expenditure
- Improved body composition
- More energy
- Improved ability to cope with stress
- Improved mood, higher self-esteem, and a greater sense of well-being
- Improved ability to fall asleep and sleep well

- Reduced risk of dying prematurely from all causes
- Reduced risk of developing and/or dying from heart disease, diabetes, high blood pressure, and colon cancer
- Reduced risk of becoming obese
- Reduced anxiety, tension, and depression
- Reduced risk of falls and fractures
- Reduced spending for health care

FIGURE 1.5 Benefits of regular physical activity.

Maintain a Healthy Body Weight
Overweight and obesity are associated with a number of disabling and potentially fatal conditions and diseases, including heart disease, cancer, and type 2 diabetes. The Centers for Disease Control and Prevention (CDC) estimates that obesity kills 112,000 Americans each year. Healthy body weight is an important part of wellness—but short-term dieting is not part of fitness or wellness. Maintaining a healthy body weight requires a lifelong commitment to regular exercise, a healthy diet, and effective stress management.

Manage Stress Effectively
Many people cope with stress by eating, drinking, or smoking too much. Others don't deal with it at all. In the short term, inappropriate stress management can lead to fatigue, sleep disturbances, and other symptoms. Over longer periods of time, poor stress management can lead to less efficient functioning of the immune system and increased susceptibility to disease. Learning to incorporate effective stress management techniques into daily life is an important part of a fit and well lifestyle.

Avoid Tobacco and Drug Use and Limit Alcohol Consumption
Tobacco use is associated with 8 of the top 10 causes of death in the United States; personal tobacco use and secondhand smoke kill nearly 500,000 Americans each year, more than any other behavioral or environmental factor. In 2012, 18% of adult Americans described themselves as current smokers. Lung cancer is the most common cause of cancer death among both men and women and one of the leading causes of death overall. On average, the direct health care costs associated with smoking exceed $133 billion per year. If the cost of lost productivity from sickness, disability, and premature death is included, the total is closer to $295 billion.

Excessive alcohol consumption is linked to 6 of the top 10 causes of death and results in about 88,000 deaths a year in the United States. The social, economic, and medical costs of alcohol abuse are estimated at more than $224 billion per year. Alcohol or drug intoxication is an especially notable factor in the death and disability of young people, particularly through **unintentional injuries** (such as drownings and car crashes caused by drunken driving) and violence.

Protect Yourself from Disease and Injury
The most effective way of dealing with disease and injury is to prevent them. Many of the lifestyle strategies discussed here help protect you against chronic illnesses. In addition, you can take specific steps to avoid infectious diseases, particularly those that are sexually transmitted.

Take Other Steps toward Wellness
Other important behaviors contribute to wellness, including these:

- Developing meaningful relationships
- Planning for successful aging
- Learning about the health care system
- Acting responsibly toward the environment

THE EVIDENCE FOR EXERCISE
Does Being Physically Active Make a Difference in How Long You Live?

How can we be sure that physical activity and exercise are good for our health? To answer this question, the U.S. Department of Health and Human Services asked a committee to review scientific literature. The committee's mission was to determine if enough evidence exists to warrant the government making physical activity recommendations to the public. The committee's report, the *Physical Activity Guidelines Advisory Committee Report, 2008,* summarizes the scientific evidence for the health benefits of regular physical activity and the risks of sedentary behavior. The report provides the rationale for the federal government's physical activity guidelines, and its findings were confirmed in the *Scientific Report of the 2015 Dietary Guidelines Committee.*

The Physical Activity Guidelines Advisory committee started by asking whether physical activity actually helps people live longer. The committee investigated the link between physical activity and all-cause mortality—deaths from all causes—by looking at 73 studies dating from 1995 to 2008. The studies included men and women from all age groups (16 to 65+) and from different racial and ethnic groups.

The data from these studies strongly support an *inverse relation* between physical activity and all-cause mortality; that is, physically active people were less likely to die during a study's follow-up period (ranging from 10 months to 28 years). The review found that active people have about a 30% lower risk of dying compared with inactive people. These inverse associations were found not just for healthy adults but also for older adults (age 65 and older), for people with coronary artery disease, diabetes, or impaired mobility, and for people who were overweight or obese. Poor fitness and low physical activity levels were found to be better predictors of premature death than smoking, diabetes, or obesity. Based on the evidence, the committee determined that about 150 minutes (2.5 hours) of physical activity per week is enough to reduce all-cause mortality (see Chapter 2 for more details). It appears that it is the overall volume of energy expended, no matter which kinds of activities are done, that makes a difference in risk of premature death.

The committee also looked at whether there is a *dose-response* relation between physical activity and all-cause mortality—that is, whether more activity reduces death rates even further. Again, the studies showed an inverse relation between these two variables. So, more activity above and beyond 150 minutes per week produces greater benefits. Surprisingly, for inactive people, benefits are seen at levels below 150 minutes per week. In fact, *any* increase in physical activity resulted in reduced risk of death. The committee refers to this as the "some is good; more is better" message. A target of 150 minutes per week is recommended, but any level of activity below the target is encouraged for inactive people.

Looking more closely at this relationship, the committee found that the greatest risk reduction is seen at the lower end of the physical activity spectrum (30 to 90 minutes per week). In fact, sedentary people who become more active have the greatest potential for improving health and reducing the risk of premature death. Additional risk reduction occurs as physical activity increases, but at a slower rate. For example, people who engaged in physical activity 90 minutes per week had a 20% reduction in mortality risk compared with inactive people, and those who were active 150 minutes per week, as noted earlier, had a 30% reduction in risk. But to achieve a 40% reduction in mortality risk, study participants had to be physically active 420 minutes per week (7 hours).

The message from the research is clear: It doesn't matter what activity you choose or even how much time you can devote to it per week, as long as you get moving!

SOURCE: 2015 Dietary Guidelines Advisory Committee. 2015. *Scientific Report of the 2015 Dietary Guidelines Advisory Committee.* Washington, D.C.: U.S. Department of Health and Human Services; Physical Activity Guidelines Advisory Committee. 2008. *Physical Activity Guidelines Advisory Committee Report, 2008.* Washington, D.C.: U.S. Department of Health and Human Services.

The Role of Other Factors in Wellness

Heredity, the environment, and adequate health care are other important influences on health and wellness. These factors can interact in ways that raise or lower the quality of a person's life and the risk of developing particular diseases. For example, a sedentary lifestyle combined with a genetic predisposition for diabetes can greatly increase a person's risk of developing the disease. If this sedentary, genetically predisposed person also lacks adequate health care, he or she is much more likely to suffer dangerous complications from diabetes.

Ask Yourself
QUESTIONS FOR CRITICAL THINKING AND REFLECTION
How often do you feel exuberant? Vital? Joyful? What makes you feel that way? Conversely, how often do you feel downhearted, de-energized, or depressed? What makes you feel that way? Have you ever thought about how you might increase experiences of vitality and decrease experiences of discouragement?

But in many cases, behavior can tip the balance toward health even if heredity or environment is a negative factor. Breast cancer, for example, can run in families, but it is also associated with overweight and a sedentary lifestyle. A woman with a family history of breast cancer is less likely to die from the disease if she controls her weight, exercises, performs regular breast self-exams, and consults with her physician about mammograms.

College Students and Wellness

Most college students appear to be healthy, but appearances can be deceiving. Each year, thousands of students lose productive academic time to physical and emotional health problems—some of which can continue for a lifetime. According to the Spring 2014 American College Health Association National College Health Assessment, the following were commonly reported factors affecting academic performance:

- Stress (30.3% of students affected)
- Anxiety (21.8%)
- Sleep difficulties (21.0%)
- Cold/flu/sore throat (15.1%)
- Depression (13.5%)
- Excessive use of Internet/computer games (11.6%)

Each of these factors is related to one or more dimensions of wellness, and most can be influenced by choices students make daily. For example, there are many ways to manage stress: By reducing unhealthy choices, such as using alcohol to relax, and by increasing healthy choices, such as using time management techniques, even busy students can reduce the impact of stress.

What about wellness choices in other areas? Students do not always make the best choices; the American College Health Association survey found the following:

- 63% of college students reported eating two or fewer servings of fruits and vegetables per day.
- 50% of students reported less than recommended amounts of exercise.
- 43% of students reported that they did not use a contraceptive the last time they had vaginal intercourse.
- 22% of students had seven or more drinks the last time they partied.
- 14% reported using prescription drugs that were not prescribed to them at some point in the past year.

How do your daily wellness choices compare to those of other students? What is recommended to promote wellness? Remember: It's never too late to change. The sooner you trade an unhealthy behavior for a healthier one, the longer you'll be around to enjoy the benefits.

> **behavior change** A lifestyle management process that involves cultivating healthy behaviors and working to overcome unhealthy ones. **TERMS**

REACHING WELLNESS THROUGH LIFESTYLE MANAGEMENT

Moving in the direction of wellness means cultivating healthy behaviors and working to overcome unhealthy ones. This approach to lifestyle management is called **behavior change**. As you may already know from experience, changing an unhealthy habit can be harder than it sounds. When you embark on a behavior change plan, it may seem like too much work at first. But as you make progress, you will gain confidence in your ability to take charge of your life. You will also experience the benefits of wellness—more energy, greater vitality, deeper feelings of appreciation and curiosity, and a higher quality of life.

The rest of this chapter outlines a general process for changing unhealthy behaviors that is backed by research and has worked for many people. You will also find many specific strategies and tips for change. For additional support, work through the activities in the Behavior Change Workbook at the end of the text.

Getting Serious about Your Health

Before you can start changing a wellness-related behavior, you have to know that the behavior is problematic and that you *can* change it. To make good decisions, you need information about relevant topics and issues, including what resources are available to help you change.

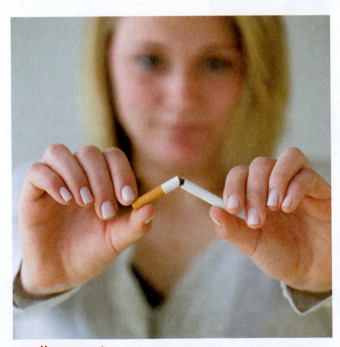

Wellness Tip Look for behavior change support if you need it. Certain health behaviors are exceptionally difficult to change. Some people can quit smoking on their own; others get help from a smoking cessation program or a nicotine replacement product.

CRITICAL CONSUMER
Evaluating Sources of Health Information

Surveys indicate that college students are smart about evaluating health information. They trust the health information they receive from health professionals and educators and are skeptical about popular information sources, such as magazine articles and websites.

How smart are you about evaluating health information? Here are some tips.

General Strategies

Whenever you encounter health-related information, take the following steps to make sure it is credible:

- **Go to the original source.** Media reports often simplify the results of medical research. Find out for yourself what a study really reported, and determine whether it was based on good science. What type of study was it? Was it published in a recognized medical journal? Was it an animal study, or did it involve people? Did the study include a large number of people? What did the study's authors actually report?

- **Watch for misleading language.** Reports that tout "breakthroughs" or "dramatic proof" are probably hype. A study may state that a behavior "contributes to" or is "associated with" an outcome, but this does not prove a cause-and-effect relationship.

- **Distinguish between research reports and public health advice.** Do not change your behavior based on the results of a single report or study. If an agency such as the National Cancer Institute urges a behavior change, however, you should follow its advice. Large, publicly funded organizations issue such advice based on many studies, not a single report.

- **Remember that anecdotes are not facts.** A friend may tell you he lost weight on some new diet, but individual success stories do not mean the plan is truly safe or effective. Check with your doctor before making any serious lifestyle changes.

- **Be skeptical.** If a report seems too good to be true, it probably is. Be wary of information contained in advertisements. An ad's goal is to sell a product, even if there is no need for it, and sometimes even if the product has not been proven to be safe or effective.

- **Make choices that are right for you.** Friends and family members can be a great source of ideas and inspiration, but you need to make health-related choices that work best for you.

Internet Resources

Online information sources pose special challenges. When reviewing a health-related website, ask these questions:

- **What is the source of the information?** Websites maintained by government agencies, professional associations, or established academic or medical institutions are likely to present trustworthy information. Many other groups and individuals post accurate information, but it is important to look at the qualifications of the people who are behind the site. (Check the home page or click the "About Us" link.)

- **How often is the site updated?** Look for sites that are updated frequently. Check the "last modified" date of any web page.

- **Is the site promotional?** Be wary of information from sites that sell specific products, use testimonials as evidence, appear to have a social or political agenda, or ask for money.

- **What do other sources say about a topic?** Be wary of claims and information that appear at only one site or come from a chat room, bulletin board, or blog.

- **Does the site conform to any set of guidelines or criteria for quality and accuracy?** Look for sites that identify themselves as conforming to some code or set of principles, such as those set forth by the Health on the Net Foundation or the American Medical Association. These codes include criteria such as use of information from respected sources and disclosure of the site's sponsors.

Examine Your Current Health Habits Have you considered how your current lifestyle is affecting your health today and how it will affect your health in the future? Do you know which of your current habits enhance your health and which ones may be harmful? Begin your journey toward wellness with self-assessment: Think about your own behavior, complete the self-assessment in Lab 1.2, and talk with friends and family members about what they've noticed about your lifestyle and your health.

Choose a Target Behavior Changing any behavior can be demanding. This is why it's a good idea to start small, by choosing one behavior you want to change—called a **target behavior**—and working on it until you succeed. Your chances of success will be greater if your first goal is simple, such as resisting the urge to snack between classes. As you change one behavior, make your next goal a little more significant, and build on your success over time.

Learn about Your Target Behavior After you've chosen a target behavior, you need to learn its risks and benefits for you—both now and in the future. As a starting point, use this text and the resources listed in the For Further Exploration section at

> **target behavior** An isolated behavior selected as the object of a behavior change program. **TERMS**

the end of each chapter; see the box "Evaluating Sources of Health Information" for additional guidelines. Ask these questions:

- How is your target behavior affecting your level of wellness today?
- Which diseases or conditions does this behavior place you at risk for?
- What effect would changing your behavior have on your health?

Find Help Have you identified a particularly challenging target behavior or mood—something like alcohol addiction, binge eating, or depression—that interferes with your ability to function or places you at a serious health risk? Help may be needed to change behaviors or conditions that are too deeply rooted or too serious for self-management. Don't be discouraged by the seriousness or extent of the problem; many resources are available to help you solve it. On campus, the student health center or campus counseling center can provide assistance. To locate community resources, consult yellowpages.com, your physician, or the Internet.

Building Motivation to Change

Knowledge is necessary for behavior change, but it isn't usually enough to make people act. Millions of people have sedentary lifestyles, for example, even though they know it's bad for their health. To succeed at behavior change, you need strong motivation.

Examine the Pros and Cons of Change Health behaviors have short-term and long-term benefits and costs. Consider the benefits and costs of an inactive lifestyle:

- *Short-term.* Such a lifestyle allows you more time to watch TV and hang out with friends, but it leaves you less fit and less able to participate in recreational activities.
- *Long-term.* This lifestyle increases the risk of heart disease, cancer, stroke, and premature death.

To successfully change your behavior, you must believe that the benefits of change outweigh the costs.

Carefully examine the pros and cons of continuing your current behavior and of changing to a healthier one. Focus on the effects that are most meaningful to you, including those tied to your personal identity and values. For example, engaging in regular physical activity and adequate sleep can support an image of yourself as an active person who is a good role model for others. To work toward being independent and taking control over your life, quitting smoking can be one way to eliminate a dependency. To complete your analysis, ask friends and family members about the effects of your behavior on them.

For example, a younger sister may tell you that your smoking habit influenced her decision to take up smoking.

The short-term benefits of behavior change can be an important motivating force. Although some people are motivated by long-term goals, such as avoiding a disease that may hit them in 30 years, most are more likely to be moved to action by shorter-term, more personal goals. Feeling better, doing better in school, improving at a sport, reducing stress, and increasing self-esteem are common short-term benefits of health behavior change. Many wellness behaviors are associated with immediate improvements in quality of life. For example, surveys of Americans have found that nonsmokers feel healthy and full of energy more days each month than do smokers, and they report fewer days of sadness and troubled sleep. The same is true when physically active people are compared with sedentary people. Over time, these types of differences add up to a substantially higher quality of life for people who engage in healthy behaviors.

Boost Self-Efficacy When you start thinking about changing a health behavior, a big factor in your eventual success is whether you have confidence in yourself and in your ability to change. **Self-efficacy** refers to your belief in your ability to successfully take action and perform a specific task. Strategies for boosting self-efficacy include developing an internal locus of control, using visualization and self-talk, and getting encouragement from supportive people.

LOCUS OF CONTROL Who do you believe is controlling your life? Is it your parents, friends, or school? Is it "fate"? Or is it you? **Locus of control** refers to the figurative place a person designates as the source of responsibility for the events in his or her life. People who believe they are in control of their own lives are said to have an *internal locus of control.* Those who believe that factors beyond their control determine the course of their lives are said to have an *external locus of control.*

For lifestyle management, an internal locus of control is an advantage because it reinforces motivation and commitment. An external locus of control can sabotage efforts to change

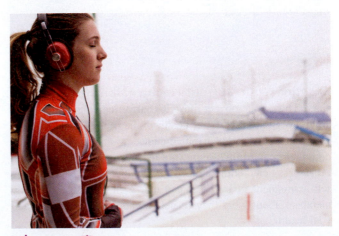

Fitness Tip Visualization is such a powerful technique that Olympic athletes learn how to harness it for peak performance. It works for average people, too. Set a small fitness goal, then imagine yourself doing it—as clearly and as often as you can. Visualization can help you believe in yourself, and belief can be a step toward success!

behavior. For example, if you believe that you are destined to die of breast cancer because your mother died from the disease, you may view monthly breast self-exams and regular checkups as a waste of time. In contrast, if you believe that you can take action to reduce your risk of breast cancer in spite of hereditary factors, you will be motivated to follow guidelines for early detection of the disease.

If you find yourself attributing too much influence to outside forces, gather more information about your wellness-related behaviors. List all the ways that making lifestyle changes will improve your health. If you believe you'll succeed, and if you recognize that you are in charge of your life, you're on your way to wellness.

VISUALIZATION AND SELF-TALK   One of the best ways to boost your confidence and self-efficacy is to visualize yourself successfully engaging in a new, healthier behavior. Imagine yourself going for an afternoon run three days a week or no longer smoking cigarettes. Also visualize yourself enjoying all the short-term and long-term benefits that your lifestyle change will bring. Create a new self-image: What will you and your life be like when you become a regular exerciser or a nonsmoker?

You can also use **self-talk**, the internal dialogue you carry on with yourself, to increase your confidence in your ability to change. Counter any self-defeating patterns of thought with more positive or realistic thoughts: "I am a strong, capable person, and I can maintain my commitment to change." See Chapter 10 for more on self-talk.

ROLE MODELS AND OTHER SUPPORTIVE INDIVIDUALS Social support can make a big difference in your level of motivation and your chances of success. Perhaps you know people who have reached the goal you are striving for; they could be role models or mentors, providing information and support for your efforts. Gain strength from their experiences, and tell yourself, "If they can do it, so can I." In addition, find a buddy who wants to make the same changes you do and who can take an active role in your behavior change program. For example, an exercise partner can provide companionship and encouragement when you might be tempted to skip your workout.

Identify and Overcome Barriers to Change Don't let past failures at behavior change discourage you; they can be a great source of information you can use to boost your chances of future success. Make a list of the problems and challenges you faced in any previous behavior change attempts. To this list, add the short-term costs of behavior change that you identified in your analysis of the pros and cons of change. After you've listed these key barriers to change, develop a practical plan for overcoming each one. For example, if you always smoke when you're with certain friends, decide in advance how you will turn down the next cigarette you are offered.

Enhancing Your Readiness to Change

The transtheoretical, or "stages-of-change," model is an effective approach to lifestyle self-management. According to this model, you move through distinct stages as you work to change

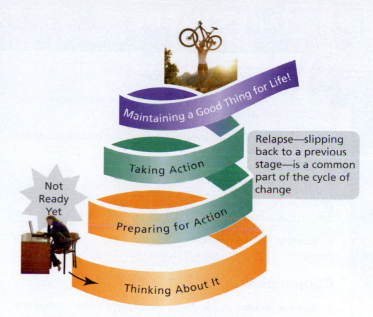

FIGURE 1.6   The stages of change: A spiral model.

SOURCE: Adapted from Centers for Disease Control and Prevention. (n.d.) *PEP guide: Personal empowerment plan for improving eating and increasing physical activity.* Dallas, TX: The Cooper Institute.

your target behavior. It is important to determine what stage you are in now so that you can choose appropriate strategies for progressing through the cycle of change. (Figure 1.6) This approach can help you enhance your readiness and intention to change. Read the following sections to determine what stage you are in for your target behavior.

Precontemplation   People at this stage do not think they have a problem and do not intend to change their behavior. They may be unaware of the risks associated with their behavior or may deny them. They may have tried unsuccessfully to change in the past and may now think the situation is hopeless. They may also blame other people or external factors for their problems. People in the precontemplation stage believe that there are more reasons or more important reasons not to change than there are reasons to change.

Contemplation   People at this stage know they have a problem and intend to take action within six months. They acknowledge the benefits of behavior change but worry about the costs of changing. To be successful, people must believe that the benefits of change outweigh the costs. People in the contemplation stage wonder about possible courses of action but don't know how to proceed. There may also be specific barriers to change that appear too difficult to overcome.

Preparation   People at this stage plan to take action within a month or may already have begun to make small changes in their behavior. They may be engaging in their new, healthier

self-talk   A person's internal dialogue.   **TERMS**

TAKE CHARGE
Tips for Moving Forward in the Cycle of Behavior Change

Precontemplation

- **Raise your awareness.** Research your target behavior and its effects.

- **Be self-aware.** Look at the mechanisms you use to resist change, such as denial or rationalization. Find ways to counteract these mechanisms.

- **Seek social support.** Friends and family members can help you identify target behaviors and understand their impact on the people around you.

- **Identify helpful resources.** These might include exercise classes or stress-management workshops offered by your school.

Contemplation

- **Keep a journal.** A record of your target behavior and the circumstances that elicit the behavior can help you plan a change program.

- **Do a cost-benefit analysis.** Identify the costs and benefits (both current and future) of maintaining your behavior and of changing it. Costs can be monetary, social, emotional, and so on.

- **Identify barriers to change.** Knowing these obstacles can help you overcome them.

- **Engage your emotions.** Watch movies or read books about people with your target behavior. Imagine what your life will be like if you don't change.

- **Create a new self-image.** Imagine what you'll be like after changing your target behavior. Try to think of yourself in new terms right now.

- **Think before you act.** Learn why you engage in the target behavior. Determine what "sets you off" and train yourself not to act reflexively.

Preparation

- **Create a plan.** Include a start date, goals, rewards, and specific steps you will take to change your behavior.

- **Make change a priority.** Create and sign a contract with yourself.

- **Practice visualization and self-talk.** These techniques can help prepare you mentally for challenging situations.

- **Take short steps.** Successfully practicing your new behavior for a short time—even a single day—can boost your confidence and motivation.

Action

- **Monitor your progress.** Keep up with your journal entries.

- **Change your environment.** Make changes that will discourage the target behavior—for example, getting rid of snack foods or not stocking the refrigerator with beer.

- **Find alternatives to your target behavior.** Make a list of things you can do to replace the behavior.

- **Reward yourself.** Rewards should be identified in your change plan. Give yourself lots of praise, and focus on your success.

- **Involve your friends.** Tell them you want to change, and ask for their help.

- **Don't get discouraged.** Real change is difficult.

Maintenance

- **Keep going.** Continue using the positive strategies that worked in earlier stages.

- **Be prepared for lapses.** Don't let slip-ups set you back.

- **Be a role model.** After you have successfully changed your behavior, you may be able to help someone else do the same thing.

If relapses keep occurring or if you can't seem to control them, you may need to return to a previous stage of the behavior change process. If this is necessary, reevaluate your goals and your strategy. A different or less stressful approach may help you avoid setbacks when you try again.

---

behavior but not yet regularly or consistently. They may have created a plan for change but may be worried about failing.

Action During the action stage, people outwardly modify their behavior and their environment. The action stage requires the greatest commitment of time and energy, and people in this stage are at risk for reverting to old, unhealthy patterns of behavior.

Maintenance People at this stage have maintained their new, healthier lifestyle for at least six months. Lapses may have occurred, but people in maintenance have been successful in quickly reestablishing the desired behavior. The maintenance stage can last for months or years.

Termination People at the termination stage have exited the cycle of change and are no longer tempted to lapse back into their old behavior. They have a new self-image and total self-efficacy with regard to their target behavior. For ideas on changing stages, see the box "Tips for Moving Forward in the Cycle of Behavior Change."

Dealing with Relapse

People seldom progress through the stages of change in a straightforward, linear way. Rather, they tend to move to a new stage and then slip back to a previous stage before resuming their forward progress. Research suggests that most people make several attempts before they successfully change a behavior; four out of five people experience some degree of backsliding. For this reason, the stages of change are best conceptualized as a spiral in which people cycle back through previous stages but are further along in the process each time they renew their commitment.

If you experience a lapse—a single slip—or a relapse—a return to old habits—don't give up. Relapse can be demoralizing, but it is not the same as failure. Failure means stopping before you reach your goal and never changing your target behavior. During the early stages of the change process, it's a good idea to plan for relapse so you can avoid guilt and self-blame and get back on track quickly. Follow these steps:

1. *Forgive yourself.* A single setback isn't the end of the world, but abandoning your efforts to change could have negative effects on your life.

2. *Give yourself credit for the progress you have already made.* You can use that success as motivation to continue.

3. *Move on.* You can learn from a relapse and use that knowledge to deal with potential setbacks in the future.

Developing Skills for Change: Creating a Personalized Plan

Once you are committed to making a change, it's time to put together a plan of action. Your key to success is a well-thought-out plan that sets goals, anticipates problems, and includes rewards. This plan includes the following steps:

1. *Monitor your behavior and gather data.* Keep a record of your target behavior and the circumstances surrounding it. Record this information for at least a week or two. Keep your notes in a health journal or notebook or on your computer (see the sample journal entries in Figure 1.7). Record each occurrence of your behavior, noting the following:

- What the activity was
- When and where it happened
- What you were doing
- How you felt at that time

If your goal is to start an exercise program, track your activities to determine how to make time for workouts. A blank log is provided in Activity 3 in the Behavior Change Workbook at the end of this text.

2. *Analyze the data and identify patterns.* After you have collected data on the behavior, analyze the data to identify patterns. When are you most likely to overeat? To skip a meal? What events trigger your appetite? Perhaps you are especially hungry at midmorning or when you put off eating dinner until 9:00 P.M. Perhaps you overindulge in food and drink when you go to a particular restaurant or when you're with certain friends. Note the connections between your feelings and such external cues as time of day, location, situation, and the actions of others around you.

3. *Be "SMART" about setting goals.* If your goals are too challenging, you will have trouble making steady progress and will be more likely to give up altogether. If, for example, you are in poor physical condition, it will not make sense to set a goal of being ready to run a marathon within two months. If you set goals you can live with, it will be easier to stick with your behavior change plan and be successful.

Date November 5					Day M [TU] W TH F SA SU					
Time of day	M/S	Food eaten	Cals.	H	Where did you eat?	What else were you doing?	How did someone else influence you?	What made you want to eat what you did?	Emotions and feelings?	Thoughts and concerns?
7:30	M	1 C Crispix cereal 1/2 C skim milk coffee, black 1 C orange juice	110 40 — 120	3	home	looking at news headlines on my phone	alone	I always eat cereal in the morning	a little keyed up & worried	thinking about quiz in class today
10:30	S	1 apple	90	1	hall outside classroom	studying	alone	felt tired & wanted to wake up	tired	worried about next class
12:30	M	1 C chili 1 roll 1 pat butter 1 orange 2 oatmeal cookies 1 soda	290 120 35 60 120 150	2	campus food court	talking	eating w/ friends; we decided to eat at the food court	wanted to be part of group	excited and happy	interested in hearing everyone's plans for the weekend
	M/S = Meal or snack			H = Hunger rating (0–3)						

FIGURE 1.7 Sample health journal entries.

Experts suggest that your goals meet the "SMART" criteria. That is, your behavior change goals should be

- *Specific.* Avoid vague goals like "eat more fruits and vegetables." Instead, state your objectives in specific terms, such as "eat two cups of fruit and three cups of vegetables every day."

- *Measurable.* Recognize that your progress will be easier to track if your goals are quantifiable, so give your goal a number. You might measure your goal in terms of time (such as "walk briskly for 20 minutes a day"), distance ("run two miles, three days per week"), or some other amount ("drink eight glasses of water every day").

- *Attainable.* Set goals that are within your physical limits. For example, if you are a poor swimmer, it might not be possible for you to meet a short-term fitness goal by swimming laps. Walking or biking might be better options.

- *Realistic.* Manage your expectations when you set goals. For example, it may not be possible for a long-time smoker to quit cold turkey. A more realistic approach might be to use nicotine replacement patches or gum for several weeks while getting help from a support group.

- *Time frame–specific.* Give yourself a reasonable amount of time to reach your goal, state the time frame in your behavior change plan, and set your agenda to meet the goal within the given time frame.

Using these criteria, a sedentary person who wants to improve his health and build fitness might set a goal of being able to run three miles in 30 minutes, to be achieved within a time frame of six months. To work toward that goal, he might set a number of smaller, intermediate goals that are easier to achieve. For example, his list of goals might look like this:

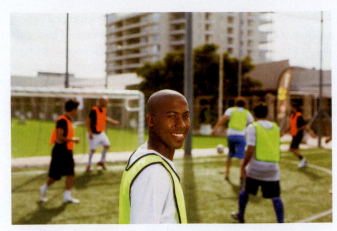

Wellness Tip Your environment contains powerful cues for both positive and negative lifestyle choices. The presence of parks and running/bike paths encourages physical activity, even in an urban setting. Examine your environment for cues that can support your behavior change efforts.

WEEK	FREQUENCY (DAYS/WEEK)	ACTIVITY	DURATION (MINUTES)
1	3	Walk < 1 mile	10–15
2	3	Walk 1 mile	15–20
3	4	Walk 1–2 miles	20–25
4	4	Walk 2–3 miles	25–30
5–7	3–4	Walk/run 1 mile	15–20
21–24	4–5	Run 2–3 miles	25–30

It may not be possible to meet these goals, but you never know until you try. As you work toward meeting your long-term goal, you may find it necessary to adjust your short-term goals. For example, you may find that you can start running sooner than you thought, or you may be able to run farther than you originally estimated. In such cases, it may be reasonable to make your goals more challenging. Otherwise, you may want to make them easier in order to stay motivated.

For some goals and situations, it may make more sense to focus on something other than your outcome goal. If your goal involves a long-term lifestyle change, such as reaching a healthy weight, it is better to focus on developing healthy habits than to target a specific weight loss. Your goal in this case might be exercising 30 minutes every day, reducing portion sizes, or eliminating late-night snacks.

4. *Devise a plan of action.* Develop a strategy that will support your efforts to change. Your plan of action should include the following steps:

- *Get what you need.* Identify resources that can help you. For example, you can join a community walking club or sign up for a smoking cessation program. You may also need to buy some new running shoes or nicotine replacement patches. Get the items you need right away; waiting can delay your progress.

- *Modify your environment.* If there are cues in your environment that trigger your target behavior, try to control them. For example, if you normally have alcohol at home, getting rid of it can help prevent you from indulging. If you usually study with a group of friends in an environment that allows smoking, try moving to a nonsmoking area. If you always buy a snack at a certain vending machine, change your route to avoid it.

- *Control related habits.* You may have habits that contribute to your target behavior; modifying these habits can help change the behavior. For example, if you usually plop down on the sofa while watching TV, try putting an exercise bike in front of the set so you can burn calories while watching your favorite programs.

- *Reward yourself.* Giving yourself instant, real rewards for good behavior will reinforce your efforts. Plan your rewards; decide in advance what each one will be and how you will earn it. Tie rewards to achieving specific goals or subgoals. For example, you might treat yourself to a movie after a week of avoiding snacks. Make a list of items or events to use as rewards. They should be special to you and preferably unrelated to food or alcohol.

- *Involve the people around you.* Ask family and friends to help you with your plan. To help them respond appropriately to your needs, create a specific list of dos and don'ts. For example, ask them to support you when you set aside time to exercise or when you avoid second helpings at dinner.

- *Plan for challenges.* Think about situations and people that might derail your program and develop ways to cope with them. For example, if you think it will be hard to stick to your usual exercise program during exams, schedule short bouts of physical activity (such as a brisk walk) as stress-reducing study breaks.

5. *Make a personal contract.* A serious personal contract—one that commits you to your word—can result in a higher chance of follow-through than a casual, offhand promise. Your contract can help prevent procrastination by specifying important dates and can also serve as a reminder of your personal commitment to change.

Your contract should include a statement of your goal and your commitment to reaching it. The contract should also include details, such as the following:

- The date you will start
- The steps you will take to measure your progress
- The strategies you plan to use to promote change
- The date you expect to reach your final goal

Have someone—preferably someone who will be actively helping you with your program—sign your contract as a witness.

Figure 1.8 shows a sample behavior change contract for someone committing to eating more fruit every day. A blank contract is included as Activity 8 in the Behavior Change Workbook at the end of this text.

Putting Your Plan into Action

The starting date has arrived, and you are ready to put your plan into action. This stage requires commitment, the resolve to stick with the plan no matter what temptations you encounter. Remember all the reasons you have to make the change—and remember that *you* are the boss. Use all your strategies to make your plan work. Make sure your environment is change friendly, and get as much support and encouragement from others as possible. Keep track of your progress in your health journal, and give yourself regular rewards. And don't forget to give yourself a pat on the back—congratulate yourself, notice how much better you look or feel, and feel good about how far you've come and how you've gained control of your behavior.

Staying with It

As you continue with your program, don't be surprised when you run up against obstacles; they're inevitable. In fact, it's a good idea to expect problems and give yourself time to step

Behavior Change Contract

1. I, __Tammy Lau__, agree to __increase my consumption of fruit from 1 cup per week to 2 cups per day.__

2. I will begin on ____10/5____ and plan to reach my goal of __2 cups of fruit per day__ by __12/7__

3. To reach my final goal, I have devised the following schedule of mini-goals. For each step in my program, I will give myself the reward listed.

I will begin to have ½ cup of fruit with breakfast	10/5	see movie
I will begin to have ½ cup of fruit with lunch	10/26	new cd
I will begin to substitute fruit juice for soda 1 time per day	11/16	concert

My overall reward for reaching my goal will be __trip to beach__

4. I have gathered and analyzed data on my target behavior and have identified the following strategies for changing my behavior: __Keep the fridge stocked with easy-to-carry fruit. Pack fruit in my backpack every day. Buy lunch at place that serves fruit.__

5. I will use the following tools to monitor my progress toward my final goal: __Chart on fridge door__ __Health journal__

I sign this contract as an indication of my personal commitment to reach my goal: _____Tammy Lau_____ _____9/28_____

I have recruited a helper who will witness my contract and __also increase his consumption of fruit; eat lunch with me twice a week.__
_____Eric March_____ _____9/28_____

FIGURE 1.8 **A sample behavior change contract.**

back, see how you're doing, and make some changes before going on. If your program is grinding to a halt, identify what is blocking your progress. It may come from one of the sources described in the following sections.

Social Influences Take a hard look at the reactions of the people you're counting on, and see if they're really supporting you. If they come up short, connect with others who will be more supportive. A related trap is trying to get your friends or family members to change *their* behaviors. The decision to make a major behavior change is something people come to only after intensive self-examination. You may be able to influence someone by tactfully providing facts or support, but that's all. Focus on yourself. When you succeed, you may become a role model for others.

Levels of Motivation and Commitment You won't make real progress until an inner drive leads you to the stage of change at which you are ready to make a personal commitment to the goal. If commitment is your problem, you may need to wait until the behavior you're dealing with makes you unhappier or unhealthier; then your desire to change it will be stronger. Or you may find that changing your goal will inspire you to keep going. For more ideas, refer to Activity 9 in the Behavior Change Workbook.

Choice of Techniques and Level of Effort If your plan is not working as well as you thought it would, make changes where you're having the most trouble. If you've lagged on your running schedule, for example, maybe it's because you don't like running. An aerobics class might suit you better. There are many ways to move toward your goal. Or you may not be trying hard enough. You do have to push toward your goal. If it were easy, you wouldn't need a plan.

Stress Barrier If you hit a wall in your program, look at the sources of stress in your life. If the stress is temporary, such as catching a cold or having a term paper due, you may want to wait until it passes before strengthening your efforts. If the stress is ongoing, find healthy ways to manage it (see Chapter 10). You may even want to make stress management your highest priority for behavior change.

Procrastinating, Rationalizing, and Blaming Be alert to games you might be playing with yourself, so you can stop them. Such games include the following:

• *Procrastinating.* If you tell yourself, "It's Friday already; I might as well wait until Monday to start," you're procrastinating. Break your plan into smaller steps that you can accomplish one day at a time.

• *Rationalizing.* If you tell yourself, "I wanted to go swimming today but wouldn't have had time to wash my hair afterward," you're making excuses.

• *Blaming.* If you tell yourself, "I couldn't exercise because Dave was hogging the elliptical trainer," you're blaming others for your own failure to follow through. Blaming is a way of taking your focus off the real problem and denying responsibility for your own actions.

Being Fit and Well for Life

Your first attempts at making behavior changes may never go beyond the contemplation or preparation stage. Those that do may not all succeed. But as you experience some success, you'll start to have more positive feelings about yourself. You may discover new physical activities and sports you enjoy, and you may encounter new situations and meet new people. Perhaps you'll surprise yourself by accomplishing things you didn't think were possible—breaking a long-standing nicotine habit, competing in a race, climbing a mountain, or developing a leaner body. Most of all, you'll discover the feeling of empowerment that comes from taking charge of your health. Being healthy takes effort, but the paybacks in energy and vitality are priceless.

TIPS FOR TODAY AND THE FUTURE

You are in charge of your health. Many of the decisions you make every day have an impact on the quality of your life, both now and in the future.

RIGHT NOW YOU CAN

■ Go for a 15-minute walk.
■ Have a piece of fruit for a snack.
■ Call a friend and arrange for a time to catch up with each other.
■ Start thinking about whether you have a health behavior you'd like to change. If you do, consider the elements of a behavior change strategy. For example, begin a mental list of the pros and cons of the behavior, or talk to someone who can support you in your attempts to change.

IN THE FUTURE YOU CAN

■ Stay current on health and wellness news and issues.
■ Participate in health awareness and promotion campaigns in your community—for example, support smoking restrictions in local venues.
■ Be a role model for someone else who is working on a health behavior you have successfully changed.

Once you've started, don't stop. Assume that health improvement is forever. Take on the easier problems first, and then use what you learn to tackle more difficult problems later. When you feel challenged, remind yourself that you are creating a lifestyle that minimizes your health risks and maximizes your enjoyment of life. You *can* take charge of your health in a dramatic and meaningful way. *Fit and Well* will show you how.

SUMMARY

• Wellness is the ability to live life fully, with vitality and meaning. Wellness is dynamic and multidimensional; it incorporates physical, emotional, intellectual, interpersonal, cultural, spiritual, environmental, financial, and occupational dimensions.

• People today have greater control over and greater responsibility for their health than ever before.

• Behaviors that promote wellness include being physically active, choosing a healthy diet, maintaining a healthy body weight, managing stress effectively, avoiding tobacco and limiting alcohol use, and protecting yourself from disease and injury.

• Although heredity, environment, and health care all play roles in wellness and disease, behavior can mitigate their effects.

• To make lifestyle changes, you need information about yourself, your health habits, and resources available to help you change.

- You can increase your motivation for behavior change by examining the benefits and costs of change, boosting self-efficacy, and identifying and overcoming key barriers to change.

- The stages-of-change model describes six stages that people may move through as they try to change their behavior: precontemplation, contemplation, preparation, action, maintenance, and termination.

- A specific plan for change can be developed by (1) collecting data on your behavior and recording it in a journal; (2) analyzing the recorded data; (3) setting specific goals; (4) devising strategies for modifying the environment, rewarding yourself, and involving others; and (5) making a personal contract.

- To start and maintain a behavior change program, you need commitment, a well-developed and manageable plan, social support, and strong stress-management techniques. It is also important to monitor the progress of your program, revising it as necessary.

FOR FURTHER EXPLORATION

The Internet addresses listed here were accurate at the time of publication.

Centers for Disease Control and Prevention. Through phone, fax, and the Internet, the CDC provides a wide variety of health information.
http://www.cdc.gov

Federal Deposit Insurance Corporation: Money Smart. A free source of information, unaffiliated with commercial interests, that includes eight modules on topics such as "borrowing basics" and "paying for college and cars."
https://www.fdic.gov/consumers/consumer/moneysmart/mscbi/mscbi.html

Federal Trade Commission: Consumer Protection—Health. Includes online brochures about a variety of consumer health topics, including fitness equipment, generic drugs, and fraudulent health claims.
http://www.ftc.gov/bcp/menus/consumer/health.shtm

Healthfinder. A gateway to online publications, websites, support and self-help groups, and agencies and organizations that produce reliable health information.
http://www.healthfinder.gov

Health.gov. A portal for online information from a wide variety of federal agencies.
http://health.gov/

Healthy Campus. The American College Health Association's introduction to the Healthy Campus program.
http://www.achancha.org/

Healthy People. Provides information on Healthy People objectives and priority areas.
http://www.healthypeople.gov

MedlinePlus. Provides links to news and reliable information about health from government agencies and professional associations; also includes a health encyclopedia and information on prescription and over-the-counter drugs.
http://www.nlm.nih.gov/medlineplus/

National Health Information Center (NHIC). Puts consumers in touch with the organizations that are best able to provide answers to health-related questions.
http://www.health.gov/nhic/

National Institutes of Health. Provides information about all NIH activities as well as consumer publications, hotline information, and an A-to-Z listing of health issues with links to the appropriate NIH institute.
http://www.nih.gov

National Wellness Institute. Serves professionals and organizations that promote optimal health and wellness.
http://www.nationalwellness.org

National Women's Health Information Center. Provides information and answers to frequently asked questions.
http://www.womenshealth.gov

Office of Minority Health. Promotes improved health among racial and ethnic minority populations.
http://minorityhealth.hhs.gov

Surgeon General. Includes information on activities of the Surgeon General and the text of many key reports on such topics as tobacco use, physical activity, and mental health.
http://www.surgeongeneral.gov

World Health Organization (WHO). Provides information about health topics and issues affecting people around the world.
http://www.who.int/en

SELECTED BIBLIOGRAPHY

American Cancer Society. 2014. *Cancer Facts and Figures—2014.* Atlanta: American Cancer Society.

American College Health Association. 2014. *American College Health Association—National College Health Assessment II: Reference Group Executive Summary Spring 2014.* Hanover, MD: American College Health Association.

American Heart Association. 2014. *Heart Disease and Stroke Statistics—2015 Update.* Dallas: American Heart Association.

Centers for Disease Control and Prevention. 2008. Racial/Ethnic Disparities in Self-Rated Health Status among Adults with and without Disabilities—United States, 2004–2006. *Morbidity and Mortality Weekly Report* 57(39): 1069–1073.

Centers for Disease Control and Prevention. 2013. *Racial and Ethnic Approaches to Community Health (REACH)* (http://www.cdc.gov/nccdphp/dch/programs/reach/; retrieved April 7, 2015).

Everett, B. G., et al. 2013. The nonlinear relationship between education and mortality: An examination of cohort, race/ethnic, and gender differences. *Population Research and Policy Review* 32(6).

Fisher, E. G., et al. 2011. Behavior matters. *American Journal of Preventive Medicine* 40(5): e15–30.

Flegal, K. M., et al. 2010. Prevalence and trends in obesity among U.S. adults, 1999–2008. *Journal of the American Medical Association* 303(3): 235–241.

Jepsen, R., et al. 2015. Physical activity and quality of life in severely obese adults during a two-year lifestyle intervention programme. *Journal of Obesity,* vol. 2015, Article ID 314194.

Mokdad, A. H., et al. 2004. Actual causes of death in the United States, 2000. *Journal of the American Medical Association* 291(10): 1238–1245.

Mokdad, A. H., et al. 2005. Correction: Actual causes of death in the United States, 2000. *Journal of the American Medical Association* 293(3): 293–294.

National Center for Health Statistics. 2012. *Health, United States, 2011 with Special Feature on Socioeconomic Status and Health.* Hyattsville, Md.: National Center for Health Statistics.

National Center for Health Statistics. 2013. National health interview survey. Centers for Disease Control and Prevention. Hyattsville, MD.

National Center for Health Statistics. 2015. Deaths: Final data for 2013. *National Vital Statistics Report* 64(2), http://www.cdc.gov/nchs/data/nvsr/nvsr64/nvsr64_02.pdf, retrieved August 19, 2015.

Participants at the 6th Global Conference on Health Promotion. The Bangkok Charter for health promotion in a globalized world. Geneva: World Health Organization, August 11, 2005.

Persky, Susan, et al. 2013. The role of weight, race, and health care experiences in care use among young men and women. *Obesity* 10.1002/oby.20677. [Epub ahead of print]

Pinkhasov, R. M., et al. 2010. Are men shortchanged on health? Perspective on health care utilization and health risk behavior in men and women in the United States. *International Journal of Clinical Practice* 64(4): 475–487.

Rotimi, C. N. 2012. Health disparities in the genomic era: The case for diversifying ethnic representation. *Genomic Medicine* 4(8): 65.

U.C. Berkeley. 2010 Update. *Evaluating Web Pages: Techniques to Apply and Questions to Ask* (http://www.lib.berkeley.edu/TeachingLib/Guides/Internet/ Evaluate.html; retrieved June 26, 2011).

U.S. Department of Health and Human Services, Public Health Service, Office of the Surgeon General. 2014. *The health consequences of smoking-50 years of progress: A report of the surgeon general, 2014.*

Vaccaro, J. A., and F. G. Huffman. 2012. Reducing health disparities: Medical advice received for minorities with diabetes. *Journal of Health and Human Services Administration* 34(4): 389–417.

Williams, D. R. 2012. Miles to go before we sleep: Racial inequities in health. *Journal of Health and Social Behavior* 53(3): 279–295.

Wojno, Marc A. 2013. 12 Things College Students Don't Need. *Kiplinger,* August 29, 2013.

World Health Organization. 2011. *Why Gender and Health?* (http://www.who.int/ gender/genderandhealth/en; retrieved March 21, 2013).

Name _____ **Section** _____ **Date** _____

LAB 1.1   Your Wellness Profile

Consider how your lifestyle, attitudes, and characteristics relate to each of the dimensions of wellness. Fill in at least three strengths for each dimension (examples of strengths are listed with each dimension). Once you've completed your lists, choose what you believe are your five most important strengths and circle them.

Physical wellness: To maintain overall physical health and engage in appropriate physical activity (e.g., stamina, strength, flexibility, healthy body composition).

_____

_____

_____

Emotional wellness: To have a positive self-concept, deal constructively with your feelings, and develop positive qualities (e.g., optimism, trust, self-confidence, determination).

_____

_____

_____

Intellectual wellness: To pursue and retain knowledge, think critically about issues, make sound decisions, identify problems, and find solutions (e.g., common sense, creativity, curiosity).

_____

_____

_____

Interpersonal/social wellness: To develop and maintain meaningful relationships with a network of friends and family members, and to contribute to your community (e.g., friendly, good-natured, compassionate, supportive, good listener).

_____

_____

_____

Cultural Wellness: To accept, value, and even celebrate personal and cultural differences (e.g., refuse to stereotype based on ethnicity, gender, religion, or sexual orientation; create relationships with those who are different from you; maintain and value your own cultural identity).

_____

_____

_____

Spiritual wellness: To develop a set of beliefs, principles, or values that gives meaning or purpose to your life; to develop faith in something beyond yourself (e.g., religious faith, service to others).

_____

_____

_____

Environmental wellness: To protect yourself from environmental hazards and to minimize the negative impact of your behavior on the environment (e.g., carpooling, recycling).

_____

_____

_____

Financial wellness: Your ability to live within your means and manage your money in a way that gives you peace of mind.

_____

_____

_____

Occupational Wellness: To gain a measure of happiness and fulfillment through your work (e.g., enjoy what you do, feel valued by your manager, build positive relationships with co-workers, take advantage of opportunities to learn and be challenged).

_____

_____

_____

LABORATORY ACTIVITIES

Next, think about where you fall on the wellness continuum for each of the dimensions of wellness. Indicate your placement for each—physical, emotional, intellectual, interpersonal/social, cultural spiritual, environmental, financial, and occupational—by placing Xs on the continuum below.

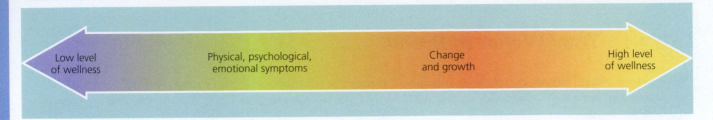

Based on both your current lifestyle and your goals for the future, what do you think your placement on the wellness continuum will be in 10 years? What new health behaviors will you have to adopt to achieve your goals? Which of your current behaviors will you need to change to maintain or improve your level of wellness in the future?

Does the description of wellness given in this chapter encompass everything you believe is part of wellness for you? Write your own definition of wellness, including any additional dimensions that are important to you. Then rate your level of wellness based on your own definition.

Using Your Results

How did you score? Are you satisfied with your current level of wellness—overall and in each dimension? In which dimension(s) would you most like to increase your level of wellness?

What should you do next? As you consider possible target behaviors for a behavior change program, choose things that will maintain or increase your level of wellness in one of the dimensions you listed as an area of concern. Remember to consider health behaviors such as smoking or eating a high-fat diet that may threaten your level of wellness in the future. Below, list several possible target behaviors and the wellness dimensions that they influence.

For additional guidance in choosing a target behavior, complete the lifestyle self-assessment in Lab 1.2.

Name _____ **Section** _____ **Date** _____

LAB 1.2   Lifestyle Evaluation

How does your current lifestyle compare with the lifestyle recommended for wellness? For each question, choose the answer that best describes your behavior. Then add up your score for each section.

Exercise/Fitness

	Almost Always	Sometimes	Never
1. I engage in moderate exercise, such as brisk walking or swimming, for the equivalent of at least 150 minutes per week.	4	1	0
2. I do exercises to develop muscular strength and endurance at least twice a week.	2	1	0
3. I spend some of my leisure time participating in individual, family, or team activities, such as gardening, bowling, or softball.	2	1	0
4. I maintain a healthy body weight, avoiding overweight and underweight.	2	1	0

Exercise/Fitness Score: _____

Nutrition

	Almost Always	Sometimes	Never
1. I eat a variety of foods each day, including seven or more servings of fruits and/or vegetables.	3	1	0
2. I limit the amount of saturated and trans fat in my diet.	3	1	0
3. I avoid skipping meals.	2	1	0
4. I limit the amount of salt and added sugars I eat.	2	1	0

Nutrition Score: _____

Tobacco Use

	Almost Always	Sometimes	Never
1. I avoid smoking cigarettes.	4	1	0
2. I avoid using a pipe or cigars.	2	1	0
3. I avoid spit tobacco.	2	1	0
4. I limit my exposure to environmental tobacco smoke.	2	1	0

Tobacco Use Score: _____

Alcohol and Drugs

	Almost Always	Sometimes	Never
1. I avoid alcohol, or I drink no more than one (women) or two (men) drinks a day.	4	1	0
2. I avoid using alcohol or other drugs as a way of handling stressful situations or the problems in my life.	2	1	0
3. I am careful not to drink alcohol when taking medications (such as cold or allergy medications) or when pregnant.	2	1	0
4. I read and follow the label directions when using prescribed and over-the-counter drugs.	2	1	0

Alcohol and Drugs Score: _____

Emotional Health

	Almost Always	Sometimes	Never
1. I enjoy being a student, and I have a job or do other work that I enjoy.	2	1	0
2. I find it easy to relax and express my feelings freely.	2	1	0
3. I manage stress well.	2	1	0
4. I have close friends, relatives, or others whom I can talk to about personal matters and call on for help when needed.	2	1	0
5. I participate in group activities (such as community or church organizations) or hobbies that I enjoy.	2	1	0

Emotional Health Score: _____

LABORATORY ACTIVITIES

	Almost Always	Sometimes	Never

Safety

1. I wear a safety belt while riding in a car.	2	1	0
2. I avoid driving while under the influence of alcohol or other drugs.	2	1	0
3. I obey traffic rules and the speed limit when driving.	2	1	0
4. I read and follow instructions on the labels of potentially harmful products or substances, such as household cleaners, poisons, and electrical appliances.	2	1	0
5. I avoid using a cell phone while driving.	2	1	0

Safety Score: _____

Disease Prevention

1. I know the warning signs of cancer, heart attack, and stroke.	2	1	0
2. I avoid overexposure to the sun and use sunscreen.	2	1	0
3. I get recommended medical screening tests (such as blood pressure and cholesterol checks and Pap tests), immunizations, and booster shots.	2	1	0
4. I practice monthly skin and breast/testicle self-exams.	2	1	0
5. I am not sexually active, *or* I have sex with only one mutually faithful, uninfected partner, *or* I always engage in safer sex (using condoms), and I do not share needles to inject drugs.	2	1	0

Disease Prevention Score: _____

Scores of 9 and 10 Excellent! Your answers show that you are aware of the importance of this area to your health. More important, you are putting your knowledge to work for you by practicing good health habits. As long as you continue to do so, this area should not pose a serious health risk.

Scores of 6 to 8 Your health practices in this area are good, but there is room for improvement.

Scores of 3 to 5 Your health risks are showing.

Scores of 0 to 2 You may be taking serious and unnecessary risks with your health.

Using Your Results

How did you score? In which areas did you score the lowest? Are you satisfied with your scores in each area? In which areas would you most like to improve your scores?

What should you do next? To improve your scores, look closely at any item to which you answered "sometimes" or "never." Identify and list at least three possible targets for a health behavior change program. (If you are aware of other risky health behaviors you currently engage in, but that were not covered by this assessment, you may include those in your list.) For each item on your list, identify your current "stage of change" and one strategy you could adopt to move forward (see pp. 15–20). Possible strategies might be obtaining information about the behavior, completing an analysis of the pros and cons of change, or beginning a written record of your target behavior.

Behavior	Stage	Strategy
1. _____	_____	_____
2. _____	_____	_____
3. _____	_____	_____

SOURCE: Adapted from *Healthstyle: A Self-Test,* developed by the U.S. Public Health Service. The behaviors covered in this test are recommended for most Americans, but some may not apply to people with certain chronic diseases or disabilities or to pregnant women, who may require special advice from their physician.

Principles of Physical Fitness

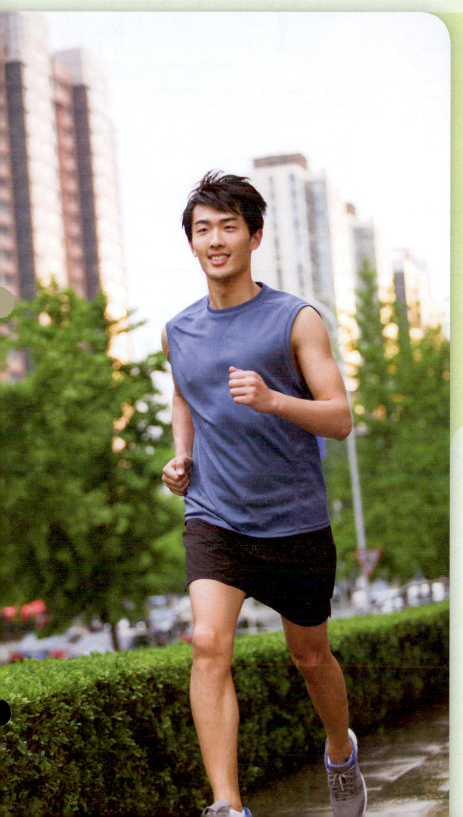

LOOKING AHEAD...

After reading this chapter, you should be able to

- Describe how much physical activity is recommended for developing health and fitness.

- Identify the components of physical fitness and the way each component affects wellness.

- Explain the goal of physical training and the basic principles of training.

- Describe the principles involved in designing a well-rounded exercise program.

- List the steps that can be taken to make an exercise program safe, effective, and successful.

TEST YOUR KNOWLEDGE

1. To improve your health, you must exercise vigorously for at least 30 minutes straight, 5 or more days per week. True or false?

2. Which of the following activities uses about 150 calories?
   a. washing a car for 45–60 minutes
   b. shooting a basketball for 30 minutes
   c. jumping rope for 15 minutes

3. Regular exercise can make a person smarter. True or false?

See answers on the next page.

Any list of the benefits of physical activity is impressive. Although people vary greatly in physical fitness and performance ability, the benefits of regular physical activity are available to everyone. Much of the increased health benefits from exercise occur when going from no activity (sedentary) to some moderate-intensity activity (Figure 2.1). Further health benefits occur when exercising harder or longer. The relative risk of death from all causes and the risk of heart disease decrease by as much as 65% when comparing the least and most active men and women. In Figure 2.1, relative risk of death refers to the risk of death per year of sedentary people compared to people in various activity levels.

This chapter provides an overview of physical fitness. It explains how both lifestyle physical activity and more formal exercise programs contribute to wellness. It also describes the components of fitness, the basic principles of physical training, and the essential elements of a well-rounded exercise program. Chapters 3–6 provide an in-depth look at each of the elements of a fitness program; Chapter 7 puts these elements together in a complete, personalized program.

PHYSICAL ACTIVITY AND EXERCISE FOR HEALTH AND FITNESS

Almost any kind of physical activity promotes health. Try to be more active during the day, regardless of whether you can fit in a formal workout. Short periods of intense exercise do not compensate for hours of inactivity. So try to get up and move around each hour when you are studying, working on the computer, or watching TV (see the box "Move More, Sit Less"). Physical activity and exercise are points along a continuum.

Physical Activity on a Continuum

Physical activity is movement that is carried out by the skeletal muscles and requires energy. Different types of physical activity can vary by ease or intensity. Standing up or walking down a hallway requires little energy or effort, but each is a higher level of activity than sitting or lying down. More intense sustained activities, such as cycling five miles or running in a race, require considerably more effort.

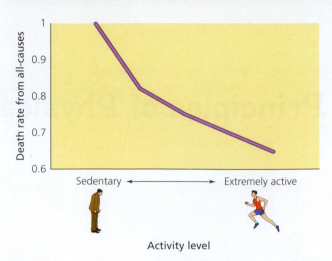

FIGURE 2.1 Exercise promotes longevity. The risk of death each year from all causes decreases with increased amounts and intensities of weekly physical activity.

SOURCE: Adapted from a composite of 12 studies involving more than 200,000 men and women. Wen, M., et al. 2014. Physical activity and mortality among middle-aged and older adults in the United States. *Journal Physical Activity & Health* 11: 303–312.: Physical Activity Guidelines Advisory Committee. *Physical Activity Guidelines Advisory Committee Report, 2008.* Washington, D.C.: U.S. Department of Health and Human Services, 2008. Schnohr, P., et al. 2015. Dose of jogging and long-term mortality: the Copenhagen City Heart Study. *Journal American College of Cardiology* 65(5): 411–419.

Exercise refers to planned, structured, repetitive movement intended specifically to improve or maintain physical fitness. As discussed in Chapter 1, physical fitness is a set of physical attributes that allows the body to respond or adapt to the demands and stress of physical effort—to perform moderate to vigorous levels of physical activity without becoming overly tired. Levels of fitness depend on such physiological factors as the heart's ability to pump blood and the energy-generating capacity of the cells. These factors in turn depend both on *genetics*—a person's inborn potential for physical fitness—and *behavior*—getting enough physical activity to stress the body and cause long-term physiological changes.

Physical activity is essential to health and confers wide-ranging health benefits, but exercise is necessary to significantly improve physical fitness. This important distinction between physical activity, which improves health and wellness, and exercise, which improves fitness, is a key concept in understanding the guidelines discussed in this section.

Increasing Physical Activity to Improve Health and Wellness According to the U.S. Surgeon General's Office (USSGO), "Engaging in regular physical activity is one of the most important things that people of all ages can do to improve their health." Physical activity is central to the national prevention strategy to improve health by promoting community design to support active lifestyles, encouraging exercise in young people, providing safe and accessible places for sports and exercise, and supporting physical activity in the workplace. The U.S. Department of Health and Human Services, American College of Sports Medicine, the American Heart Association,

A regular exercise program provides huge wellness benefits, but it does not cancel out all the negative effects of too much sitting during the day. Advances in technology promote sedentary behavior—we can now work or study at a desk, watch TV or play video games in our leisure time, order take-out and delivery for meals, and shop and bank online. To avoid the negative health effects of too little daily activity, you may need a plan to reduce your sitting time. Try some of the following strategies:

• Stand up and/or walk when you are on work or personal phone calls.

• Take the stairs whenever and wherever you can; walk up and down escalators instead of just riding them.

• At work, walk to a co-worker's desk rather than emailing or calling; take the long route to the restroom; and take a walk break whenever you take a coffee or snack break. Drink plenty of water so you'll have to take frequent restroom breaks.

• Set reminders to get up and move: Use commercial breaks while watching TV; at work or while using a digital device, use the clock function on your computer or phone to make sure you don't sit for longer than an hour at a time.

• Engage in active chores and leisure activities.

• Track your sedentary time to get a baseline, and then continue monitoring to note any improvements. You can also use a step counter to track your general activity level.

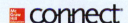

and USSGO have made specific exercise recommendations for promoting health. Their reports stress the importance of regular physical activity and emphasize that some physical activity is better than none. They also present evidence that regular activity promotes health and prevents premature death and a variety of diseases (Figure 2.1). The reports include the following key guidelines for adults:

• For substantial health benefits, adults should do at least 150 minutes (2 hours and 30 minutes) a week of moderate-intensity aerobic physical activity, or 75 minutes (1 hour and 15 minutes) a week of vigorous-intensity aerobic physical activity, or an equivalent combination of moderate- and vigorous-intensity aerobic activity. Activity should preferably be spread throughout the week.

• For additional and more extensive health benefits, adults should increase their aerobic physical activity to 300 minutes (5 hours) a week of moderate-intensity activity, or 150 minutes a week of vigorous-intensity activity, or an equivalent combination of moderate- and vigorous-intensity activity. Adults can enjoy additional health benefits by engaging in physical activity beyond this amount. The Health and Retirement Study—a long-term study of older adults sponsored by the National Institute on Aging—found that people who exercised vigorously had a lower death rate than those who exercised at moderate intensities or did no physical activity. After 16 years, the survival rate was 84% in those doing vigorous exercise, 78% in those doing moderate-intensity physical activity, and only 65% in those doing no physical activity.

• Adults should also do muscle-strengthening activities, such as weight training or calisthenics, that are moderate or high intensity and involve all major muscle groups on two or more days a week, because these activities provide additional health benefits.

• Everyone should avoid inactivity. Adults, teenagers, and children should spend less time in front of a television or computer screen because such inactivity decreases metabolic health and contributes to a sedentary lifestyle and increases the risk of obesity.

The reports state that physical activity benefits people of all ages and of all racial and ethnic groups, including people with disabilities. The reports emphasize that the benefits of activity outweigh the dangers.

These levels of physical activity promote health and wellness by lowering the risk of high blood pressure, stroke, heart disease, type 2 diabetes, colon cancer, and osteoporosis and by reducing feelings of mild to moderate depression and anxiety.

What exactly is moderate physical activity? Activities such as brisk walking, dancing, swimming, cycling, and yard work can all count toward the daily total. A moderate amount of activity uses about 150 calories of energy and causes a noticeable increase in heart rate, such as would occur with a brisk walk. Examples of activities that use about 150 calories in 15 to 60 minutes are shown in Figure 2.2. You can burn the same number of calories by doing a lower-intensity activity for a longer time or a higher-intensity activity for a shorter time. People are more likely to participate in physical activities they enjoy, such as dancing.

In contrast to moderate-intensity activity, *vigorous* physical activity—such as jogging—causes rapid breathing and a substantial increase in heart rate (Table 2.1). Physical activity and exercise recommendations for promoting general health, fitness, and weight management are shown in Table 2.2.

The daily total of physical activity can be accumulated in multiple bouts of 10 or more minutes per day—for example, two

physical activity Body movement that is carried out by the skeletal muscles and requires energy.

exercise Planned, structured, repetitive movement intended to improve or maintain physical fitness.

TERMS

Common Activities	Duration (min.)	
Washing and waxing a car	45–60	
Washing windows or floors	45–60	Less Vigorous, More Time
Gardening	30–45	
Wheeling self in wheelchair	30–40	
Pushing a stroller 1½ miles	30	
Raking leaves	30	
Walking 2 miles	30 (15 min/mile)	
Shoveling snow	15	
Stairwalking	15	
Sporting Activities		
Playing volleyball	45–60	
Playing touch football	45	
Walking 1¾ miles	35 (20 min/mile)	
Basketball (shooting baskets)	30	
Bicycling 5 miles	30	
Dancing fast (social)	30	
Water aerobics	30	
Swimming laps	20	
Basketball (playing game)	15–20	
Bicycling 4 miles	15	More Vigorous, Less Time
Jumping rope	15	
Running 1½ miles	15 (10 min/mile)	

FIGURE 2.2 Examples of moderate-intensity physical activity. Each example uses about 150 calories.
SOURCE: National Heart, Lung, and Blood Institute. 2010. *Why Is Exercise Important?* (www.nhlbi.nih.gov/health/public/heart/obesity/lose_wt/physical/htm; September 1, 2015).

10-minute bike rides to and from class and a brisk 10-minute walk to the store. In this lifestyle approach to physical activity, people can choose activities that they find enjoyable and that fit into their daily routine; everyday tasks at school, work, and home can be structured to contribute to the daily activity total. If Americans who are currently sedentary were to increase their lifestyle physical activity to 30 minutes per day, both public health and their individual well-being would benefit enormously (see the box "Exercise Is Good for Your Brain").

Increasing Physical Activity to Manage Weight

Because two-thirds of Americans are overweight, the U.S. Department of Health and Human Services has also published physical activity guidelines focusing on weight management. These guidelines recognize that for people who need to prevent weight gain, lose weight, or maintain weight loss, 150 minutes per week of physical activity may not be enough. Instead, they recommend up to 90 minutes of physical activity per day. Unfortunately, exercise alone will seldom promote long-term weight loss; but exercise has many health benefits, even in the absence of substantial weight loss.

Exercising to Improve Physical Fitness As mentioned earlier, moderate physical activity confers significant health and wellness benefits, especially for those who are currently sedentary and become moderately active. However, people can obtain even greater health and wellness benefits by increasing the duration and intensity of physical activity. With

Table 2.1	Examples of Moderate- and Vigorous-Intensity Exercise

MODERATE-INTENSITY ACTIVITY	VIGOROUS-INTENSITY ACTIVITY
Uses 3.5 to 7 calories per minute and causes your breathing and heart rate to increase but still allows for comfortable conversation.	Uses more than 7 calories per minute and increases your heart and breathing rates considerably. These exercises cause larger increases in physical fitness.
• Actively playing with children or pets	• Aerobic dancing: high-impact step aerobics
• Archery	• Backpacking
• Ballroom dancing	• Basketball, recreational
• Bicycling or stationary bike, moderate pace	• Bicycling, high intensity
• Downhill skiing, moderate intensity	• Calisthenics, vigorous: jumping jacks, burpees, air squats
• Figure skating, recreational	• Circuit weight training
• Fly fishing or walking along stream	• Cross-country skiing or snowshoeing
• Gardening or yard work, moderate pace	• Cross-training, such as CrossFit
• Golf	• Downhill skiing, vigorous intensity
• Hiking, leisurely pace	• Football, recreational
• Horseback riding, recreational	• Gardening or yard work, shoveling heavy snow, digging ditches
• Housework, moderate intensity	• Hand cycling
• Skateboarding	• Horseback riding, galloping or jumping
• Softball	• In-line skating
• Using stair-climber, elliptical trainer, or rowing machine, moderate pace	• Interval training: running, elliptical trainer, swimming, cycling
• Table tennis	• Jogging
• Tennis, doubles	• Kayaking, whitewater
• Walking at a moderate pace: walking to school or work; walking for pleasure	• Pushing a car
• Water aerobics	• Running up stairs
• Waxing the car	• Soccer, recreational
• Weight training and bodybuilding	• Tennis, singles
• Yoga	• Wheelchair wheeling

SOURCE: Adapted from the Centers for Disease Control and Prevention, 2015, http://www.cdc.gov/nccdphp/dnpa/physical/pdf/PA_Intensity_table_2_1.pdf

Table 2.2	Physical Activity and Exercise Recommendations for Promoting General Health, Fitness, and Weight Management

GOAL	RECOMMENDATION
General health	Perform moderate-intensity aerobic physical activity for at least 150 minutes per week or 75 minutes of vigorous-intensity physical activity per week. Also, be more active in your daily life: Walk instead of driving, take the stairs instead of the elevator, and watch less television.
Increased health benefits	Exercise at moderate intensity for 300 minutes per week or at vigorous intensity for 150 minutes per week.
Achieve or maintain weight loss	Exercise moderately for 60–90 minutes per day on most days of the week.
Muscle strength and endurance	Perform 1 or more sets of resistance exercises that work the major muscle groups for 8–12 repetitions (10–15 reps for older adults) on at least two nonconsecutive days per week. Examples include weight training and exercises that use body weight as resistance (such as core stabilizing exercises, pull-ups, push-ups, lunges, and squats).
Flexibility	Perform range-of-motion (stretching) exercises at least two days per week. Hold each stretch for 10–30 seconds.
Neuromuscular training	Older adults should do balance training two–three days per week. Examples include yoga, tai chi, and balance exercises (standing on one foot, step-ups, and walking lunges). These exercises are probably beneficial for young and middle-aged adults, as well.

SOURCES: Garber, C. E., et al. 2011. Quantity and quality of exercise for developing and maintaining cardiorespiratory, musculoskeletal, and neuromotor fitness in apparently healthy adults: Guidance for prescribing exercise. *Medicine and Science in Sports and Exercise* 43(7): 1334–1359; Physical Activity Guidelines Advisory Committee. 2008. *Physical Activity Guidelines Advisory Committee Report, 2008.* Washington, D.C.: U.S. Department of Health and Human Services; U.S. Surgeon General's Office. 2014. National prevention strategy: active living. http: www.surgeongeneral.gov.

increased activity, they will see more improvements in quality of life and greater reductions in disease and mortality risk.

More vigorous activity, as in a structured, systematic exercise program, also improves physical fitness. Moderate physical activity alone is not enough. Physical fitness requires more intense movement that poses a substantially greater challenge to the body. The American College of Sports Medicine has issued guidelines for creating a formal exercise program that will develop physical fitness. These guidelines are described in detail later in the chapter.

How Much Physical Activity Is Enough?

Some experts believe that people get most of the health benefits of physical activity simply by becoming more active over the course of the day; the amount of activity needed depends on an individual's health status and goals. Other experts believe that leisure-time physical activity is not enough; they argue that people should exercise long enough and intensely enough to improve the body's capacity for exercise—that is, to improve physical fitness. There is probably some truth in both of these positions.

Regular physical activity, regardless of the intensity, makes you healthier and can help protect you from many chronic diseases. Although you get many of the health benefits of exercise by being more active, you obtain even more benefits when you are physically fit. In addition to long-term health benefits, fitness also contributes significantly to quality of life. Fitness can give you freedom to move your body the way you want. Fit people have more energy and better body control. They can enjoy a more active lifestyle than their more sedentary counterparts. Even if you don't like sports, you need physical energy and stamina in your daily life and for many non-sport leisure activities, such as visiting museums, playing with children, and gardening.

Where does this leave you? Most experts agree that some physical activity is better than none, but that more—as long as it does not result in injury—is better than some. To set a personal goal for physical activity and exercise, consider your current activity level, your health status, and your overall goals. At the very least, strive to become more active and do 30 minutes of moderate-intensity activity at least five days per week. Choose to be active whenever you can. If weight management is a concern for you, begin by achieving the goal of 30 minutes of activity per day and then try to raise your activity level further, to 60–90 minutes per day or more. For even better health and well-being, participate in a structured exercise program that develops physical fitness. Any increase in physical activity will contribute to your health and well-being, now and in the future.

COMPONENTS OF PHYSICAL FITNESS

Some components of fitness relate to specific skill activities, such as tennis and skiing, and others to general health. **Health-related fitness** includes the following components:

- Cardiorespiratory endurance
- Muscular strength

THE EVIDENCE FOR EXERCISE
Exercise Is Good for Your Brain

Some scientists call exercise the new "brain food." Studies show that even moderate physical activity can improve brain health and function and may delay the decline in cognitive function that occurs for many people as they age. Regular physical activity has the following positive effects on the brain:

- Exercise improves cognitive function—the brain's ability to learn, remember, think, and reason.

- Exercise can help overcome the negative effects of a poor diet on brain health.

- Exercise promotes the creation of new nerve cells (neurons) throughout the nervous system. By promoting this process (called *neurogenesis*), exercise provides protection against injury and degenerative conditions that destroy neurons. Physical activity is less effective for promoting brain health when exercising in polluted air.

- Exercise enhances the nervous system's *plasticity*—its ability to change and adapt. In the brain, spinal cord, and nerves, this can mean developing new pathways for transmitting sensory information or motor commands.

- Exercise appears to have a protective effect on the brain as people age, helping to delay or even prevent the onset of neurodegenerative disorders such as Alzheimer's disease.

Although most people consider brain health to be a concern for the elderly, it is vital to wellness throughout life. For this reason, many studies on exercise and brain health include children as well as older adults. Targeted research has also focused on the impact of exercise on people with disorders such as cerebral palsy, multiple sclerosis, and developmental disabilities. Generally speaking, these studies all reach a similar conclusion: Exercise enhances brain health, at least to some degree, in people of all ages and a wide range of health statuses.

Along with the brain's physical health, mental health is enhanced by exercise. Even modest activity, such as taking a daily walk, can help combat a variety of mental health disorders and improve mood.

It's hard to understate the impact of physical and mental disorders related to brain health. According to the Alzheimer's Association, 5.3 million Americans currently suffer from Alzheimer's disease, and the number is increasing at a rate of 70 people per second. People with depression, anxiety, or other mental disorders are more likely to suffer from chronic physical conditions. Taken together, these and other brain-related disorders cost untold millions of dollars in health care costs and lost productivity, as well as thousands of years of productive lifetime lost.

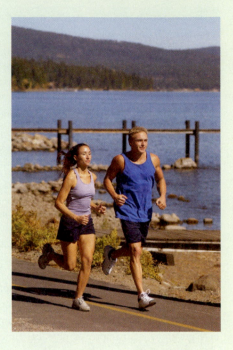

So, for the sake of your brain—as well as your muscles, bones, and heart—start creating your exercise program soon. You'll be healthier, and you may even feel a little smarter.

SOURCES: Szuhany, K. L., et al. 2015. A meta-analytic review of the effects of exercise on brain-derived neurotrophic factor. *Journal of Psychiatric Research* 60: 56–64. Garber, C. E., et al. 2011. Quantity and quality of exercise for developing and maintaining cardiorespiratory, musculoskeletal, and neuromotor fitness in apparently healthy adults: guidance for prescribing exercise. *Medicine and Science in Sports and Exercise* 43(7): 1334–1359; Bos, I., et al. 2013. Subclinical effects of aerobic training in urban environment. *Medicine Science in Sports and Exercise* 45(3): 439–447; Siette, J., et al. 2013. Age-specific effects of voluntary exercise on memory and the older brain. *Biological Psychiatry* 73(5): 435–442.

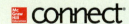

- Muscular endurance
- Flexibility
- Body composition

> **health-related fitness** Physical capacities that contribute to health: cardiorespiratory endurance, muscular strength, muscular endurance, flexibility, and body composition.
>
> **cardiorespiratory endurance** The ability of the body to perform prolonged, large-muscle, dynamic exercise at moderate to high levels of intensity.

TERMS

Health-related fitness helps you withstand physical challenges and protects you from diseases.

Cardiorespiratory Endurance

Cardiorespiratory endurance is the ability to perform prolonged, large-muscle, dynamic exercise at moderate to high levels of intensity. It depends on such factors as the ability of the lungs to deliver oxygen from the environment to the bloodstream, the capacity of the heart to pump blood, the ability of the nervous system and blood vessels to regulate blood flow, and the capability of the cells' chemical systems to use oxygen and process fuels for exercise and rest.

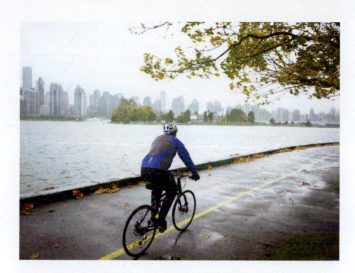

When cardiorespiratory fitness is low, the heart has to work hard during normal daily activities and may not be able to work hard enough to sustain high-intensity physical activity in an emergency. As cardiorespiratory fitness improves, related physical functions also improve. For example:

- The heart pumps more blood per heartbeat.
- Resting heart rate slows.
- Blood volume increases.
- Blood supply to tissues improves.
- The body can cool itself better.
- Blood vessels become more pliable.
- Resting blood pressure decreases.
- Metabolism in skeletal muscle is enhanced, which improves fuel use.
- The level of antioxidant chemicals in the body increases and oxidative stress decreases. During metabolism, the body naturally produces chemicals called free radicals (oxidative stress) that cause cell damage. Exercise training increases the production of antioxidants that help neutralize free radicals.

A healthy heart can better withstand the strains of everyday life, the stress of occasional emergencies, and the wear and tear of time.

Cardiovascular endurance training also improves the functioning of the body's chemical systems, particularly in the muscles and liver. These changes enhance the body's ability to derive energy from food, allow the body to perform more exercise with less effort, increase sensitivity to insulin, and prevent type 2 diabetes. Exercise reduces blood vessel inflammation, which is linked to coronary artery disease, heart attack, and stroke.

Physically fit people also have healthier, more resilient genes. Exercise preserves gene structures called telomeres, which form the ends of the DNA strands and hold them together. Over time the telomeres shorten, reducing their effectiveness, which triggers illness and death. Exercise helps to keep them from getting too short.

Cardiorespiratory endurance is a central component of health-related fitness because heart and lung function is so essential to overall good health. A person can't live very long or very well without a healthy heart or healthy lungs. Poor cardiorespiratory fitness is linked with heart disease, type 2 diabetes, colon cancer, stroke, depression, and anxiety. A moderate level of cardiorespiratory fitness can help compensate for certain health risks, including excess body fat: People with higher levels of body fat but who are otherwise fit have been found to have lower death rates than those who are lean but have low cardiorespiratory fitness.

You can develop cardiorespiratory endurance through activities that involve continuous, rhythmic movements of large-muscle groups, such as the legs. Such activities include walking, jogging, cycling, and group aerobics.

Muscular Strength

Muscular strength is the amount of force a muscle can produce with a single maximum effort. It depends on such factors as the size of muscle cells and the ability of nerves to activate muscle cells. Strong muscles are important for everyday activities, such as climbing stairs, as well as for emergency situations. They help keep the skeleton in proper alignment, preventing back and leg pain and providing the support necessary for good posture. Muscular strength has obvious importance in recreational activities. Strong people can hit a tennis ball harder, kick a soccer ball farther, and ride a bicycle uphill more easily.

Muscle tissue is an important element of overall body composition. Greater muscle mass means faster energy use and a higher rate of **metabolism,** and the sum of all the vital processes by which food energy and nutrients are made available to and used by the body. Greater muscle mass reduces markers of oxidative stress and maintains mitochondria (the "powerhouses" of the cell); both of these benefits are important for metabolic health and long life. Training to build muscular strength can also help people manage stress and boost their self-confidence.

Maintaining strength and muscle mass is vital for healthy aging. Stronger people live longer. Older people tend to experience a decrease in both number and size of muscle cells, a condition called *sarcopenia*. Many of the remaining muscle cells become slower, and some become nonfunctional because they lose their attachment to the nervous system. Strength training (also known as *resistance training* or *weight training*) increases antioxidant enzymes and lowers oxidative stress. It also helps maintain muscle mass and function and possibly helps decrease the risk of osteoporosis (bone loss) in older people, greatly enhancing their quality of life and preventing life-threatening injuries.

Muscular Endurance

Muscular endurance is the ability to resist fatigue and sustain a given level of muscle tension—that is, to hold a muscle contraction for a long time or to contract a muscle over and over again. It depends on such factors as the size of muscle cells, the ability of muscles to store fuel, blood supply, and the metabolic capacity of muscles.

Muscular endurance is important for good posture and for injury prevention. For example, if abdominal and back muscles cannot support and stabilize the spine correctly when you sit or stand for long periods, the chances of low back pain and back injury are increased. Good muscular endurance in the trunk muscles is more important than muscular strength for preventing back pain. Muscular endurance helps people cope with daily physical demands and enhances performance in sports and work.

Flexibility

Flexibility is the ability to move the joints through their full ranges of motion. It depends on joint structure, the length and elasticity of connective tissue, and nervous system activity. Flexible, pain-free joints are important for good health and well-being. Inactivity causes the joints to become stiffer with age. Stiffness, in turn, often causes people to assume unnatural body postures that can stress joints and muscles. Stretching exercises can help ensure a healthy range of motion for all major joints.

Body Composition

Body composition refers to the proportion of fat and **fat-free mass** (muscle, bone, and water) in the body. Healthy body composition involves a high proportion of fat-free mass and an acceptably low level of body fat, adjusted for age and gender. A person with excessive body fat—especially excess fat in the abdomen—is more likely to experience health problems, including heart disease, insulin resistance, high blood pressure, stroke, joint problems, type 2 diabetes, gallbladder disease, blood vessel inflammation, some types of cancer, back pain, and premature death.

The best way to lose fat is through a lifestyle that includes a sensible diet and exercise. The best way to add muscle mass is through strength training. Large changes in body composition are not necessary to improve health; even a small increase in physical activity and a small decrease in body fat can lead to substantial health improvements.

Somatotype, or body build, affects a person's choice of exercise. *Endomorphs* are round and pear-shaped. They often excel at weight lifting and weight-supported aerobic exercises such as swimming or cycling. Conversely, they might find distance running difficult and painful. *Mesomorphs* are lean and muscular and usually excel at almost any kind of physical activity or sport. *Ectomorphs* are thin and linear. Their light frame helps them succeed in activities such as distance running and gymnastics. No matter what body type you have, you can benefit from some form of physical activity.

Skill (Neuromuscular)-Related Components of Fitness

In addition to the five health-related components of physical fitness, the ability to perform a particular sport or activity may depend on **skill (neuromuscular)-related fitness**. Neuromuscular refers to the complex control of muscles and movement by the brain and spinal column. The components of skill-related fitness include the following:

- *Speed*—the ability to perform a movement in a short period of time
- *Power*—the ability to exert force rapidly, based on a combination of strength and speed
- *Agility*—the ability to change the position of the body quickly and accurately
- *Balance*—the ability to maintain equilibrium while moving or while stationary
- *Coordination*—the ability to perform motor tasks accurately and smoothly using body movements and the senses
- *Reaction and movement time*—the ability to respond and react quickly to a stimulus

TERMS

muscular endurance   The ability of a muscle to remain contracted or to contract repeatedly for a long period of time.

flexibility   The ability to move joints through their full ranges of motion.

body composition   The proportion of fat and fat-free mass (muscle, bone, and water) in the body.

fat-free mass   The nonfat component of the human body, consisting of skeletal muscle, bone, and water.

somatotype   A body-type classification system that describes people as predominantly muscular (mesomorph), tall and thin (ectomorph), or round and heavy (endomorph).

skill (neuromuscular)-related fitness   Physical capacities that contribute to performance in a sport or an activity, including speed, power, agility, balance, coordination, and reaction time; neuromuscular fitness refers specifically to maintaining performance levels of balance, agility, coordination, and gait through the control of muscles and movement by the brain and spinal column.

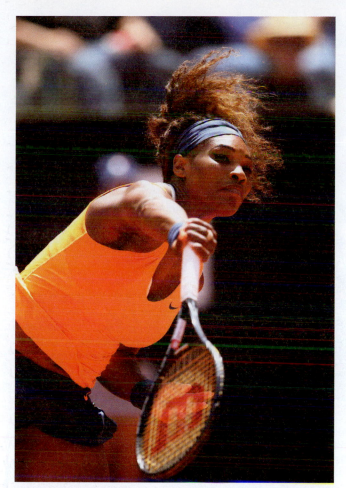

Fitness Tip You don't need to develop the skills of a professional athlete to participate in sports, but boosting sport-specific skills such as speed, power, coordination, and reaction time can make participating in sports more fun. And if you enjoy yourself, you are more likely to stick with the activity!

Skill-related fitness tends to be sport-specific and is best developed through practice. For example, playing basketball can develop the speed, coordination, and agility needed to engage in the sport. Participating in sports is fun, can help build fitness, and contributes to other areas of wellness. Young adults often find it easier to exercise regularly when they participate in sports and activities they enjoy, such as dancing, tennis, snowboarding, or basketball. Older adults can develop balance by practicing exercises such as yoga and tai chi. Skill-related activities are particularly important for older adults to help prevent life-threatening falls.

PRINCIPLES OF PHYSICAL TRAINING: ADAPTATION TO STRESS

The human body is very adaptable. The greater the demands made on it, the more it adjusts to meet those demands. Over time, immediate, short-term adjustments (**adaptations**) translate into long-term changes and improvements. When breathing

and heart rate increase during exercise, for example, the heart gradually develops the ability to pump more blood with each beat. Then, during exercise, it doesn't have to beat as fast to meet the cells' demands for oxygen. The goal of **physical training** is to produce these long-term changes and improvements in the body's functioning and fitness. Although people differ in the maximum levels of physical fitness and performance they can achieve through training, the wellness benefits of exercise are available to everyone (see the box "Fitness and Disability").

Particular types and amounts of exercise are most effective in developing the various components of fitness. To put together an effective exercise program, you should first understand the basic principles of physical training, including the following:

- Specificity
- Progressive overload
- Reversibility
- Individual differences

All of these rest on the larger principle of adaptation.

Specificity—Adapting to Type of Training

To develop a particular fitness component, you must perform exercises designed specifically for that component. This is the principle of **specificity**. Weight training, for example, develops muscular strength but is less effective for developing cardiorespiratory endurance or flexibility. Specificity also applies to the skill-related fitness components (to improve at tennis, you must practice tennis) and to the different parts of the body (to develop stronger arms, you must exercise your arms). A well-rounded exercise program includes exercises geared to each component of fitness, to different parts of the body, and to specific activities or sports.

Sports science pioneer Franklin Henry from the University of California, Berkeley, developed the principle of specificity of training. His studies showed that a specific movement performed at a specific speed develops a unique skill. Motor control studies have shown that practice reinforces motor patterns in the brain that are specific to a given movement. In other words, there is no general coordination, agility, balance, and accuracy. The balance required in skiing is different from the balance required to stand on one foot or do tricks on a skateboard. Each requires its own specific training.

> **TERMS**
>
> **adaptation** The physiological changes that occur with exercise training.
>
> **physical training** The performance of different types of activities that cause the body to adapt and improve its level of fitness.
>
> **specificity** The training principle that developing a particular fitness component requires performing exercises specifically designed for that component.

Physical fitness and athletic achievement are not limited to the able-bodied. People with disabilities can also attain high levels of fitness and performance. Elite athletes compete in the Paralympics, the premier event for athletes with disabilities that is held in the same year and city as the Olympics. The performance of these skilled athletes makes it clear that people with disabilities can be active, healthy, and extraordinarily fit. Just like able-bodied athletes, athletes with disabilities strive for excellence and can serve as role models.

According to the U.S. Census Bureau, about 54 million Americans have some type of chronic disability. Some disabilities are the result of injury, such as spinal cord injuries sustained in car crashes or war. Other disabilities result from illness, such as the blindness that sometimes occurs as a complication of diabetes or the joint stiffness that accompanies arthritis. And some disabilities are present at birth, as in the case of congenital limb deformities or cerebral palsy.

Exercise and physical activity are as important for people with disabilities as for able-bodied individuals—if not *more* important. Being active helps prevent secondary conditions that may result from prolonged inactivity, such as circulatory or muscular problems. Currently, about 19% of people with disabilities engage in regular moderate-intensity activity.

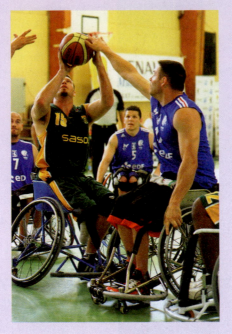

People with disabilities don't have to be elite athletes to participate in sports and lead an active life. Some health clubs, fitness centers, city recreation centers, and universities offer activities and events geared for people of all ages and types of disabilities. They may have modified aerobics classes, special weight training machines, classes for mild exercise in warm water, and other activities adapted for people with disabilities. Popular sports and recreational activities include adapted horseback riding, golf, swimming, and skiing. Competitive sports are also available—for example, there are wheelchair versions of billiards, tennis, weight lifting, hockey, and basketball, as well as sports for people with hearing, visual, or mental impairments. For those who prefer to get their exercise at home, special videos are geared to individuals who use wheelchairs or who have arthritis, hearing impairments, metabolic diseases, or many other disabilities.

The Department of Education's Office for Civil Rights has issued guidelines for providing equal opportunities for sports and exercise to students with disabilities. Schools and universities must make reasonable modifications to insure that students with disabilities have equal access to sports and physical education.

If you have a disability and want to be more active, check with your physician about what's appropriate for you. Call your local community center, university, YMCA/YWCA, hospital, independent living center, or fitness center to locate facilities. Look for a facility with experienced personnel and appropriate adaptive equipment. For specialized videos, check with hospitals and health associations that address specific disabilities, such as the Arthritis Foundation.

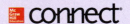

Progressive Overload—Adapting to the Amount of Training and the FITT Principle

The body adapts to the demands of exercise by improving its functioning. When the amount of exercise (also called *overload* or *stress*) is increased progressively, fitness continues to improve. This is the principle of **progressive overload**.

The amount of overload is important. Too little exercise will have no effect on fitness (although it may improve health); too much may cause injury and problems with the body's immune or endocrine (hormone) systems. The point at which exercise becomes excessive is highly individual; it occurs at a much higher level in an Olympic athlete than in a sedentary person. For every type of exercise, there is a training threshold at which fitness benefits begin to occur, a zone within which maximum fitness benefits occur, and an upper limit of safe training.

The amount of exercise needed depends on the individual's current level of fitness, the person's genetically determined capacity to adapt to training, his or her fitness goals, and the component being developed. A novice, for example, might experience fitness benefits from jogging a mile in 10 minutes, but this level of exercise would not benefit a trained distance runner. Beginners should start at the lower end of the fitness benefit zone; fitter individuals will make more rapid gains by exercising at the higher end of the fitness benefit zone. Progressive overload is critical. Exercising

TERMS **progressive overload** The training principle that progressively increasing amounts of stress on the body causes adaptation that improves fitness.

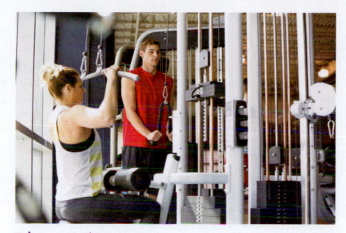

Fitness Tip Progressive overload is important because the body adapts to overload (increased volume and intensity of exercise) by becoming more fit. This is true even if your starting level of fitness is low. At the gym, don't be intimidated by people who seem to be in better shape than you are. Remember: they got in shape by focusing on themselves, not by worrying about what other people thought about them.

at the same intensity every training session will maintain fitness but will not increase it because the training stress is below the threshold required to produce adaptation. Fitness increases only if the volume and intensity of workouts increase.

The amount of overload needed to maintain or improve a particular level of fitness for a particular fitness component is determined through four dimensions, represented by the acronym FITT:

- *Frequency*—how often
- *Intensity*—how hard
- *Time*—how long (duration)
- *Type*—mode of activity

Chapters 3, 4, and 5 show you how to apply the FITT principle to exercise programs for cardiorespiratory endurance, muscular strength and endurance, and flexibility, respectively.

Frequency Developing fitness requires regular exercise. Optimum exercise frequency, expressed in number of days per week, varies with the component being developed and the individual's fitness goals. For most people, a frequency of three to five days per week for cardiorespiratory endurance exercise and two or more days per week for resistance and flexibility training are appropriate for a general fitness program.

An important consideration in determining appropriate exercise frequency is recovery time. The amount of time required to recover from exercise is highly individual and depends on factors such as training experience, age, and intensity of training. For example, 24 hours of rest between highly intense workouts involving heavy weights or track sprints is not enough recovery time for safe and effective training in most cases. Intense workouts need to be spaced out during the week to allow for sufficient recovery time. On the other hand, you can exercise every day if your program consists of moderate-intensity walking or cycling. Learn to "listen to your body" to get enough rest between workouts. Chapters 3–5 provide more

detailed information about training techniques and recovery periods for workouts focused on different fitness components.

Intensity Fitness benefits occur when a person exercises harder than his or her normal level of activity. The appropriate exercise intensity varies with each fitness component. To develop cardiorespiratory endurance, for example, you must raise your heart rate above normal. To develop muscular strength, you must lift a heavier weight than normal. To develop flexibility, you must stretch muscles beyond their normal length.

Time (Duration) Fitness benefits occur when you exercise for an extended period of time. For cardiorespiratory endurance exercise, 20–60 minutes per exercise session is recommended. Exercise can take place in a single session or in several sessions of 10 or more minutes. The greater the intensity of exercise, the less time needed to obtain fitness benefits. For high-intensity exercise, such as running, 20–30 minutes is appropriate. For moderate-intensity exercise, such as walking, 45–60 minutes may be needed. High-intensity exercise poses a greater risk of injury than low-intensity exercise, so if you are a nonathletic adult, it's best to first emphasize low- to moderate-intensity activity of longer duration.

To build muscular strength, muscular endurance, and flexibility, similar amounts of time are advisable, but training for these health components is more commonly organized in terms of a specific number of *repetitions* of a particular exercise. For resistance training, for example, a recommended program includes one or more sets of 8–12 repetitions of 8–10 different exercises that work the major muscle groups. Older adults should do 10–15 repetitions per set with lighter weights.

Type (Mode of Activity) The type of exercise in which you should engage varies with each fitness component and with your personal fitness goals. To develop cardiorespiratory endurance, you need to engage in continuous activities involving large-muscle groups—walking, jogging, cycling, or swimming, for example. Resistance exercises develop muscular strength and endurance, and stretching exercises build flexibility. The frequency, intensity, and time of the exercise will be different for each type of activity. (See pp. 38–41 for more on choosing appropriate activities for your fitness program.)

Reversibility—Adapting to a Reduction in Training

Fitness is a reversible adaptation. The body adjusts to lower levels of physical activity the same way it adjusts to higher levels. This is the principle of **reversibility**. When a person stops exercising, up to 50% of fitness improvements are lost within two months. However, not all fitness levels reverse at the same rate. Strength fitness is very resilient, so a person can maintain strength fitness

reversibility The training principle that fitness improvements are lost when demands on the body are lowered.

by doing resistance exercise as infrequently as once a week. On the other hand, cardiovascular and cellular fitness reverse themselves more quickly—sometimes within just a few days or weeks. If you must temporarily reduce the frequency or duration of your training, you can maintain much of your fitness improvement by keeping the intensity of your workouts constant.

Individual Differences—Limits on Adaptability

Anyone watching the Olympics can see that, from a physical standpoint, we are not all created equal. There are large individual differences in our ability to improve fitness, achieve a desirable body composition, and learn and perform sports skills. Some people are able to run longer distances, lift more weight, or kick a soccer ball more skillfully than others will ever be able to, no matter how much they train. People respond to training at different rates, so a program that works for one person may not be right for another person.

There are limits on the adaptability—the potential for improvement—of any human body. The body's ability to transport and use oxygen, for example, can be improved by only about 5–30% through training. An endurance athlete must therefore inherit a large metabolic capacity to reach competitive performance levels. In the past few years, scientists have identified specific genes that influence body fat, strength, and endurance. For example, more than 800 genes are associated with endurance performance, and 100 of those determine individual differences in exercise capacity. However, physical training improves fitness regardless of heredity. The average person's body can improve enough to achieve reasonable fitness goals.

DESIGNING YOUR OWN EXERCISE PROGRAM

Physical training works best when you have a plan. A plan helps you make gradual but steady progress toward your goals. First, determine that exercise is safe for you; then assess how fit you are, decide what your goals are, and choose the right activities to help you get there.

Getting Medical Clearance

Participating in exercise and sports is usually a wonderful experience that improves wellness in both the short and the long term. In rare instances, however, vigorous exertion is associated with sudden death. It may seem difficult to understand that

although regular exercise protects people from heart disease, exercise also increases the risk of sudden death for some.

Exercise and Cardiac Risk Overall, the risk of death from exercise is small—and people are much safer exercising than engaging in many other common activities, including driving a car. One study of joggers found one death for every 396,000 hours of jogging; another study of men involved in a variety of physical activities found one death per 1.5 million hours of exercise.

In people under 35, congenital heart defects (heart abnormalities present at birth) are the most common cause of exercise-related sudden death. In nearly all other cases, coronary artery disease is responsible. In this condition, fat and other substances build up in the arteries that supply blood to the heart. Death can result if an artery becomes blocked or if the heart's rhythm and pumping action are disrupted. Exercise, particularly intense exercise, may trigger a heart attack in someone with underlying heart disease. The riskiest scenario may involve the middle-aged or older individual who suddenly begins participating in a vigorous sport or activity after being sedentary for a long time. Engaging in very vigorous exercise over the long term can also be risky for some individuals, due to the stress on the cardiovascular system. For example, study of joggers in Denmark found the lowest mortality rate among those who jogged a moderate amount (2–3 workouts for a total of 60 to 150 minutes per week); higher rates of death were found among non-joggers and those who jogged at a very intense level and/or for long distances (even moderate jogging is high-intensity exercise).

Where does this leave you? Overall, exercise causes many positive changes in the body—in healthy people as well as those with heart disease—that more than make up for the slightly increased short-term risk of sudden death. People who exercise regularly have an overall risk of sudden death only about two-thirds that of non-exercisers. Active people who stop exercising can expect their heart attack risk to increase by 300%. The risk of heart-related sudden death in middle-aged and older adults is least in people who exercise approximately 150 minutes per week—the activity level recommended by the U.S. Department of Health and Human Services.

Medical Clearance Recommendations People of any age who are not at high risk for serious health problems can safely exercise at a moderate intensity (60% or less of maximum heart rate) without a prior medical evaluation (see Chapter 3 for a discussion of maximum heart rate). Likewise, if you are male and under 40 or female and under 50 and in good health, exercise is probably safe for you. If you do not fit into these age groups, or if you have health problems—especially high blood pressure, heart disease, muscle or joint problems, or obesity—see your physician before starting a vigorous exercise program. The Canadian Society for Exercise Physiology has developed the Physical Activity Readiness Questionnaire (PAR-Q) to help evaluate exercise safety; it is included in Lab 2.1. Completing it should alert you to any potential problems you may have. If a physician isn't sure whether exercise is safe for you, she or he may recommend an **exercise stress test** or a **graded exercise test (GXT)** to see whether you

---

TERMS

exercise stress test   A test usually administered on a treadmill or cycle ergometer using an electrocardiogram (EKG or ECG) to analyze changes in electrical activity in the heart during exercise; used to determine if any heart disease is present and to assess current fitness level.

graded exercise test (GXT)   An exercise test that starts at an easy intensity and progresses to maximum capacity.

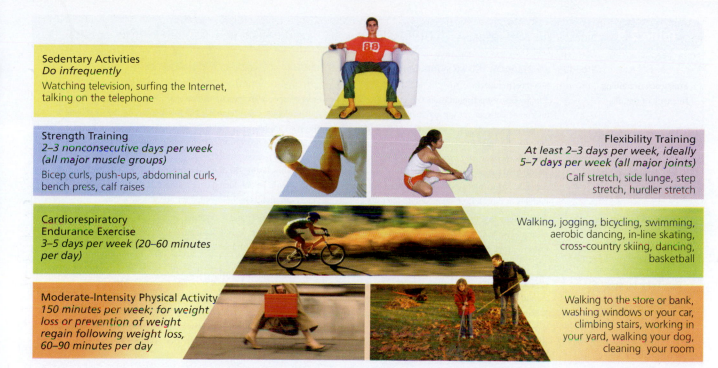

FIGURE 2.3 Physical activity pyramid.

show symptoms of heart disease during exercise. For most people, however, it's far safer to exercise than to remain sedentary.

Assessing Yourself

The first step in creating a successful fitness program is to assess your current level of physical activity and fitness for each of the five health-related fitness components. The results of the assessment tests will help you set specific fitness goals and plan your fitness program. Lab 2.3 gives you the opportunity to assess your current overall level of activity and determine if it is appropriate. Assessment tests in Chapters 3–6 will help you evaluate your cardiorespiratory endurance, muscular strength, muscular endurance, flexibility, and body composition.

Setting Goals

The ultimate general goal of every health-related fitness program is the same—wellness that lasts a lifetime. That life-long goal might include the specific goals of walking 30 to 60 minutes every day or doing a few callisthenic exercises every morning. Whatever your specific goals, they must be important enough to you to keep you motivated. Most sports psychologists believe that setting and achieving goals is the most effective way to stay motivated about exercise. (Refer to Chapter 1 for more on goal setting, as well as Common Questions Answered at the end of this chapter.) After you complete the assessment tests in Chapters 3–6, you will be able to set goals directly related to each fitness component, such as working toward a three-mile jog or doing 20 push-ups. First, though, think carefully about your overall goals, and be clear about why you are starting a program.

Choosing Activities for a Balanced Program

An ideal fitness program combines a physically active life-style with systematic exercise to develop and maintain physical fitness. This overall program is shown in the physical activity pyramid in Figure 2.3. If you are currently sedentary, your goal should be to focus on activities at the bottom of the pyramid and gradually increase the amount of moderate-intensity physical activity in your daily life. Appropriate activities include walking briskly, climbing stairs, doing yard work, and washing your car. You don't have to exercise vigorously, but you should experience a moderate increase in your heart and breathing rates. As described earlier, your activity time can be broken up into small blocks over the course of a day.

The next two levels of the pyramid illustrate parts of a formal exercise program. The principles of this program are consistent with those of the American College of Sports Medicine (ACSM), the professional organization for people involved in sports medicine and exercise science. The ACSM has established guidelines for creating an exercise program that will develop physical fitness (Table 2.3). A balanced program includes activities to develop all the health-related components of fitness:

- *Cardiorespiratory endurance* is developed by continuous rhythmic movements of large-muscle groups in activities such as walking, jogging, cycling, swimming, aerobic dance, and other forms of group exercise. High intensity interval training (HIIT)—short bouts of high-intensity exercise

Table 2.3   ACSM Exercise Recommendations for Fitness Development in Healthy Adults

EXERCISE TO DEVELOP AND MAINTAIN CARDIORESPIRATORY ENDURANCE AND BODY COMPOSITION

Frequency of training	3–5 days per week.
Intensity of training	55/65–90% of maximum heart rate or 40/50–85% of heart rate reserve or oxygen uptake reserve. (Reserve refers to the difference between resting and maximum values of heart rate or oxygen consumption.) The lower-intensity values (55–64% of maximum heart rate and 40–49% of heart rate reserve plus rest) are most applicable to unfit individuals. For average individuals, intensities of 70–85% of maximum heart rate or 60–80% of heart rate reserve plus rest are appropriate. These methods increase exercise intensity within the limits of each person's reserve capacity.
Time (duration) of training	20–60 total minutes per day of continuous or intermittent (in sessions lasting 10 or more minutes) aerobic activity. Duration depends on the intensity of activity; thus, low-intensity activity should be conducted over a longer period of time (30 minutes or more). Low- to moderate-intensity activity of longer duration is recommended for nonathletic adults.
Type (mode) of activity	Any activity that uses large-muscle groups, can be maintained continuously and is rhythmic and aerobic in nature—for example, walking-hiking, running-jogging, bicycling, cross-country skiing, aerobic dancing and other forms of group exercise, rope-skipping, rowing, stair-climbing, swimming, skating, and endurance game activities.

EXERCISE TO DEVELOP AND MAINTAIN MUSCULAR STRENGTH AND ENDURANCE, FLEXIBILITY, AND BODY COMPOSITION

Resistance training	One set of 8–10 exercises that condition the major muscle groups, performed at least two days per week. Most people should complete 8–12 repetitions of each exercise to the point of fatigue; practicing other repetition ranges (for example, 3–5 or 12–15) also builds strength and endurance; for older and frailer people (approximately 50–60 and older), 10–15 repetitions with a lighter weight may be more appropriate. Multiple-set regimens will provide greater benefits if time allows. Any mode of exercise that is comfortable throughout the full range of motion is appropriate (for example, free weights, kettlebells, calisthenics, elastic bands, or weight machines).
Flexibility training	Static stretches, performed for the major muscle groups at least 2–3 days per week, ideally 5–7 days per week. Stretch to the point of tightness, holding each stretch for 10–30 seconds; perform 2–4 repetitions of each stretch.

*Chapter 3 provides instructions for calculating target heart rate intensity for cardiorespiratory endurance exercise.

SOURCE: Adapted from American College of Sports Medicine. 2013. *ACSM's Guidelines for Exercise Testing and Prescription,* 9th ed. Philadelphia: Wolters Kluwer/Lippincott Williams & Wilkins Health; Garber, C. E., et al. 2011. Quantity and quality of exercise for developing and maintaining cardiorespiratory, musculoskeletal, and neuromotor fitness in apparently healthy adults: guidance for prescribing exercise. *Medicine and Science in Sports and Exercise* 43(7): 1334–1359.

followed by rest—also builds endurance quickly. The advantage of HIIT is that it does not take as much time as traditional endurance training. The disadvantage is that it can be painful and uncomfortable. The safety of HIIT has not been determined.

Choose activities that you enjoy and are convenient. Popular choices are in-line skating, skiing, dancing, cycling, and backpacking. Start-and-stop activities such as tennis, racquetball, and soccer can also develop cardiorespiratory endurance if your skill level is sufficient to enable periods of continuous play. Training for cardiorespiratory endurance is discussed in Chapter 3.

- *Muscular strength and endurance* can be developed through resistance training—training with weights or performing calisthenics such as push-ups, planks, and curl-ups. Training for muscular strength and endurance is discussed in Chapter 4.
- *Flexibility* is developed by stretching the major muscle groups regularly and with proper technique. Flexibility is discussed in Chapter 5.
- *Healthy body composition* can be developed through a sensible diet and a program of regular exercise. Cardiorespiratory endurance exercise is best for reducing body fat; resistance training builds muscle mass, which, to a small extent, helps increase metabolism. Body composition is discussed in Chapter 6.

Chapter 7 contains guidelines to help you choose activities and put together a complete exercise program that will suit your goals and preferences. (Refer to Figure 2.4 for a summary of the health and fitness benefits of different levels of physical activity and exercise programs.)

What about the tip of the activity pyramid? Although sedentary activities are often unavoidable—attending class, studying, working in an office, and so on—many people *choose* inactivity over activity during their leisure time. Change sedentary patterns by becoming more active whenever you can.

Guidelines for Training

The following guidelines will make your exercise program more effective and successful.

Train the Way You Want Your Body to Change
Stress your body so it adapts in the desired manner. To have a more muscular build, lift weights. To be more flexible, do stretching exercises. To improve performance in a particular sport, practice that sport or its movements.

Train Regularly
Consistency is the key to improving fitness. Fitness improvements are lost if too much time passes between exercise sessions.

	Lifestyle physical activity	Moderate exercise program	Vigorous exercise program
Description	Moderate physical activity (150 minutes per week; muscle-strengthening exercises 2 or more days per week)	Cardiorespiratory endurance exercise (20–60 minutes, 3–5 days per week); strength training (2–3 nonconsecutive days per week); and stretching exercises (2 or more days per week)	Cardiorespiratory endurance exercise (20–60 minutes, 3–5 days per week); interval training; strength training (3–4 nonconsecutive days per week); and stretching exercises (5–7 days per week)
Sample activities or program	• Walking to and from work, 15 minutes each way • Cycling to and from class, 10 minutes each way • Doing yard work for 30 minutes • Dancing (fast) for 30 minutes • Playing basketball for 20 minutes • Muscle exercises such as push-ups, squats, or back exercises	• Jogging for 30 minutes, 3 days per week • Weight training, 1 set of 8 exercises, 2 days per week • Stretching exercises, 3 days per week	• Running for 45 minutes, 3 days per week • Intervals, running 400 m at high effort, 4 sets, 2 days per week • Weight training, 3 sets of 10 exercises, 3 days per week • Stretching exercises, 6 days per week
Health and fitness benefits	Better blood cholesterol levels, reduced body fat, better control of blood pressure, improved metabolic health, and enhanced glucose metabolism; improved quality of life; reduced risk of some chronic diseases Greater amounts of activity can help prevent weight gain and promote weight loss	All the benefits of lifestyle physical activity, plus improved physical fitness (increased cardiorespiratory endurance, muscular strength and endurance, and flexibility) and even greater improvements in health and quality of life and reductions in chronic disease risk	All the benefits of lifestyle physical activity and a moderate exercise program, with greater increases in fitness and somewhat greater reductions in chronic disease risk Participating in a vigorous exercise program may increase risk of injury and overtraining

FIGURE 2.4 **Health and fitness benefits of different amounts of physical activity and exercise.**

Start Slowly, and Get in Shape Gradually As Figure 2.5 shows, an exercise program can be divided into three phases:

- *Beginning phase.* The body adjusts to the new type and level of activity.

- *Progress phase.* Fitness increases.

- *Maintenance phase.* The targeted level of fitness is sustained over the long term.

When beginning a program, start slowly to give your body time to adapt to the stress of exercise. Choose activities carefully according to your fitness status. If you have been sedentary or are overweight, try an activity such as walking or swimming that won't jar the body or strain the joints.

As you progress, increase duration and frequency before increasing intensity. If you train too much or too intensely, you are more likely to suffer injuries or become **overtrained**, a condition characterized by lack of energy, aching muscles and joints, and decreased physical performance. Injuries and overtraining slow down an exercise program and impede motivation. The goal is not to get in shape as quickly as possible but to gradually become and then remain physically fit.

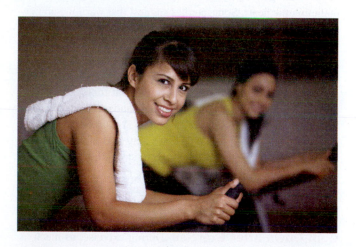

Wellness Tip Moderation is Important, especially if you're just starting to get physically active. Work at a pace that's comfortable and enjoyable, with a goal of making gradual improvements. This will help you get into the habit of being active and will help you avoid burnout.

overtraining A condition caused by training too much or too intensely, characterized by lack of energy, decreased physical performance, and aching muscles and joints. **TERMS**

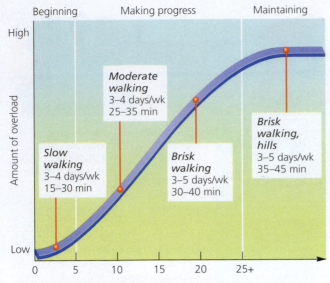

Beginning   Making progress   Maintaining

Moderate walking
3–4 days/wk
25–35 min

Slow walking
3–4 days/wk
15–30 min

Brisk walking
3–5 days/wk
30–40 min

Brisk walking, hills
3–5 days/wk
35–45 min

High

Low

Amount of overload

0   5   10   15   20   25+

Time since beginning an exercise program (in weeks)

FIGURE 2.5   Progression of an exercise program. This figure shows how the amount of overload is increased gradually over time in a walking and running program. Regardless of the activity chosen, it is important that an exercise program begin slowly and progress gradually. After you achieve the desired level of fitness, you can maintain it by exercising 3–5 days a week.

SOURCE: Progression data from American College of Sports Medicine. 2009. *ACSM's Guidelines for Exercise Testing and Prescription,* 8th ed. Philadelphia: Lippincott Williams and Wilkins.

Warm Up before Exercise Warming up can decrease your chances of injury by helping your body gradually progress from rest to activity. A good warm-up can increase muscle temperature, reduce joint stiffness, bathe the joint surfaces in lubricating fluid, and increase blood flow to the muscles, including the heart. Some studies suggest that warming up may also enhance muscle metabolism and mentally prepare you for a workout.

A warm-up should include low-intensity, whole-body movements similar to those used in the activity. For example, runners may walk and jog slowly prior to running at full speed. A tennis player might hit forehands and backhands at a low intensity before playing a vigorous set of tennis. A warm-up is not the same as a stretching workout. For safety and effectiveness, it is best to stretch *after* an endurance or strength training workout, when muscles are warm—and not as part of a warm-up. (Appropriate and effective warm-ups are discussed in greater detail in Chapters 3–5.)

Cool Down after Exercise During exercise, as much as 90% of circulating blood is directed to the muscles and skin, up from as little as 20% during rest. If you suddenly stop moving after exercise, the amount of blood returning to your heart and brain may be insufficient, and you may experience dizziness, a drop in blood pressure, or other problems. Cooling down at the end of a workout helps safely restore circulation to its normal resting condition. So, after you exercise, cool down before you sit or lie down or jump into the shower. Cool down by continuing to move at a slow pace—walking for 5–10 minutes, for

example, as your heart and breathing rate and blood pressure slowly return to normal. At the end of the cool-down period, do stretching exercises while your muscles are still warm. Cool down longer after intense exercise sessions.

Exercise Safely Physical activity can cause injury or even death if you don't consider safety. For example, you should always:

- Wear a helmet when biking, skiing, or rock climbing.
- Wear eye protection when playing racquetball or squash.
- Wear bright clothing when exercising on a public street.
- Walk or run with a partner on a deserted track or in a park.
- Give vehicles plenty of leeway, even when you have the right of way.
- In the weight room, be aware of people exercising near you, and use spotters and collars when appropriate.

Overloading your muscles and joints can lead to serious injury, so train within your capacity. Use high-quality equipment and keep it in good repair. Report broken gym equipment to the health club manager or physical education instructor. (See Appendix A for more information on personal safety.)

Listen to Your Body and Get Adequate Rest Rest can be as important as exercise for improving fitness. Fitness reflects an adaptation to the stress of exercise. Building fitness involves a series of exercise stresses, recuperation, and adaptation leading to improved fitness, followed by further stresses. Build rest into your training program, and don't exercise if it doesn't feel right. Sometimes you need a few days of rest to recover enough to train with the intensity required for improving fitness. Getting enough sleep is an important part of the recovery process. On the other hand, don't train sporadically, either. If you listen to your body and it always tells you to rest, you won't make any progress.

Cycle the Volume and Intensity of Your Workouts To add enjoyment and variety to your program and to further improve fitness, don't train at the same intensity during every workout. Train intensely on some days and train lightly on others. Proper management of workout intensity is a key to improving physical fitness. Use cycle training, also known as *periodization,* to provide enough recovery for intense training: By training lightly one workout, you can train harder the next. However, take care to increase the volume and intensity of your program gradually—never more than 10% per week.

Vary Your Activities Change your exercise program from time to time to keep things fresh and help develop a higher degree of fitness. The body adapts quickly to an exercise stress, such as walking, cycling, or swimming. Gains in fitness in a particular activity become more difficult with time. Varying the exercises in your program allows you to adapt to many types of exercise and develops fitness in a variety of activities (see the box "Vary Your Activities"). Changing activities may also help reduce your risk of injury. This is a central principle in

Do you have a hard time thinking of new activities to try? Check the boxes next to the activities listed here that interest you. Then look for resources and facilities on your campus or in your community.

OUTDOOR EXERCISES

☐ Walking	☐ In-line skating	☐ Hiking
☐ Running	☐ Skateboarding	☐ Backpacking
☐ Cycling	☐ Rowing	☐ Ice skating
☐ Swimming	☐ Horseback riding	☐ Fly fishing

SPORTS AND GAMES

☐ Basketball	☐ Softball	☐ Bowling
☐ Tennis	☐ Water skiing	☐ Surfing
☐ Volleyball	☐ Windsurfing	☐ Dancing
☐ Golf	☐ Badminton	☐ Snow skiing
☐ Soccer	☐ Ultimate Frisbee	☐ Gymnastics

EXERCISES YOU CAN DO AT HOME AND WORK

☐ Desk exercises	☐ Yard work	☐ Painting walls
☐ Calisthenics	☐ Sweeping	☐ Walking the dog
☐ Gardening	☐ Exploring on foot	☐ Shopping
☐ Housework	☐ Doing a walk-a-thon	☐ Doing errands

HEALTH CLUB EXERCISES

☐ Weight training	☐ Ski machine	☐ Elliptical trainer
☐ Circuit training	☐ Supine bike	☐ Medicine ball
☐ Group exercise	☐ Rowing machine	☐ Rope skipping
☐ Treadmill	☐ Plyometrics	☐ Punching bag
☐ Stationary bike	☐ Water aerobics	☐ Racquetball

cross-training exercise techniques such as CrossFit. CrossFit is a commercial exercise program that uses a variety of training methods to improve fitness, including running, swimming, climbing, gymnastics, functional training, Olympic weight lifting, kettlebells, rope climbing, and calisthenics.

Train with a Partner People who train together can motivate and encourage each other through rough spots and help each other develop proper exercise techniques. Training with a partner can make exercising seem easier and more fun. It can also help you keep motivated and on track. A commitment to a friend is a powerful motivator. If you can afford it, you may benefit from a certified personal trainer who can give you instruction in exercise techniques and help provide motivation.

Train Your Mind Becoming fit requires commitment, discipline, and patience. These qualities come from understanding the importance of exercise and setting clear and reachable goals. Use the lifestyle management techniques discussed in Chapter 1 to keep your program on track.

Fuel Your Activity Appropriately Good nutrition, including rehydration and resynthesis of liver and muscle carbohydrate stores, is part of optimal recuperation from exercise. Consume enough calories to support your exercise program without gaining body fat. Many studies show that consuming carbohydrates and protein before or after exercise promotes restoration of stored fuels and helps heal injured tissues so that you can exercise intensely again shortly. Nutrition for exercise is discussed in greater detail in Chapters 3 and 8.

Have Fun You are more likely to stick with an exercise program if it's fun. Choose a variety of activities that you enjoy. Some people like to play competitive sports, such as tennis, golf, or volleyball. Competition can boost motivation, but remember: Sports are competitive, whereas training for fitness is not. Other people like more solitary activities, such as jogging, walking, or swimming. Still others like high-skill individual sports, such as snowboarding, surfing, or skateboarding. Many activities can help you get fit, so choose the ones you enjoy. You can also boost your enjoyment and build your social support network by exercising with friends and family.

Track Your Progress Monitoring the progress of your program can help keep you motivated and on track. Depending on the activities you've included in your program, you may track different measures of your program—minutes of jogging, miles of cycling, laps of swimming, number of push-ups, amount of weight lifted, and so on. If your program focuses on increasing daily physical activity, consider using an inexpensive pedometer or exercise GPS app to monitor the number of steps you take each day. (See Lab 2.3 for more information on setting goals and monitoring activity with a pedometer; see the box "Digital Workout Aids" for an introduction to products and apps that can help you track your progress.) Specific examples of program monitoring can be found in the labs for Chapters 3–5.

Get Help and Advice If You Need It One of the best places to get help starting an exercise program is an exercise class. If you join a health club or fitness center, follow the guidelines in the box "Choosing a Fitness Center." There, expert instructors can help you learn the basics of training and answer your questions. Make sure the instructor is certified by a recognized professional organization and/or has formal training in exercise physiology. Read articles by credible experts in fitness magazines (such as *Fitness Rx for Women* and *Fitness Rx for Men*). Many of these magazines include articles by leading experts in exercise science written at a layperson's level.

WELLNESS IN THE DIGITAL AGE
Digital Workout Aids

When you're just starting to get physically active, you can wind up with a lot of questions. How many miles did I walk? How many sit-ups did I do? How many minutes did I run? When your mind is completely focused on just *doing* an activity, it's easy to lose count of time, distance, and reps. But it's important to keep track of these things: Move too little and you won't see any progress; move too much and you run the risk of injury or burnout. Either outcome is bad news for your exercise program.

Luckily, we live in a digital age, and the fitness industry is providing an ever-growing array of high-tech tools and apps that can track your progress for you. If you like to walk or run, cell phone apps can track your distance, number of steps you take, and give you a detailed map of where you ran, biked, or skied. Advanced trackers can even record any hills you encounter during your workout. Heart rate monitors can help you reach and maintain the right exercise intensity. If calisthenics are your choice, there are gaming systems and smartphone apps that work for specific exercises to count reps, assess your form, and challenge you to push yourself harder.

Smart phone programs, such as Coach's Eye, Hudl Technique and Dartfish, can help you analyze your golf swing or tennis forehand in slow motion. The programs even make it possible to compare your progress by showing several performances side-by-side.

You can track more than just your exercise habits with digital assistance. Electronic devices and smart programs are available to help with many aspects of wellness, including the following:

- Dietary habits
- Calories consumed and burned
- Stress management
- Meditation and spirituality
- Heart rate and respiration
- Menstrual cycles
- Family medical history
- Journaling

And that's just to name a few. We'll introduce a variety of these digital devices and apps in later chapters, in the "Wellness in the Digital Age" feature box like this one. You may find one or more digital apps (many of which are free) that appeal to you and can help you make progress toward your own fitness and wellness goals.

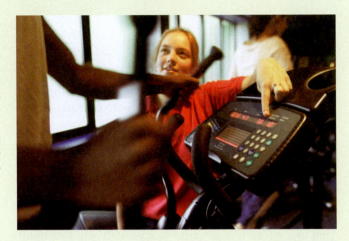

A qualified personal trainer can also help you get started in an exercise program or a new form of training. Make sure this person has proper qualifications, such as certification by the ACSM, National Strength and Conditioning Association (NSCA), or International Sports Sciences Association (ISSA). Don't seek out a person for advice simply because he or she looks fit. UCLA researchers found that 60% of the personal trainers in their study couldn't pass a basic exam on training methods, exercise physiology, or biomechanics. Trainers who performed best had college degrees in exercise physiology, physical education, or physical therapy. So choose your trainer carefully and don't get caught up with fads or appearances.

Keep Your Exercise Program in Perspective As important as physical fitness is, it is only part of a well-rounded life. You need time for work and school, family and friends, relaxation and hobbies. Some people become over-involved in exercise and neglect other parts of their lives. They think of themselves as runners, dancers, swimmers, or triathletes rather than as people who happen to participate in those activities. Balance and moderation are key ingredients of a fit and well life.

Ask Yourself

QUESTIONS FOR CRITICAL THINKING AND REFLECTION

If you were to start planning a fitness program, what would be your three most important long-term goals? What would you set as short-term goals? What rewards would be meaningful to you?

COMMON QUESTIONS ANSWERED

Q **I have asthma. Is it OK for me to start an exercise program?**

A Probably, but you should see your doctor before you start exercising, especially if you have been sedentary up to this point. Your personal physician can advise you on the type of exercise program that is best for you, given the severity of your condition, and how to avoid suffering exercise-related asthma attacks.

Q **What should my fitness goals be?**

A Begin by thinking about your general overall goals—the benefits you want to obtain by increasing your activity level and/or beginning a formal exercise program. Examples of long-term goals include reducing your risk of chronic diseases, increasing your energy level, and maintaining a healthy body weight.

To help shape your fitness program, you need to set specific, short-term goals based on measurable factors. These specific goals should be an extension of your overall goals—the specific changes to your current activity and exercise habits needed to achieve your general goals. In setting short-term goals, be sure to use the SMART criteria described in Chapter 1. As noted there, your goals should be **S**pecific, **M**easurable, **A**ttainable, **R**ealistic, and **T**ime frame–specific (SMART).

You need information about your current levels of physical activity and physical fitness in order to set appropriate goals. The labs in this chapter will help you determine your physical activity level—for example, how many minutes per day you engage in moderate or vigorous activity or how many daily steps you take. Using this information, you can set goals for lifestyle physical activity to help you meet your overall goals. For example, if your general long-term goals are to reduce the risk of chronic disease and prevent weight gain, the Dietary Guidelines recommend 60 minutes of moderate physical activity daily. If you currently engage in 30 minutes of moderate activity daily, then your behavior change goal would be to add 30 minutes of daily physical activity (or an equivalent number of additional daily steps—about 3,500–4,000); your time frame for the change might be 8–12 weeks.

Labs in Chapters 3–6 provide opportunities to assess your fitness status for all the health-related components of fitness. The results of these assessments can guide you in setting specific fitness goals. For instance, if the labs in Chapter 4 indicate that you have good muscular strength and endurance in your lower body but poor strength and endurance in your upper body, then setting a specific goal for improving upper-body muscle fitness would be an appropriate goal—increasing the number of push-ups you can do from 22 to 30, for example. Chapters 3–6 include additional advice for setting appropriate goals.

After you start your behavior change program, you may discover that your goals aren't quite appropriate; perhaps you were overly optimistic, or maybe you set the bar too low. There are limits to the amount of fitness you can achieve, but within the limits of your genes, health status, and motivation, you can make significant improvements in fitness. Adjust your goals as needed.

Q **Should I follow my exercise program if I'm sick?**

A If you have a mild head cold or feel one coming on, it is probably okay to exercise moderately. Just begin slowly and see how you feel. However, if you have symptoms of a more serious illness—fever, swollen glands, nausea, extreme tiredness, muscle aches—wait until you have recovered fully before resuming your exercise program. Continuing to exercise while suffering from an illness more serious than a cold can compromise your recovery and may even be dangerous.

CRITICAL CONSUMER
Choosing a Fitness Center

Fitness centers can provide you with many benefits—motivation and companionship are among the most important. A fitness center may also offer expert instruction and supervision as well as access to better equipment than you could afford on your own. All fitness centers, however, are not of the same overall quality, and every fitness center is not for every person. If you're thinking of joining a fitness center, here are some guidelines to help you choose a club that's right for you.

Convenience

- Look for an established facility that's within 10–15 minutes of your home or work. If it's farther away, your chances of sticking to an exercise regimen start to diminish.

- Visit the facility at the time you would normally exercise. Is there adequate parking? Will you have easy access to equipment and classes at that time?

- What child care services are available, and how are they supervised?

Atmosphere

- Look around to see if there are other members who are your age and at about your fitness level. Some clubs cater to a certain age group or lifestyle, such as hard-core bodybuilders.

- Observe how the members dress. Will you fit in, or will you be uncomfortable?

- Observe the staff. Are they easy to identify? Are they friendly, professional, and helpful?

- Check to see that the facility is clean, including showers and lockers. Make sure the facility is climate controlled, well ventilated, and well lit.

Safety

- Find out if the facility offers some type of preactivity screening as well as basic fitness testing that includes cardiovascular screening.

- Determine if personnel are trained in CPR and if there is emergency equipment such as automated external defibrillators (AEDs) on the premises. An AED can help someone who has a cardiac arrest.

- Ask if at least one staff member on each shift is trained in first aid.

Trained Personnel

- Determine if the personal trainers and fitness instructors are certified by a recognized professional association such as the ACSM, Aerobics and Fitness Association of America (AFAA), NSCA, or ISSA. All personal trainers are not equal; more than 100 organizations certify trainers, and few of these require much formal training.

- Find out if the club has a trained exercise physiologist on staff, such as someone with a degree in exercise physiology, kinesiology, or exercise science. If the facility offers nutritional counseling, it should employ someone who is a registered dietitian (RD) or has similar formal training.

- Ask how much experience the instructors have. Ideally, trainers should have both academic preparation and practical experience.

Cost

- Buy only what you need and can afford. If you want to use only workout equipment, you may not need a club that has racquetball courts and saunas.

- Check the contract. Choose the one that covers the shortest period of time possible, especially if it's your first fitness club experience. Don't feel pressured to sign a long-term contract.

- Make sure the contract permits you to extend your membership if you have a prolonged illness or go on vacation. Some clubs have exchange agreements that allow you to train in other cities while on vacation or business.

- Try out the club. Ask for a free trial workout, or a one-day pass, or an inexpensive one- or two-week trial membership.

- Find out whether there is an extra charge for the particular services you want. Get any special offers in writing.

Effectiveness

- Tour the facility. Does it offer what the brochure says it does? Does it offer the activities and equipment you want?

- Check the equipment. A good club will have treadmills, bikes, stair-climbers, resistance machines, and weights. Make sure these machines are up to date and well maintained.

- Find out if new members get a formal orientation and instruction on how to safely use the equipment. Will a staff member help you develop a program that is appropriate for your current fitness level and goals?

- Make sure the facility is certified. Look for the displayed names ACSM, American Council on Exercise (ACE), AFAA, or International Health, Racquet, and Sportsclub Association (IHRSA).

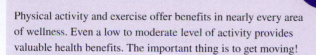

TIPS FOR TODAY AND THE FUTURE

Physical activity and exercise offer benefits in nearly every area of wellness. Even a low to moderate level of activity provides valuable health benefits. The important thing is to get moving!

RIGHT NOW YOU CAN

- Look at your calendar for the rest of the week and write in some physical activity—such as walking, running, biking, skating, swimming, hiking, or playing Frisbee—on as many days as you can. Schedule the activity for a specific time and stick to it.
- Call a friend and invite her or him to start planning a regular exercise program with you.
- Download a pedometer app on your phone and keep track of your daily activity.

IN THE FUTURE YOU CAN

- Schedule a session with a qualified personal trainer who can evaluate your current fitness level and help you set personalized fitness goals.
- Create seasonal workout programs for the spring, summer, fall, and winter. Develop programs that are varied but consistent with your overall fitness goals.

SUMMARY

- Moderate daily physical activity contributes substantially to good health. Even without a formal, vigorous exercise program, you can get many of the same health benefits just by becoming more physically active.

- If you are already active, you benefit even more by increasing the intensity or duration of your activities.

- The five components of physical fitness most important for health are cardiorespiratory endurance, muscular strength, muscular endurance, flexibility, and body composition.

- Physical training is the process of producing long-term improvements in the body's functioning through exercise. All training is based on the fact that the body adapts to physical stress.

- According to the principle of specificity, bodies change specifically in response to the type of training received.

- Bodies also adapt to progressive overload. When you progressively increase the frequency, intensity, and time (duration) of the right type of exercise, you become increasingly fit.

- Bodies adjust to lower levels of activity by losing fitness, a principle known as reversibility. To counter the effects of reversibility, it's important to keep training at the same intensity, even if you have to reduce the number or length of sessions.

- According to the principle of individual differences, people vary in the maximum level of fitness they can achieve and in the rate of change they can expect from an exercise program.

- When designing an exercise program, determine if medical clearance is needed, assess your current level of fitness, set realistic goals, and choose activities that develop all the components of fitness.

- Train regularly, get in shape gradually, warm up and cool down, maintain a structured but flexible program, get enough rest, exercise safely, vary activities, consider training with a partner or personal trainer, train your mind, eat sensibly, have fun, monitor your progress, and keep exercise in perspective.

FOR FURTHER EXPLORATION

American Alliance for Health, Physical Education, Recreation, and Dance (AAHPERD). A professional organization dedicated to promoting quality health and physical education programs.
http://www.aahperd.org

American College of Sports Medicine (ACSM). The principal professional organization for sports medicine and exercise science. Provides brochures, publications, and videos.
http://www.acsm.org

American Council on Exercise (ACE). Promotes exercise and fitness; the website features fact sheets on many consumer topics, including choosing shoes, cross-training, and steroids.
http://www.acefitness.org

American Heart Association: Start! Walking for a Healthier Lifestyle. Provides practical advice for people of all fitness levels plus an online fitness diary.
http://startwalkingnow.org

CDC Physical Activity Information. Provides information on the benefits of physical activity and suggestions for incorporating moderate physical activity into daily life.
http://www.cdc.gov/physicalactivity

CrossFit. A cross-training method involving a variety of exercises and unaccustomed physical challenges. The program includes franchised health clubs and training facilities. The website provides extensive information on cross training, nutrition, exercise techniques, and sports psychology.
http://www.crossfit.com

Disabled Sports USA. Provides sports and recreation services to people with physical or mobility disorders.
http://www.dsusa.org

Health and Retirement Study. A website describing a study of 20,000 people begun in 1992 at the University of Michigan and updated every two years. Included is an extensive reference list of published studies.
hrsonline.isr.umich.edu.

International Health, Racquet, and Sportsclub Association (IHRSA): Health Clubs. Provides guidelines for choosing a health or fitness facility and links to clubs that belong to IHRSA.
http://www.healthclubs.com

International Sports Sciences Association (ISSA). Trains and certifies personal trainers.
http://www.issaonline.com

MedlinePlus: Exercise and Physical Fitness. Provides links to news and reliable information about fitness and exercise from government agencies and professional associations.

http://www.nlm.nih.gov/medlineplus/exerciseandphysicalfitness.html

President's Council on Fitness, Sports and Nutrition. Provides information on programs and publications, including fitness guides and fact sheets.

http://www.fitness.gov
http://www.presidentschallenge.org

Shape Up America! A nonprofit organization that provides information and resources on exercise, nutrition, and weight loss.

http://www.shapeup.org

StrongFirst: A school of strength, directed by kettlebell master Pavel Tsatsouline, that teaches men and women how to reach high levels of strength and fitness without interfering with work, school, family, or sport. The program offers clinics and web-based information.

http://www.strongfirst.com

SELECTED BIBLIOGRAPHY

Alzheimer's Association. 2015. *2015 Alzheimer's Disease Facts and Figures.* Chicago: Alzheimer's Association.

American College of Sports Medicine. 2012. *ACSM's Health/Fitness Facility Standards and Guidelines,* 4th ed. Champaign, Ill.: Human Kinetics.

American College of Sports Medicine. 2011. The recommended quantity and quality of exercise for developing and maintaining cardiorespiratory and muscular fitness, and flexibility in healthy adults. ACSM position stand. *Medicine and Science in Sports and Exercise* 43(7): 1334–1359.

American College of Sports Medicine. 2013. *ACSM's Resource Manual for Guidelines for Exercise Testing and Prescription,* 7th ed. Philadelphia: Wolters Kluwer/Lippincott Williams & Wilkins Health.

American College of Sports Medicine, Pescatello, S., ed. 2013. *ACSM's Guidelines for Exercise Testing and Prescription,* 9th ed. Philadelphia: Wolters Kluwer/Lippincott Williams & Wilkins Health.

American College of Sports Medicine. 2011. *ACSM's Complete Guide to Fitness & Health.* Champaign, Ill.: Human Kinetics.

Ascensao, A., et al. 2011. Mitochondria as a target for exercise-induced cardioprotection. *Current Drug Targets* 12(6): 860–871.

Bigley, A. B., et al. 2013. Can exercise-related improvements in immunity influence cancer prevention and prognosis in the elderly? *Maturitas* 76(1): 51–56.

Biswas, A., et al. 2015. Sedentary time and its association with risk for disease incidence, mortality, and hospitalization in adults: a systematic review and meta-analysis. *Annals of Internal Medicine* 162(2): 123–132.

Bouchard, C., et al. 2015. Personalized preventive medicine: Genetics and the response to regular exercise in preventive interventions. *Progress in Cardiovascular Diseases* 57(4): 337–346.

Bos, I., et al. 2013. Subclinical effects of aerobic training in urban environment. *Medicine and Science in Sports and Exercise* 45(3): 439–447.

Casazza, K., et al. 2013. Myths, presumptions, and facts about obesity. *New England Journal of Medicine* 368 (5): 446–454.

Centers for Disease Control and Prevention. 2014. State Indicator Report on Physical Activity, 2014. Atlanta, GA: U.S. Department of Health and Human Services.

Dietary Guidelines Advisory Committee. 2015. Scientific Report of the 2015 Dietary Advisory Committee. Washington, D.C.: U.S. Department of Agriculture, Agricultural Research Service.

Donnelly, J. E., et al. 2009. Appropriate physical activity intervention strategies for weight loss and prevention of weight regain for adults (ACSM position stand). *Medicine and Science in Sports and Exercise.* 41(2): 459–471.

Duvivier, B., et al. 2013. Minimal-intensity physical activity (standing and walking) of longer duration improves insulin action and plasma lipids more than shorter periods of moderate to vigorous exercise (cycling) in sedentary subjects when energy expenditure is comparable. *PlosOne* 8(2): e55542.

Ekblom-Bak, E., et al. 2014. The importance of non-exercise physical activity for cardiovascular health and longevity. *British Journal Sports Medicine* 48(3): 233–238.

Fahey, T., and M. Fahey. 2014. Nutrition, Physical Activity, and the Obesity Epidemic: Issues, Policies, and Solutions (1960s-Present). *The Guide to U.S. Health and Health Care Policy.* T. Oliver (ed.). New York, DWJ Books: 363–374.

Fontes, E. B., et al. 2015. Brain activity and perceived exertion during cycling exercise: An fMRI study. *British Journal Sports Medicine* 49(8): 556–560.

Howley, E., and D. Thompson. 2012. *Fitness Professional's Handbook,* 6th ed. Champaign, Ill.: Human Kinetics.

John, D. 2013. *Intervention: Course Correction for the Athlete and Trainer.* Santa Cruz, Ca: On Target.

McArdle, W.D., et al. 2014. *Exercise Physiology: Nutrition, Energy, and Human Performance.* Wolters Kluwer.

Pate, R. and D. Buchner. 2014. *Implementing Physical Activity Strategies.* Champaign, IL: Human Kinetics.

Physical Activity Guidelines Advisory Committee. 2008. *Physical Activity Guidelines Advisory Committee Report, 2008.* Washington, D.C.: U.S. Department of Health and Human Services.

Puterman, E., et al. 2015. Determinants of telomere attrition over 1 year in healthy older women: stress and health behaviors matter. *Molecular Psychiatry* 20(4): 529–535.

Szuhany, K. L., et al. 2015. A meta-analytic review of the effects of exercise on brain-derived neurotrophic factor. *Journal of Psychiatric Research* 60: 56–64.

Thompson, W.R. 2014. Worldwide survey of fitness: Trends for 2015. *ACSM's Health & Fitness Journal* 18(6): 8–17.

U.S. Department of Health and Human Services. 1996. *Physical Activity and Health: A Report of the Surgeon General.* Atlanta: U.S. Department of Health and Human Services.

U.S. Department of Health and Human Services. 2008. *Physical Activity Guidelines for Americans.* Washington, D.C.: U.S. Department of Health and Human Services.

U.S. Department of Health and Human Services. 2010. *The Surgeon General's Vision for a Healthy and Fit Nation.* Rockville, Md.: U.S. Department of Health and Human Services, Office of the Surgeon General.

U.S. Department of Health and Human Services. 2013. *Physical Activity Guidelines for Americans Midcourse Report.* Washington, D.C.: U.S. Department of Health and Human Services.

Wen, M., et al. 2013. Physical activity and mortality among middle-aged and older adults in the United States. *Journal Physical Activity & Health.* Published online.

Name _____ Section _____ Date _____

LAB 2.1 Safety of Exercise Participation

Physical Activity Readiness
Questionnaire - PAR-Q
(revised 2002)

PAR-Q & YOU

(A Questionnaire for People Aged 15 to 69)

Regular physical activity is fun and healthy, and increasingly more people are starting to become more active every day. Being more active is very safe for most people. However, some people should check with their doctor before they start becoming much more physically active.

If you are planning to become much more physically active than you are now, start by answering the seven questions in the box below. If you are between the ages of 15 and 69, the PAR-Q will tell you if you should check with your doctor before you start. If you are over 69 years of age, and you are not used to being very active, check with your doctor.

Common sense is your best guide when you answer these questions. Please read the questions carefully and answer each one honestly: check YES or NO.

YES	NO		
☐	☐	1.	Has your doctor ever said that you have a heart condition <u>and</u> that you should only do physical activity recommended by a doctor?
☐	☐	2.	Do you feel pain in your chest when you do physical activity?
☐	☐	3.	In the past month, have you had chest pain when you were not doing physical activity?
☐	☐	4.	Do you lose your balance because of dizziness or do you ever lose consciousness?
☐	☐	5.	Do you have a bone or joint problem (for example, back, knee or hip) that could be made worse by a change in your physical activity?
☐	☐	6.	Is your doctor currently prescribing drugs (for example, water pills) for your blood pressure or heart condition?
☐	☐	7.	Do you know of <u>any other reason</u> why you should not do physical activity?

If

you

answered

YES to one or more questions

Talk with your doctor by phone or in person BEFORE you start becoming much more physically active or BEFORE you have a fitness appraisal. Tell your doctor about the PAR-Q and which questions you answered YES.

- You may be able to do any activity you want — as long as you start slowly and build up gradually. Or, you may need to restrict your activities to those which are safe for you. Talk with your doctor about the kinds of activities you wish to participate in and follow his/her advice.
- Find out which community programs are safe and helpful for you.

NO to all questions

If you answered NO honestly to <u>all</u> PAR-Q questions, you can be reasonably sure that you can:
- start becoming much more physically active — begin slowly and build up gradually. This is the safest and easiest way to go.
- take part in a fitness appraisal – this is an excellent way to determine your basic fitness so that you can plan the best way for you to live actively. It is also highly recommended that you have your blood pressure evaluated. If your reading is over 144/94, talk with your doctor before you start becoming much more physically active.

DELAY BECOMING MUCH MORE ACTIVE:
- if you are not feeling well because of a temporary illness such as a cold or a fever — wait until you feel better; or
- if you are or may be pregnant — talk to your doctor before you start becoming more active.

PLEASE NOTE: If your health changes so that you then answer YES to any of the above questions, tell your fitness or health professional. Ask whether you should change your physical activity plan.

<u>Informed Use of the PAR-Q</u>: The Canadian Society for Exercise Physiology, Health Canada, and their agents assume no liability for persons who undertake physical activity, and if in doubt after completing this questionnaire, consult your doctor prior to physical activity.

No changes permitted. You are encouraged to photocopy the PAR-Q but only if you use the entire form.

NOTE: If the PAR-Q is being given to a person before he or she participates in a physical activity program or a fitness appraisal, this section may be used for legal or administrative purposes.

"I have read, understood and completed this questionnaire. Any questions I had were answered to my full satisfaction."

NAME _____

SIGNATURE _____   DATE _____

SIGNATURE OF PARENT _____   WITNESS _____
or GUARDIAN (for participants under the age of majority)

Note: This physical activity clearance is valid for a maximum of 12 months from the date it is completed and becomes invalid if your condition changes so that you would answer YES to any of the seven questions.

 CSEP SCPE © Canadian Society for Exercise Physiology

Supported by: 🍁 Health Canada Santé Canada

Physical Activity Readiness Questionnaire (PAR-Q) © 2002. Reprinted with permission from the Canadian Society for Exercise Physiology. http://www.csep.ca/forms.asp.

LABORATORY ACTIVITIES

General Health Profile

To help further assess the safety of exercise for you, complete as much of this health profile as possible.

General Information

Age: _____

Height: _____

Weight: _____

Total cholesterol: _____

HDL: _____

LDL: _____

Blood pressure: _____ / _____

Triglycerides: _____

Blood glucose: _____

Are you currently trying to _____ gain or _____ lose weight? (check one if appropriate)

Medical Conditions/Treatments

Check any of the following that apply to you, and add any other conditions that might affect your ability to exercise safely.

_____ heart disease

_____ lung disease

_____ diabetes

_____ allergies

_____ asthma

_____ depression, anxiety, or other psychological disorder

_____ eating disorder

_____ back pain

_____ arthritis

_____ other injury to joint problem: _____

_____ substance abuse problem

_____ other: _____

_____ other: _____

_____ other: _____

_____ Do you have a family history of cardiovascular disease (CVD) (a parent, sibling, or child who had a heart attack or stroke before age 55 for men or 65 for women)?

List any medications or supplements you are taking or any medical treatments you are undergoing. Include the name of the substance or treatment and its purpose. Include both prescription and over-the-counter drugs and supplements.

_____   _____

_____   _____

Lifestyle Information

Check any of the following that is true for you, and fill in the requested information.

_____ I usually eat high-fat foods (fatty meats, cheese, fried foods, butter, full-fat dairy products) every day.

_____ I consume fewer than 5 servings of fruits and vegetables on most days.

_____ I smoke cigarettes or use other tobacco products. If true, describe your use of tobacco (type and frequency): _____

_____ I regularly drink alcohol. If true, describe your typical weekly consumption pattern: _____

_____ I often feel as if I need more sleep. (I need about _____ hours per day; I get about _____ hours per day.)

_____ I feel as though stress has adversely affected my level of wellness during the past year.

Describe your current activity pattern. What types of moderate physical activity do you engage in on a daily basis? Are you involved in a formal exercise program, or do you regularly participate in sports or recreational activities?

_____

_____

Using Your Results

Are you ready to exercise? Did the PAR-Q indicate that exercise is likely to be safe for you? Is there anything in your health profile that you think may affect your ability to exercise safely? Have you had any problems with exercise in the past?

What should you do next? If the assessments in this lab indicate that you should see your physician before beginning an exercise program, or if you have any questions about the safety of exercise for you, make an appointment to talk with your health care provider to address your concerns.

Name _____ Section _____ Date _____

LAB 2.2   Overcoming Barriers to Being Active

Barriers to Being Active Quiz

Directions: Listed below are reasons that people give to describe why they do not get as much physical activity as they think they should. Please read each statement and circle the number that describes how likely you are to say each of the following statements.

How likely are you to say this?	Very likely	Somewhat likely	Somewhat unlikely	Very unlikely
1. My day is so busy now, I just don't think I can make the time to include physical activity in my regular schedule.	3	2	1	0
2. None of my family members or friends like to do anything active, so I don't have a chance to exercise.	3	2	1	0
3. I'm just too tired after work to get any exercise.	3	2	1	0
4. I've been thinking about getting more exercise, but I just can't seem to get started.	3	2	1	0
5. I'm getting older so exercise can be risky.	3	2	1	0
6. I don't get enough exercise because I have never learned the skills for any sport.	3	2	1	0
7. I don't have access to jogging trails, swimming pools, bike paths, etc.	3	2	1	0
8. Physical activity takes too much time away from other commitments—like work, family, etc.	3	2	1	0
9. I'm embarrassed about how I will look when I exercise with others.	3	2	1	0
10. I don't get enough sleep as it is. I just couldn't get up early or stay up late to get some exercise.	3	2	1	0
11. It's easier for me to find excuses not to exercise than to go out and do something.	3	2	1	0
12. I know of too many people who have hurt themselves by overdoing it with exercise.	3	2	1	0
13. I really can't see learning a new sport at my age.	3	2	1	0
14. It's just too expensive. You have to take a class or join a club or buy the right equipment.	3	2	1	0
15. My free times during the day are too short to include exercise.	3	2	1	0
16. My usual social activities with family or friends do not include physical activity.	3	2	1	0
17. I'm too tired during the week, and I need the weekend to catch up on my rest.	3	2	1	0
18. I want to get more exercise, but I just can't seem to make myself stick to anything.	3	2	1	0
19. I'm afraid I might injure myself or have a heart attack.	3	2	1	0
20. I'm not good enough at any physical activity to make it fun.	3	2	1	0
21. If we had exercise facilities and showers at work, then I would be more likely to exercise.	3	2	1	0

LABORATORY ACTIVITIES

Scoring

- Enter the circled numbers in the spaces provided below, putting the number for statement 1 on line 1, statement 2 on line 2, and so on.
- Add the three scores on each line. Your barriers to physical activity fall into one or more of seven categories: lack of time, social influences, lack of energy, lack of willpower, fear of injury, lack of skill, and lack of resources. A score of 5 or above in any category shows that this is an important barrier for you to overcome.

_____		_____		_____		_____	
1	+	8	+	15	=		Lack of time
2	+	9	+	16	=		Social influences
3	+	10	+	17	=		Lack of energy
4	+	11	+	18	=		Lack of willpower
5	+	12	+	19	=		Fear of injury
6	+	13	+	20	=		Lack of skill
7	+	14	+	21	=		Lack of resources

Using Your Results

How did you score? How many key barriers did you identify? Are they what you expected?

What should you do next? For your key barriers, try the strategies listed on the following pages and/or develop additional strategies that work for you. Check off any strategy that you try.

Suggestions for Overcoming Physical Activity Barriers

Lack of Time

_____ Identify available time slots. Monitor your daily activities for one week. Identify at least three 30-minute time slots you could use for physical activity.

_____ Add physical activity to your daily routine. For example, walk or ride your bike to work or shopping, organize social activities around physical activity, walk the dog, exercise while you watch TV, park farther from your destination, etc.

_____ Make time for physical activity. For example, walk, jog, or swim during your lunch hour, or take fitness breaks instead of coffee breaks.

_____ Select activities requiring minimal time, such as walking, jogging, or stair climbing.

_____ Other: _____

Social Influences

_____ Explain your interest in physical activity to friends and family. Ask them to support your efforts.

_____ Invite friends and family members to exercise with you. Plan social activities involving exercise.

_____ Develop new friendships with physically active people. Join a group, such as the YMCA or a hiking club.

_____ Other: _____

Lack of Energy

_____ Schedule physical activity for times in the day or week when you feel energetic.

_____ Convince yourself that if you give it a chance, exercise will increase your energy level. Then try it.

_____ Other: _____

Lack of Willpower

_____ Plan ahead. Make physical activity a regular part of your daily or weekly schedule and write it on your calendar.

_____ Invite a friend to exercise with you on a regular basis and write it on *both* your calendars.

_____ Join an exercise group or class.

_____ Other: _____

Fear of Injury

_____ Learn how to warm up and cool down to prevent injury.

_____ Learn how to exercise appropriately considering your age, fitness level, skill level, and health status.

_____ Choose activities involving minimal risk.

_____ Other: _____

Lack of Skill

_____ Select activities requiring no new skills, such as walking, jogging, or stair climbing.

_____ Exercise with friends who are at the same skill level as you are.

_____ Find a friend who is willing to teach you some new skills.

_____ Take a class to develop new skills.

_____ Other: _____

Lack of Resources

_____ Select activities that require minimal facilities or equipment, such as walking, jogging, jumping rope, or calisthenics.

_____ Identify inexpensive, convenient resources available in your community (community education programs, park and recreation programs, worksite programs, etc.).

_____ Other: _____

LABORATORY ACTIVITIES

Are any of the following additional barriers important for you? If so, try some of the strategies listed here or invent your own.

Weather Conditions

_____ Develop a set of regular activities that are always available regardless of weather (indoor cycling, aerobic dance, indoor swimming, calisthenics, stair-climbing, rope-skipping, mall-walking, dancing, gymnasium games, etc.).

_____ Look at outdoor activities that depend on weather conditions (cross-country skiing, outdoor swimming, outdoor tennis, etc.) as "bonuses"—extra activities possible when weather and circumstances permit.

_____ Other: _____

Travel

_____ Put a jump rope in your suitcase and jump rope.

_____ Walk the halls and climb the stairs in hotels.

_____ Stay in places with swimming pools or exercise facilities.

_____ Join the YMCA or YWCA (ask about reciprocal membership agreements).

_____ Visit the local shopping mall and walk for half an hour or more.

_____ Bring a personal music player loaded with your favorite workout music.

_____ Other: _____

Family Obligations

_____ Trade babysitting time with a friend, neighbor, or family member who also has small children.

_____ Exercise *with* the kids—go for a walk together, play tag or other running games, or get an aerobic dance or exercise DVD for kids (there are several on the market) and exercise together. You can spend time together and still get your exercise.

_____ Hire a babysitter and look at the cost as a worthwhile investment in your physical and mental health.

_____ Jump rope, do calisthenics, ride a stationary bicycle, or use other home gymnasium equipment while the kids watch TV or when they are sleeping.

_____ Try to exercise when the kids are not around (e.g., during school hours or their nap time).

_____ Other: _____

Retirement Years

_____ Look on your retirement as an opportunity to become more active instead of less. Spend more time gardening, walking the dog, and playing with your grandchildren. Children with short legs and grandparents with slower gaits are often great walking partners.

_____ Learn a new skill you've always been interested in, such as ballroom dancing, square dancing, or swimming.

_____ Now that you have the time, make regular physical activity a part of every day. Go for a walk every morning or every evening before dinner. Treat yourself to an exercycle and ride every day during a favorite TV show.

_____ Other: _____

SOURCE: Adapted from CDC Division of Nutrition and Physical Activity. 2010. *Promoting Physical Activity: A Guide for Community Action,* 2nd ed. Champaign, Ill.: Human Kinetics.

Name _____ Section _____ Date _____

LAB 2.3 Using a Pedometer to Track Physical Activity

How physically active are you? Would you be more motivated to increase daily physical activity if you had an easy way to monitor your level of activity? If so, consider wearing a pedometer to track the number of steps you take each day—a rough but easily obtainable reflection of daily physical activity. Smartphone pedometer apps use sensors that can provide reasonably accurate step measure counts. These apps are either low cost or free.

Determine Your Baseline

Wear the pedometer for a week to obtain a baseline average daily number of steps.

	M	T	W	Th	F	Sa	Su	Average
Steps								

Set Goals

Set an appropriate goal for increasing steps. The goal of 10,000 steps per day is widely recommended, but your personal goal should reflect your baseline level of steps. For example, if your current daily steps are far below 10,000, a goal of walking 2,000 additional steps each day might be appropriate. If you are already close to 10,000 steps per day, choose a higher goal. Also consider the following guidelines from health experts:

- To reduce the risk of chronic disease, aim to accumulate at least 150 minutes of moderate physical activity per week.
- To help manage body weight and prevent gradual, unhealthy weight gain, engage in 60 minutes of moderate to vigorous-intensity activity on most days of the week.
- To sustain weight loss, engage daily in at least 60–90 minutes of moderate-intensity physical activity.

To help gauge how close you are to meeting these time-based physical activity goals, you might walk for 10–15 minutes while wearing your pedometer to determine how many steps correspond with the time-based goals.

Once you have set your overall goal, break it down into several steps. For example, if your goal is to increase daily steps by 2,000, set mini-goals of increasing daily steps by 500, allowing two weeks to reach each mini-goal. Smaller goals are easier to achieve and can help keep you motivated and on track. Having several interim goals also gives you the opportunity to reward yourself more frequently. Note your goals below:

Mini-goal 1: _____ Target date: _____ Reward: _____
Mini-goal 2: _____ Target date: _____ Reward: _____
Mini-goal 3: _____ Target date: _____ Reward: _____
Overall goal: _____ Target date: _____ Reward: _____

Develop Strategies for Increasing Steps

What can you do to become more active? The possibilities include walking when you do errands, getting off one stop from your destination on public transportation, parking an extra block or two away from your destination, and doing at least one chore every day that requires physical activity. If weather or neighborhood safety is an issue, look for alternative locations to walk. For example, find an indoor gym or shopping mall or even a long hallway. Check out locations that are near or on the way to your campus, workplace, or residence. If you think walking indoors will be dull, walk with friends or family members or wear headphones (if safe) and listen to music or audiobooks.

Are there any days of the week for which your baseline steps are particularly low and/or it will be especially difficult because of your schedule to increase your number of steps? Be sure to develop specific strategies for difficult situations.

Below, list at least five strategies for increasing daily steps:

_____ _____

_____ _____

_____

LABORATORY ACTIVITIES

Track Your Progress

Based on the goals you set, fill in your goal portion of the progress chart with your target average daily steps for each week. Then wear your pedometer every day and note your total daily steps. Track your progress toward each mini-goal and your final goal. Every few weeks, stop and evaluate your progress. If needed, adjust your plan and develop additional strategies for increasing steps. In addition to the chart in this worksheet, you might also want to graph your daily steps to provide a visual reminder of how you are progressing toward your goals. Make as many copies of this chart as you need.

Week	Goal	M	Tu	W	Th	F	Sa	Su	Average
1									
2									
3									
4									

Weeks 1–4 Progress Checkup

How close are you to meeting your goal? How do you feel about your program and your progress?

If needed, describe changes to your plan and additional strategies for increasing steps:

Week	Goal	M	Tu	W	Th	F	Sa	Su	Average
5									
6									
7									
8									

Weeks 5–8 Progress Checkup

How close are you to meeting your goal? How do you feel about your program and your progress?

If needed, describe changes to your plan and additional strategies for increasing steps:

Week	Goal	M	Tu	W	Th	F	Sa	Su	Average
9									
10									
11									
12									

Weeks 9–12 Progress Checkup

How close are you to meeting your goal? How do you feel about your program and your progress?

If needed, in the space below, describe changes to your plan and additional strategies for increasing steps.

Cardiorespiratory Endurance

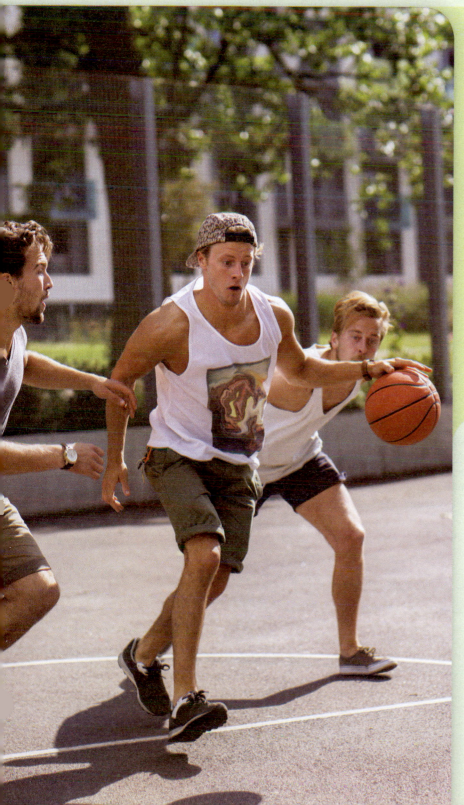

LOOKING AHEAD...

After reading this chapter, you should be able to

- Describe how the body produces the energy it needs for exercise.

- List the major effects and benefits of cardiorespiratory endurance exercise.

- Explain how cardiorespiratory endurance is measured and assessed.

- Describe how frequency, intensity, time (duration), and type of exercise (FITT) affect the development of cardiorespiratory endurance.

- Explain the best ways to prevent and treat common exercise injuries.

TEST YOUR KNOWLEDGE

1. Compared to sedentary people, those who engage in regular moderate endurance exercise are likely to:
   a. have fewer colds.
   b. be less anxious and depressed.
   c. fall asleep more quickly and sleep better.
   d. be more alert and creative.
   e. all of the above

2. About how much blood does the heart pump each minute during maximum-intensity aerobic exercise?
   a. 5 quarts
   b. 10 quarts
   c. 20 quarts

3. During an effective 30-minute cardiorespiratory endurance workout, you should lose 1–2 pounds. True or false?

See answers on the next page.

Cardiorespiratory endurance—the ability of the body to perform prolonged, large-muscle, dynamic exercise at moderate to high levels of intensity—is a key health-related component of fitness. As explained in Chapter 2, a healthy cardiorespiratory system is essential to high levels of fitness and wellness.

This chapter reviews the short- and long-term effects and benefits of cardiorespiratory endurance exercise. It then describes several tests commonly used to assess cardiorespiratory fitness. Finally, it provides guidelines for creating your own cardiorespiratory endurance training program—one that is geared to your current level of fitness and built around activities you enjoy.

BASIC PHYSIOLOGY OF CARDIORESPIRATORY ENDURANCE EXERCISE

A basic understanding of the body processes involved in cardiorespiratory endurance exercise can help you design a safe and effective fitness program.

The Cardiorespiratory System

The **cardiorespiratory system** consists of the heart, the blood vessels, and the respiratory system (the lungs). (See page T3-2 of the color transparency insert "Touring the Cardiorespiratory System" in this chapter.) The cardiorespiratory system circulates blood through the body, transporting oxygen, nutrients, and other key substances to the organs and tissues that need them. It also carries away waste products so they can be used or expelled.

The Heart   The heart is a four-chambered, fist-sized muscle located just beneath the sternum (breastbone) (Figure 3.1). It pumps oxygen-poor blood to the lungs and delivers oxygen-rich blood to the rest of the body. Blood travels through two separate circulatory systems: The right side of the heart pumps blood to the lungs through the **pulmonary circulation**, and the left side pumps blood through the rest of the body in **systemic circulation**.

The path of blood flow through the heart and cardiorespiratory system is illustrated on page T3-3 of the color transparency insert "Touring the Cardiorespiratory System" in this chapter. Refer to that illustration as you trace these steps:

1. Waste-laden, oxygen-poor blood travels through large vessels, called **venae cavae**, into the heart's right upper chamber, or **atrium**.
2. After the right atrium fills, it contracts and pumps blood into the heart's right lower chamber, or **ventricle**.
3. When the right ventricle is full, it contracts and pumps blood through the pulmonary artery into the lungs.
4. In the lungs, blood picks up oxygen and discards carbon dioxide. Oxygen moves from the lungs to the blood and carbon dioxide moves from the blood to the lungs by a process called **diffusion**. During exercise, you breathe faster to promote diffusion of these gases.
5. The cleaned, oxygenated blood flows from the lungs through the pulmonary veins into the heart's left atrium.
6. After the left atrium fills, it contracts and pumps blood into the left ventricle.
7. When the left ventricle is full, it pumps blood through the **aorta**—the body's largest artery—for distribution to the rest of the body's blood vessels.

The period of the heart's contraction is called **systole**; the period of relaxation is called **diastole**. During systole, the atria contract first, pumping blood into the ventricles. A fraction of a second later, the ventricles contract, pumping blood to the lungs and the body. During diastole, blood flows into the heart.

Blood pressure, the force exerted by blood on the walls of the blood vessels, is created by the pumping action of the heart. Blood pressure is greater during systole than during diastole. A person weighing 150 pounds has about 5 quarts of blood, which are circulated about once every minute at rest.

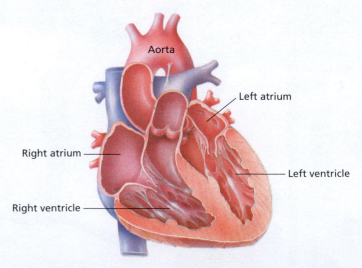

FIGURE 3.1   Chambers of the heart.

The heartbeat—the split-second sequence of contractions of the heart's four chambers—is controlled by nerve impulses. These signals originate in a bundle of specialized cells in the right atrium called the *pacemaker,* or *sinoatrial (SA) node.* The heart produces nerve impulses at a steady rate—unless it is speeded up or slowed down by the brain in response to stimuli such as exercise.

The Blood Vessels

Blood vessels are classified by size and function. **Veins** carry blood to the heart. **Arteries** carry it away from the heart. Veins have thin walls, but arteries have thick elastic walls that enable them to expand and relax with the volume of blood being pumped through them.

The blood vessels are lined with **endothelial cells** that secrete **nitric oxide**—a chemical messenger regulating blood flow. Inflammation, physical inactivity, poor diet, smoking, high blood pressure, or insulin resistance can promote blood vessel disease, which has a wide range of negative effects ranging from erectile dysfunction to heart disease. Regular physical activity helps maintain healthy blood vessels.

After leaving the heart, the aorta branches into smaller and smaller vessels. The smallest arteries branch still further into **capillaries**, tiny vessels only one cell thick. The capillaries deliver oxygen and nutrient-rich blood to the tissues and pick up oxygen-poor, waste-laden blood. From the capillaries, this blood empties into small veins (*venules*) and then into larger veins that return it to the heart to repeat the cycle.

Blood pumped through the heart doesn't reach the heart's own cells, so the organ has its own network of blood vessels. Two large vessels, the right and left **coronary arteries**, branch off the aorta and supply the heart muscle with oxygenated blood. (The coronary arteries are shown on page T3-3 of the color transparency insert "Touring the Cardiorespiratory System" in this chapter.) The fit and well lifestyle helps prevent coronary artery disease.

The Respiratory System

The **respiratory system** supplies oxygen to the body, carries off carbon dioxide—a waste product of body processes—and helps regulate acid produced during metabolism. Air passes in and out of the lungs as a result of pressure changes brought about by the contraction and relaxation of the diaphragm and rib muscles. As air is inhaled, it passes through the nasal passages, throat, larynx, trachea (windpipe), and bronchi into the lungs. The lungs consist of many branching tubes that end in tiny, thin-walled air sacs called **alveoli**.

Carbon dioxide and oxygen are exchanged between alveoli and capillaries in the lungs. Carbon dioxide passes from blood cells into the alveoli, where it is carried up and out of the lungs (exhaled). Oxygen from inhaled air is passed from the alveoli into blood cells; these oxygen-rich blood cells then return to the heart and are pumped throughout the body. Oxygen is an important component of the body's energy-producing system, so the cardiorespiratory system's ability to pick up and deliver oxygen is critical for the functioning of the body.

The Cardiorespiratory System at Rest and during Exercise

At rest and during light activity, the cardiorespiratory system functions at a fairly steady pace. Your heart beats at a rate of about 50–90 beats per minute, and you take about 12–20 breaths per minute. A typical resting blood pressure in a healthy adult, measured in millimeters of mercury, is 120 systolic and 80 diastolic (120/80).

During exercise, the demands on the cardiorespiratory system increase. Body cells, particularly working muscles, need to obtain more oxygen and fuel and to eliminate more waste

---

TERMS

cardiorespiratory system   The system that circulates blood through the body; consists of the heart, blood vessels, and respiratory system.

pulmonary circulation   The part of the circulatory system that moves blood between the heart and lungs; controlled by the right side of the heart.

systemic circulation   The part of the circulatory system that moves blood between the heart and the rest of the body; controlled by the left side of the heart.

venae cavae   The large veins through which blood is returned to the right atrium of the heart.

atrium   One of the two upper chambers of the heart in which blood collects before passing to the ventricles (pl. *atria*).

ventricle   One of the two lower chambers of the heart from which blood flows through arteries to the lungs and other parts of the body.

diffusion   The process by which oxygen moves from the lungs to the blood and carbon dioxide moves from the blood to the lungs; faster breathing concentrates oxygen and decreases carbon dioxide in the lungs and promotes diffusion.

aorta   The body's largest artery; receives blood from the left ventricle and distributes it to the body.

systole   Contraction of the heart.

diastole   Relaxation of the heart.

blood pressure   The force exerted by the blood on the walls of the blood vessels; created by the pumping action of the heart.

veins   Vessels that carry blood to the heart.

arteries   Vessels that carry blood away from the heart.

endothelial cells   Cells lining the blood vessels.

nitric oxide   A gas released by the endothelial cells to promote blood flow. The capacity of these cells to release nitric oxide is an important marker of good health.

capillaries   Very small blood vessels that distribute blood to all parts of the body.

coronary arteries   A pair of large blood vessels that branch off the aorta and supply the heart muscle with oxygenated blood.

respiratory system   The lungs, air passages, and breathing muscles; supplies oxygen to the body and removes carbon dioxide.

alveoli   Tiny air sacs in the lungs that allow the exchange of oxygen and carbon dioxide between the lungs and blood.

products. To meet these demands, your body makes the following changes:

- Heart rate increases up to 170–210 beats per minute during intense exercise.
- The heart's **stroke volume** increases, meaning that the heart pumps out more blood with each beat.
- The heart pumps and circulates more blood per minute as a result of the faster heart rate and greater stroke volume. During exercise, this **cardiac output** increases to 20 or more quarts per minute, compared to about 5 quarts per minute at rest.
- Blood flow changes, so as much as 85–90% of the blood may be delivered to working muscles. At rest, about 15–20% of blood is distributed to the skeletal muscles.
- Systolic blood pressure increases, while diastolic blood pressure holds steady or declines slightly. A typical exercise blood pressure might be 175/65.
- To oxygenate this increased blood flow, you take deeper breaths and breathe faster, up to 40–60 breaths per minute.

All of these changes are controlled and coordinated by special centers in the brain, which use the nervous system and chemical messengers to control the process.

Energy Production

Metabolism is the sum of all the chemical processes necessary to maintain the body. Energy is required to fuel vital body functions—to build and break down tissue, contract muscles, conduct nerve impulses, regulate body temperature, and so on.

The rate at which your body uses energy—its **metabolic rate**—depends on your level of activity. At rest, you have a low metabolic rate; if you begin to walk, your metabolic rate increases. If you jog, your metabolic rate may increase more than 800% above its resting level. Olympic-caliber distance runners can increase their metabolic rate by 2000% or more.

Energy from Food The body converts chemical energy from food into substances that cells can use as fuel. These fuels can be used immediately or stored for later use. The body's ability to store fuel is critical, because if all the energy from food were released immediately, much of it would be wasted.

The three classes of energy-containing nutrients in food are carbohydrates (sugar, wheat flour, honey), fats (meat, nuts, fried foods), and proteins (seafood, poultry, dairy food). During digestion, most carbohydrates are broken down into the simple sugar **glucose**. Some glucose circulates in the blood ("blood sugar"), where it can be used as a quick source of fuel to produce energy. Glucose may also be converted to **glycogen** and stored mainly in the liver and muscles. If glycogen stores are full and the body's immediate need for energy is met, the remaining glucose is converted to fat and stored in the body's fatty tissues. Excess energy from fat in the diet is also stored as body fat. Protein in the diet is used primarily to build new tissue, but it can be broken down for energy or incorporated into

fat stores. Glucose, glycogen, and fat are important fuels for the production of energy in the cells; protein is a significant energy source only when other fuels are lacking. (See Chapter 8 for more on the roles of carbohydrate, fat, and protein in the body.)

ATP: The Energy "Currency" of Cells The basic form of energy used by cells is **adenosine triphosphate**, or ATP. When a cell needs energy, it breaks down ATP, a process that releases energy in the only form the cell can use directly. Cells store a small amount of ATP; when they need more, they create it through chemical reactions that utilize the body's stored fuels—glucose, glycogen, and fat. When you exercise, your cells need to produce more energy. Consequently, your body mobilizes its stores of fuel to increase ATP production.

Exercise and the Three Energy Systems

The muscles in your body use three energy systems to create ATP and fuel cellular activity. These systems use different fuels and chemical processes and perform different, specific functions during exercise (Table 3.1).

The Immediate Energy System The **immediate ("explosive") energy system** provides energy rapidly but for only a short period of time. It is used to fuel activities that last for about 10 or fewer seconds—such as weight lifting and shot-putting or in daily life just rising from a chair or picking up a bag of groceries. The components of this energy system include existing cellular ATP stores and creatine phosphate (CP), a chemical that cells can use to make ATP. CP levels deplete rapidly during exercise, so the maximum capacity of this energy system is reached within a few seconds. Cells must then switch to the other energy systems to restore levels of ATP and CP. (Without adequate ATP, muscles will stiffen and become unusable.)

The Nonoxidative Energy System The **nonoxidative (anaerobic) energy system** is used at the start of an exercise session and for high-intensity activities lasting for about 10 seconds to 2 minutes, such as the 400-meter run. During daily activities, this system may be called on to help you run to catch a bus or dash up several flights of stairs. The nonoxidative energy system creates ATP by breaking down glucose and glycogen. This system doesn't require oxygen, which is why it is sometimes referred to as the **anaerobic** system. This system's capacity to produce energy is limited, but it can generate a great deal of ATP in a short period of time. For this reason, it is the most important energy system for very intense exercise.

There are two key limitations to the nonoxidative energy system. First, the body's supply of glucose and glycogen is limited. If these are depleted, a person may experience fatigue, dizziness, and impaired judgment. (The brain and nervous system rely on carbohydrates as fuel.) Second, the rapid metabolism caused by this energy system increases hydrogen and potassium ions that interfere with metabolism and muscle contraction and cause fatigue. During heavy exercise, such as sprinting, large

	ENERGY SYSTEM*		
	IMMEDIATE	NONOXIDATIVE	OXIDATIVE
DURATION OF ACTIVITY FOR WHICH SYSTEM PREDOMINATES	0–10 seconds	10 seconds–2 minutes	>2 minutes
INTENSITY OF ACTIVITY FOR WHICH SYSTEM PREDOMINATES	High	High	Low to moderately high
RATE OF ATP PRODUCTION	Immediate, very rapid	Rapid	Slower, but prolonged
FUEL	Adenosine triphosphate (ATP), creatine phosphate (CP)	Muscle stores of glucose and glycogen	Body stores of glycogen, glucose, fat, and protein
OXYGEN USED?	No	No	Yes
SAMPLE ACTIVITIES	Weight lifting, picking up a bag of groceries	400-meter run, running up several flights of stairs	1500-meter run, 30-minute walk, standing in line for a long time

*For most activities, all three systems contribute to energy production; the duration and intensity of the activity determine which system predominates.

SOURCE: Adapted from Brooks, G. A., et al. 2005. *Exercise Physiology: Human Bioenergetics and Its Applications,* 4th ed. New York: McGraw-Hill. Copyright © 2005 The McGraw-Hill Companies. Reproduced with permission of The McGraw-Hill Companies.

increases in hydrogen and potassium ions cause muscles to fatigue rapidly.

The anaerobic energy system also creates metabolic acids. Fortunately, exercise training increases the body's ability to cope with metabolic acid. Improved fitness allows you to exercise at higher intensities before the abrupt buildup of metabolic acids—a point that scientists call the *lactate threshold.* One metabolic acid, called **lactic acid** (lactate), is often linked to fatigue during intense exercise. Lactic acid does not last long in blood. It breaks down into lactate and hydrogen ion (acid) as soon as it is produced. Lactate is an important fuel at rest and during exercise.

The Oxidative Energy System The **oxidative (aerobic) energy system** operates during any physical activity that lasts longer than about 2 minutes, such as distance running, swimming, hiking, or even just standing in line. The oxidative system requires oxygen to generate ATP, which is why it is considered an **aerobic** system. The oxidative system cannot produce energy as quickly as the other two systems, but it can supply energy for much longer periods of time. It is the source of our energy during most daily activities.

In the oxidative energy system, ATP production takes place in cellular structures called **mitochondria**. Because mitochondria can use carbohydrates (glucose and glycogen) or fats to produce ATP, the body's stores of fuel for this system are much greater than those for the other two energy systems. The actual fuel used depends on the intensity and duration of exercise and on the fitness status of the individual. Carbohydrates are favored during more intense exercise (more than 65% of maximum capacity); fats are used for mild, low-intensity activities. During a prolonged exercise session, carbohydrates are the predominant fuel at the start of the workout, but fat utilization increases over time. Fit individuals use a greater proportion of fat as fuel because increased fitness allows people to do

TERMS

stroke volume The amount of blood the heart pumps with each beat.

cardiac output The volume of blood pumped by the heart per minute via heart rate and stroke volume.

metabolic rate The rate at which the body uses energy.

glucose A simple sugar circulating in the blood that can be used by cells to fuel adenosine triphosphate (ATP) production.

glycogen A complex carbohydrate stored principally in the liver and skeletal muscles; the major fuel source during most forms of intense exercise. Glycogen is the storage form of glucose.

adenosine triphosphate (ATP) The energy source for cellular processes.

immediate ("explosive") energy system The system that supplies very short bursts of energy to muscle cells through the breakdown of cellular stores of ATP and creatine phosphate (CP).

nonoxidative (anaerobic) energy system The system that supplies energy to muscle cells for highly intense exercise of short duration by breaking down muscle stores of glucose and glycogen; called the *anaerobic system* because chemical reactions take place without oxygen and produce lactic acid.

anaerobic Occurring in the absence of oxygen.

lactic acid A metabolic acid resulting from the metabolism of glucose and glycogen. It is broken down in the body into lactate and hydrogen ions as soon as it is produced.

oxidative (aerobic) energy system The system that supplies energy to cells for long periods of activity through the breakdown of glucose, glycogen, and fats; called the *aerobic system* because its chemical reactions require oxygen.

aerobic Dependent on the presence of oxygen.

mitochondria Cell structures that convert the energy in food to a form the body can use.

activities at lower intensities. This is an important adaptation because glycogen depletion is one of the limiting factors for the oxidative energy system. By being able to use more fat as fuel, a fit individual can exercise for a longer time before glycogen is depleted and muscles become fatigued. Aerobic exercise and high-intensity interval training increase the number and capacity of mitochondria. Increased mitochondrial capacity is the most important benefit of exercise. Mitochondrial health and fitness are linked to a reduced risk of disease and improved longevity.

Oxygen is another factor limiting exercise capacity. The oxygen requirement of this energy system is proportional to the intensity of exercise. As intensity increases, so does oxygen consumption. The body's ability to increase oxygen use is limited; this limit, known as **maximal oxygen consumption**, or $\dot{V}O_{2max}$, refers to the highest rate of oxygen consumption an individual is capable of during maximum physical effort. It is expressed in milliliters of oxygen per kilogram of body weight per minute. In the symbol, the V stands for volume, the dot over the V means per minute, the O_2 stands for oxygen, and the max means maximum. $\dot{V}O_{2max}$ determines how intensely a person can perform endurance exercise and for how long, and it is considered the best overall measure of the capacity of the cardiorespiratory system. (The assessment tests described later in the chapter are designed to help you evaluate your $\dot{V}O_{2max}$.)

The Energy Systems in Combination Your body typically uses all three energy systems when you exercise. The intensity and duration of the activity determine which system predominates. For example, when you play tennis, you use the immediate energy system when hitting the ball, but you replenish cellular energy stores by using the nonoxidative and oxidative systems. When cycling, the oxidative system predominates. However, if you must suddenly exercise intensely—by riding up a steep hill, for example—the other systems become important because the oxidative system is unable to supply ATP fast enough to sustain high-intensity effort.

> **maximal oxygen consumption ($\dot{V}O_{2max}$)** TERMS
> The highest rate of oxygen consumption an individual is capable of during maximum physical effort, reflecting the body's ability to transport and use oxygen; measured in milliliters of oxygen used per minute per kilogram of body weight.

Ask Yourself

QUESTIONS FOR CRITICAL THINKING AND REFLECTION

When you think about the types of physical activity you engage in during your typical day or week, which ones use the immediate energy system? The nonoxidative energy system? The oxidative energy system? How can you increase activities that use the oxidative energy system?

Physical Fitness and Energy Production Physically fit people can increase their metabolic rate substantially, generating the energy needed for powerful or sustained exercise. People who are not fit cannot respond to exercise in the same way. Their bodies are less capable of delivering oxygen and fuel to exercising muscles, they can't burn as many calories during or after exercise, and they are less able to cope with lactic acid and other substances produced during intense physical activity that contribute to fatigue. Because of this, they become fatigued more rapidly; their legs hurt and they breathe heavily walking up a flight of stairs, for example. Regular physical training can substantially improve the body's ability to produce energy and meet the challenges of increased physical activity.

In designing an exercise program, focus on the energy system most important to your goals. Because improving the functioning of the cardiorespiratory system is critical to overall wellness, endurance exercise that utilizes the oxidative energy system—activities performed at moderate to high intensities for a prolonged duration—is a key component of any health-related fitness program.

BENEFITS OF CARDIORESPIRATORY ENDURANCE EXERCISE

Cardiorespiratory endurance exercise helps the body become more efficient and better able to cope with physical challenges. It also lowers risk for many chronic diseases.

Improved Cardiorespiratory Functioning

Earlier, this chapter described some of the major changes that occur in the cardiorespiratory system when you exercise, such as increases in cardiac output and blood pressure, breathing rate, and blood flow to the skeletal muscles. In the short term, all these changes help the body respond to the challenge of exercise. When performed regularly, endurance exercise also leads to permanent adaptation in the cardiorespiratory system (Figure 3.2). This improvement reduces the effort required to perform everyday tasks and enables the body to respond to physical challenges. This, in a nutshell, is what it means to be physically fit.

Endurance exercise enhances the heart's health by doing the following:

- Maintaining or increasing the heart's own blood and oxygen supply.
- Improving the heart muscle's function, so it pumps more blood per beat. This improved function keeps the heart rate lower both at rest and during exercise. The resting heart rate of a fit person is often 10–20 beats per minute lower than that of an unfit person. This translates into as many as 10 million fewer beats in the course of a year.
- Strengthening the heart's contractions.
- Increasing the heart's cavity size (in young adults).

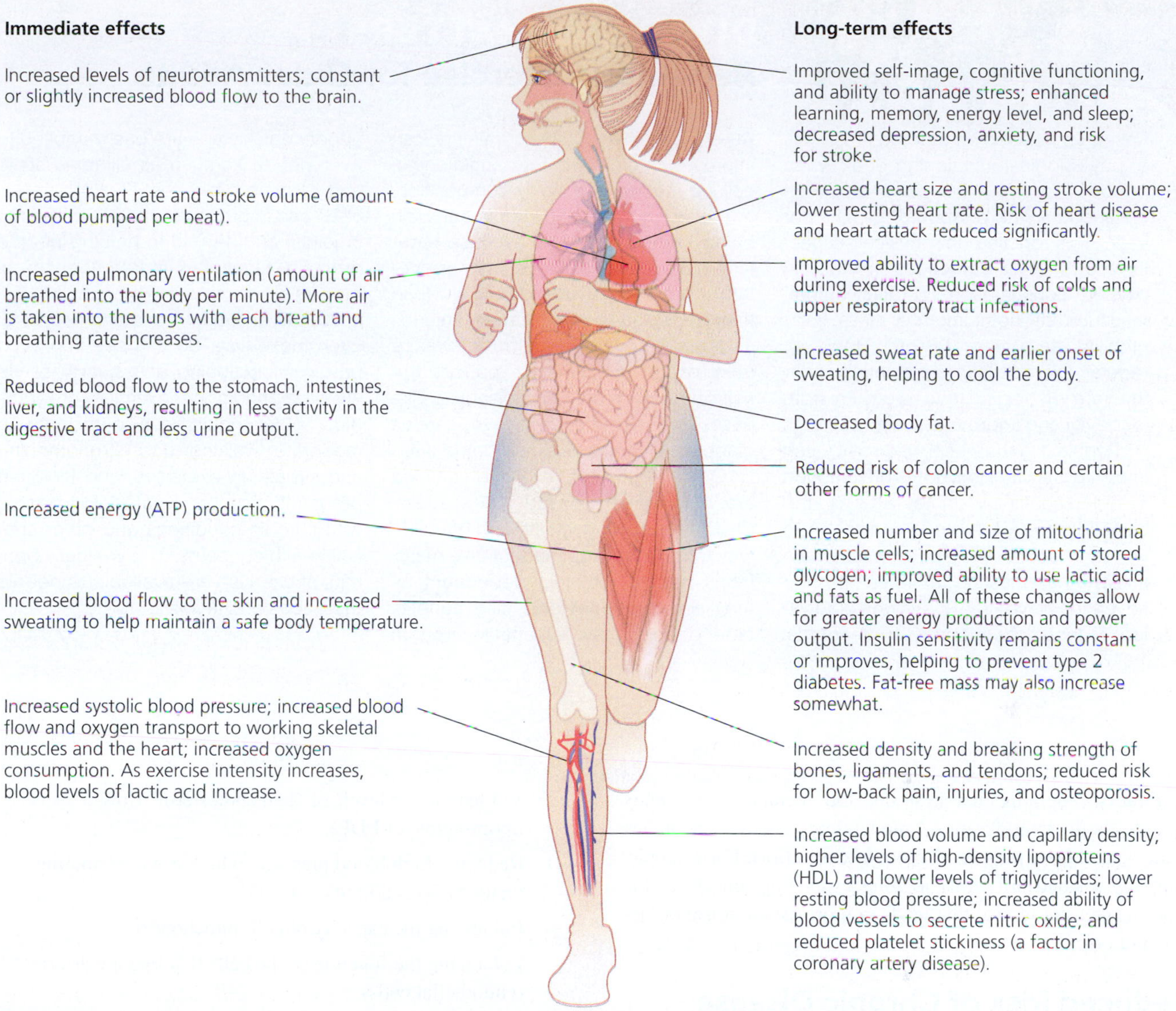

Immediate effects

Increased levels of neurotransmitters; constant or slightly increased blood flow to the brain.

Increased heart rate and stroke volume (amount of blood pumped per beat).

Increased pulmonary ventilation (amount of air breathed into the body per minute). More air is taken into the lungs with each breath and breathing rate increases.

Reduced blood flow to the stomach, intestines, liver, and kidneys, resulting in less activity in the digestive tract and less urine output.

Increased energy (ATP) production.

Increased blood flow to the skin and increased sweating to help maintain a safe body temperature.

Increased systolic blood pressure; increased blood flow and oxygen transport to working skeletal muscles and the heart; increased oxygen consumption. As exercise intensity increases, blood levels of lactic acid increase.

Long-term effects

Improved self-image, cognitive functioning, and ability to manage stress; enhanced learning, memory, energy level, and sleep; decreased depression, anxiety, and risk for stroke.

Increased heart size and resting stroke volume; lower resting heart rate. Risk of heart disease and heart attack reduced significantly.

Improved ability to extract oxygen from air during exercise. Reduced risk of colds and upper respiratory tract infections.

Increased sweat rate and earlier onset of sweating, helping to cool the body.

Decreased body fat.

Reduced risk of colon cancer and certain other forms of cancer.

Increased number and size of mitochondria in muscle cells; increased amount of stored glycogen; improved ability to use lactic acid and fats as fuel. All of these changes allow for greater energy production and power output. Insulin sensitivity remains constant or improves, helping to prevent type 2 diabetes. Fat-free mass may also increase somewhat.

Increased density and breaking strength of bones, ligaments, and tendons; reduced risk for low-back pain, injuries, and osteoporosis.

Increased blood volume and capillary density; higher levels of high-density lipoproteins (HDL) and lower levels of triglycerides; lower resting blood pressure; increased ability of blood vessels to secrete nitric oxide; and reduced platelet stickiness (a factor in coronary artery disease).

FIGURE 3.2   Immediate and long-term effects of regular cardiorespiratory endurance exercise. When endurance exercise is performed regularly, short-term changes in the body develop into more permanent adaptations; these include improved ability to exercise, reduced risk of many chronic diseases, and improved psychological and emotional well-being.

- Increasing blood volume so the heart pushes more blood into the circulatory system during each contraction (larger stroke volume). Increased blood volume also improves temperature regulation, which reduces the load on the heart.
- Reducing blood pressure.

Improved Cellular Metabolism

Regular endurance exercise improves the body's metabolism, down to the cellular level, enhancing your ability to produce and use energy efficiently. Cardiorespiratory training improves metabolism by doing the following (see Figure 3.2):

- Increasing the number of capillaries in the muscles. Additional capillaries supply the muscles with more fuel

and oxygen and more quickly eliminate waste products. Greater capillary density also helps heal injuries and reduce muscle aches.

- Training muscles to make the most of oxygen and fuel so they work more efficiently.
- Increasing the size and number of mitochondria in muscle and brain cells, thereby increasing the cells' energy capacity.
- Preventing glycogen depletion and increasing the muscles' ability to use lactate and fat as fuels.

Regular exercise may also help protect cells from chemical damage caused by agents called *free radicals*. (See Chapter 8 for details on free radicals and the special enzymes the body uses to fight them.)

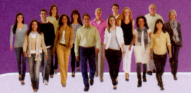
Fitness programs that best develop metabolic efficiency include both long-duration, moderately intense endurance exercise and brief periods of more intense effort. For example, climbing a small hill while jogging or cycling introduces the kind of intense exercise that leads to more efficient use of lactate and fats.

Reduced Risk of Chronic Disease

Regular endurance exercise lowers your risk of many chronic, disabling diseases. It can also help people with those diseases improve their health (see the box "Benefits of Exercise for Older Adults"). The most significant health benefits occur when someone who is sedentary becomes moderately active.

Cardiovascular Diseases Sedentary living is a key contributor to cardiovascular disease (CVD). CVD is a general category that encompasses several diseases of the heart and blood vessels, including coronary heart disease (which can cause heart attacks), stroke, and high blood pressure (see the box "Combine Aerobic Exercise with Strength Training"). Sedentary people are significantly more likely to die of CVD than are fit individuals.

Cardiorespiratory endurance exercise lowers your risk of CVD by doing the following:

- Promoting a healthy balance of fats in the blood. High concentrations of blood fats such as cholesterol and triglycerides are linked to CVD. Exercise raises levels of "good cholesterol" (high-density lipoproteins, or HDL) and may lower levels of "bad cholesterol" (low-density lipoproteins, or LDL).

- Reducing high blood pressure, which is a contributing factor to several kinds of CVD.

- Enhancing the capacity of cell mitochondria.

- Enhancing the function of the cells that line the arteries (endothelial cells).

- Reducing chronic inflammation.

- Preventing obesity and type 2 diabetes, both of which contribute to CVD.

Details on various types of CVD, their associated risk factors, and a lifestyle that can reduce your risk for developing CVD are discussed in Chapter 11. To learn more about atherosclerosis, the underlying disease process in CVD, see page T3-4 of the color transparency insert "Touring the Cardiorespiratory System" in this chapter.

Cancer Although the findings are not conclusive, some studies have shown a relationship between increased physical activity and a reduction in a person's risk of cancer. Exercise reduces the risk of colon cancer, and it may reduce the risk of cancers of the breast and reproductive organs. Physical activity during the high school and college years may be particularly important for preventing breast cancer later in life. Exercise may also reduce the risk of lung cancer, endometrial cancer, pancreatic cancer, and prostate cancer. (See Chapter 12 for more information on various types of cancer.)

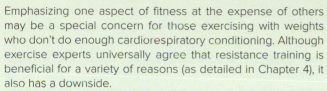

THE EVIDENCE FOR EXERCISE
Combine Aerobic Exercise with Strength Training

Emphasizing one aspect of fitness at the expense of others may be a special concern for those exercising with weights who don't do enough cardiorespiratory conditioning. Although exercise experts universally agree that resistance training is beneficial for a variety of reasons (as detailed in Chapter 4), it also has a downside.

A number of global studies have tracked the impact of weight training exercises on the cardiovascular system to find out if such training helps or harms the heart and blood vessels. These studies have shown that strength training poses short- and long-term risks to cardiovascular health and especially to arterial health. Aside from the risk of injury, lifting weights has been shown to have the following adverse effects on the cardiovascular system:

- Weight training promotes short-term stiffness of the blood vessels, which could promote hypertension (high blood pressure) over time and increase the load on the heart.

- Lifting weights (especially heavy weights) causes extreme short-term boosts in blood pressure; a Canadian study revealed that blood pressure can reach 480/350 millimeters of mercury during heavy lifting. Over the long term, sharp elevations in blood pressure can damage arteries, even if each pressure increase lasts only a few seconds.

- Weight training places stress on the endothelial cells that line blood vessels. Because these cells secrete nitric oxide (a chemical messenger involved in a variety of bodily functions), this stress can contribute to a wide range of negative effects, from erectile dysfunction to heart disease.

A variety of studies have shown that the best way to offset cardiovascular stress caused by strength training is to do cardiorespiratory endurance exercise (such as brisk walking or using an elliptical machine) immediately after a weight training session. Groundbreaking Japanese research showed that following resistance training with aerobic exercise prevents the stiffening of blood vessels and its associated damage. In this eight-week study, participants did aerobics before lifting weights, after lifting weights, or not at all. The group that did aerobics *after* weight training saw the greatest positive impact on arterial health;

participants who did aerobics before lifting weights did not see any improvement in the health of their blood vessels.

Strength training does promote endurance fitness by improving nervous control of the muscles, increasing type IIa motor units (muscle fibers have a blend of strength and endurance capacity), and increasing tendon strength. These changes increase muscle strength and the rate of force development, enhance the economy of movement, and increase the speed that blood cells travel through the muscles.

The bottom line of all this research? Resistance training and cardiorespiratory exercise are both good for you, if you do them in the right order. So, when you plan your workouts, be sure to do 15–60 minutes of aerobic exercise after each weight training session.

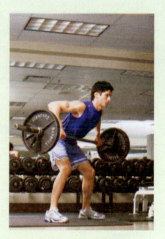

SOURCES: Ashor, A. W., et al. 2014. Effects of exercise modalities on arterial stiffness and wave reflection: A systematic review and meta-analysis of randomized controlled trials. *PLoS ONE* 9(10): e110034; Okamoto, T., M. Masuhara, and K. Ikuta. 2006. Effects of eccentric and concentric resistance training on arterial stiffness. *Journal of Human Hypertension* 20(5): 348–354; Okamoto, T., M. Masuhara, and K. Ikuta. 2007. Combined aerobic and resistance training and vascular function: Effect of aerobic exercise before and after resistance training. *Journal of Applied Physiology* 103(5): 1655–1661; Physical Activity Guidelines Advisory Committee. 2008. *Physical Activity Guidelines Advisory Committee Report, 2008.* Washington, D.C.: U.S. Department of Health and Human Services.

Type 2 Diabetes Regular exercise helps prevent the development of type 2 diabetes, the most common form of diabetes. Physical activity is also an important part of treating the disease. Obesity is a key risk factor for diabetes, and exercise helps keep body fat at healthy levels. But even without fat loss, exercise improves control of blood sugar levels in many people with diabetes. Exercise metabolizes (burns) excess sugar and makes cells more sensitive to the hormone insulin, which helps regulate blood sugar levels. (See Chapter 6 for more on diabetes and insulin resistance.)

Osteoporosis A special benefit of exercise, especially for women, is protection against osteoporosis, a disease that results in loss of bone density and strength. Weight-bearing exercise—particularly weight training—helps build bone during the teens

and twenties. People with denser bones can better endure the bone loss that occurs with aging. With stronger bones and muscles and better balance, fit people are less likely to experience debilitating falls and bone fractures. (See Chapter 8 for more on osteoporosis.)

Inflammation Inflammation is the body's response to tissue and cell damage (from injury, high blood pressure, or intense exercise), environmental poisons (e.g., cigarette smoke), or poor metabolic health (high blood fats, poor blood

> **inflammation** The body's response to tissue and cell damage, environmental poisons, or poor metabolic health.   **TERMS**

sugar control). Acute inflammation is a short-term response to exercise and is an important way that the body improves physical fitness. For example, short-term inflammation triggers increased muscle protein synthesis that promotes muscle fitness and recovery from exercise. Chronic inflammation, on the other hand, is a prolonged, abnormal process that causes tissue breakdown and diseases such as atherosclerosis, cancer, and rhematoid arthritis.

While exercise increases acute inflammation during and shortly after a workout, it reduces chronic levels of inflammation—if the training program is not too severe. For example, practicing endurance training three to five days a week will reduce inflammation. Training excessively, such as running a marathon several times a month or doing severe cross-training workouts five to seven days per week, will cause overtraining and chronic inflammation. We could call this the Goldilocks effect: the training program should not be too much or too little; it should be just right.

Deaths from All Causes Physically active people have a reduced risk of dying prematurely from all causes, with the greatest benefits found for people with the highest levels of physical activity and fitness (Figure 3.3). Physical inactivity is a predictor of premature death and is as important of a risk factor as smoking, high blood pressure, obesity, and diabetes.

Better Control of Body Fat

Too much body fat is linked to a variety of health problems, including cardiovascular disease, cancer, and type 2

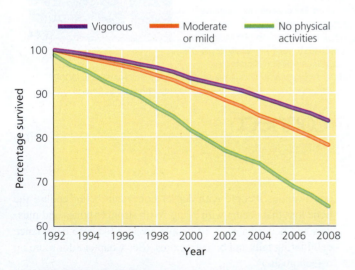

FIGURE 3.3 Survival rates for older adults doing vigorous, moderate, or no exercise, 1992–2008. The Health and Retirement Study—a long-term study of older adults—found that people who exercised vigorously over a 16-year period (1992–2008) had a lower death rate than those who exercised at moderate intensities or did no physical activity. After 16 years, the survival rate was 84% for those doing vigorous exercise, 78% for those doing moderate intensity physical activity, and only 65% for those doing no physical activity. Exercising longer or more intensely reduces the risk of dying prematurely from a variety of causes.

SOURCE: Wen, M., et al. 2014. Physical activity and mortality among middle-aged and older adults in the United States. *Journal Physical Activity & Health.* 11(2): 303–312.

diabetes. Healthy body composition can be difficult to achieve and maintain—especially for someone who is sedentary—because a diet that contains all essential nutrients can be relatively high in calories. Excess calories are stored in the body as fat. Regular exercise increases daily calorie expenditure, which means that a healthy diet is less likely to lead to weight gain. Endurance exercise burns calories directly and, if intense enough, continues to do so by raising resting metabolic rate for several hours following an exercise session. A higher metabolic rate makes it easier for a person to maintain a healthy weight or to lose weight. However, exercise alone cannot ensure a healthy body composition. As described in Chapters 6 and 9, you will lose more weight more rapidly and keep it off longer if you decrease your calorie intake and boost your calorie expenditure through exercise.

Improved Immune Function

Exercise can have either positive or negative effects on the **immune system**, the physiological processes that protect us from diseases such as colds, bacterial infections, and even cancer. Moderate endurance exercise boosts immune function, whereas overtraining (excessive training) depresses it, at least temporarily. Physically fit people get fewer colds and upper respiratory tract infections than people who are not fit.

Exercise affects immune function by influencing levels of specialized cells and chemicals involved in the immune response. As discussed in Chapter 2, physically active people also have healthier, more resilient genes, which promotes immunity. Exercise preserves the telomeres, which form the ends of the DNA strands and holds them together. Without exercise, the telomeres shorten over time, eventually reducing the effectiveness of the immune system. In addition to getting regular moderate exercise, you can further strengthen your immune system by eating a well-balanced diet, managing stress, and getting 7 to 8 hours of sleep every night.

Improved Psychological and Emotional Well-Being

Most people who participate in regular endurance exercise experience social, psychological, and emotional benefits. Skill mastery and self-control enhance one's self-image. Recreational sports provide an opportunity to socialize, have fun, and strive to excel. Endurance exercise lessens anxiety, depression, stress, anger, and hostility, thereby improving mood while boosting cardiovascular health. Regular exercise also improves sleep.

ASSESSING CARDIORESPIRATORY FITNESS

The body's ability to maintain a level of exertion (exercise) for an extended time is a direct reflection of cardiorespiratory fitness. One's level of fitness is determined by the body's ability to take up, distribute, and use oxygen during physical activity. As explained earlier, the best quantitative measure of cardiorespiratory endurance is maximal oxygen consumption, expressed as $\dot{V}O_{2max}$, the amount of oxygen the body uses when a person reaches his or her maximum ability to supply oxygen during exercise. Maximal oxygen consumption can be measured precisely in an exercise physiology laboratory through analysis of the air a person inhales and exhales when exercising to a level of exhaustion (maximum intensity). This procedure can be expensive and time-consuming, however, making it impractical for the average person.

Choosing an Assessment Test

Fortunately, several simple assessment tests provide reasonably good estimates of maximal oxygen consumption (within 10–15% of the results of a laboratory test). Four commonly used assessments are the following:

- *The 1-Mile Walk Test.* This test measures the amount of time it takes you to complete 1 mile of brisk walking and your heart rate at the end of your walk. A fast time and a low heart rate indicate a high level of cardiorespiratory endurance.

- *The 3-Minute Step Test.* In the step test, you step continually at a steady rate for 3 minutes and then monitor your heart rate during recovery. The rate at which the pulse returns to normal is a good measure of cardiorespiratory capacity; heart rate remains lower and recovers faster in people who are more physically fit.

- *The 1.5-Mile Run-Walk Test.* Oxygen consumption increases with speed in distance running, so a fast time on this test indicates high maximal oxygen consumption.

- *The Beep Test.* This test predicting maximal oxygen consumption is excellent for people who are physically fit and wish to measure their capacity for high-intensity exercise, such as sprints. A prerecorded series of "beeps" (tones) sound off at faster and faster intervals. Your task is to keep up with the beeps during the exercise.

Lab 3.1 provides detailed instructions for each of these tests. An additional assessment, the 12-Minute Swim Test, is also provided. To assess yourself, choose one of these methods based on your access to equipment, your current physical condition, and your own preference.

Don't take any of these tests without checking with your physician if you are ill or have any of the risk factors for exercise discussed in Chapter 2 and Lab 2.1.

Monitoring Your Heart Rate

Each time your heart contracts, it pumps blood into your arteries. You can measure your heart rate—the number of heart contractions per minute—by using a heart rate monitor or counting your pulse beats. Modern heart rate monitors are inexpensive and accurate. Several companies make heart rate monitor apps that are used with smart phones to measure heart rate, distances, route maps, running or cycling speed, and calories burned. Counting your pulse is the traditional method of measuring heart rate. Each contraction of the heart produces a

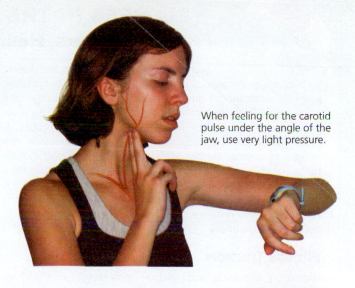

When feeling for the carotid pulse under the angle of the jaw, use very light pressure.

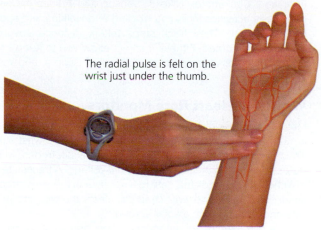

The radial pulse is felt on the wrist just under the thumb.

FIGURE 3.4 **Checking your pulse.** The pulse can be taken at the carotid artery in the neck (top) or at the radial artery in the wrist (bottom).

surge of blood that causes a pulse you can feel by holding your fingers against an artery. Heart rate is a good way to monitor exercise intensity during a workout. (Intensity is described in more detail in the next section.)

The two most common sites for monitoring heart rate are the carotid artery in the neck and the radial artery in the wrist (Figure 3.4). To take your pulse, press your index and middle fingers gently on the correct site. You may have to shift position several times to find the best place to feel your pulse. Don't use your thumb to check your pulse; it has a pulse of its own that can confuse your count. (Use your middle and ring finger if you have a strong pulse in your index finger.) Be careful not to push too hard, particularly when taking your pulse in the carotid artery (strong pressure on this artery may cause a reflex that slows the heart rate).

immune system The physiological processes that protect us from diseases such as colds, bacterial infections, and even cancer. **TERMS**

WELLNESS IN THE DIGITAL AGE
Fitness Trackers, Heart Rate Monitors, and GPS Devices

Technology has transformed the market for trackers and monitors. It is difficult to keep up with the latest exercise monitors designed as stand-alone units, smart phone apps, and GPS accessories. A heart rate monitor is an electronic device that checks the user's pulse, either continuously or on demand. These devices make it easy to monitor your heart rate before, during, and after exercise. Some include global positioning system (GPS) receivers that help you track the distance you walk, run, or bike. Wearable fitness trackers, made by Adidas, Nike, Fitbit, Withings, and BodyMedia, among others, measure distance and steps covered, calories burned, and exercise intensity.

Fitness Trackers

High-tech monitors and phone apps such as the Nike Fuelband, Cyclemeter, Nike + Sensor, and Adidas miCoach track daily activities including running and walking and sports like basketball. They track steps taken, distance covered, and calories burned. Fitness trackers allow you to keep track of your progress, compete against other people, and meet challenges.

Wearable Heart Rate Monitors

Most consumer-grade heart rate monitors have two pieces—a strap that wraps around the user's chest and a wrist strap. The chest strap contains one or more small electrodes, which detect changes in the heart's electrical voltage. A transmitter in the chest strap sends the data to a receiver in the wrist strap. A small computer in the wrist strap calculates the wearer's heart rate and displays it on a small screen.

In a few low-cost monitors, the chest and wrist straps are connected by a wire, but the most popular monitors use wireless technology to transmit data to the heart rate monitor display. In advanced wireless monitors, data are encoded so they cannot be read by other monitors that may be nearby, as is often the case in a crowded gym. A one-piece (or "strapless") heart rate monitor does not include a chest strap; the wrist-worn device contains sensors that detect a pulse in the wearer's hand.

Monitors in Gym Equipment

Many pieces of workout equipment—including newer-model treadmills, stationary bikes, and elliptical trainers—feature built-in heart rate monitors. The monitor is usually mounted into the device's handles. To check your heart rate at any time while working out, simply grip the handles in the appropriate place; within a few seconds, your current heart rate will appear on the device's console.

Other Features

Heart rate monitors can do more than just check your pulse. Most can also tell you the following:

- Highest and lowest heart rate during a session
- Average heart rate
- Target heart rate range, based on your age, weight, and other factors
- Time spent within the target range
- Number of calories burned during a session

Some monitors can upload their data to a computer, so information can be stored and analyzed. The analytical software can help you track your progress over a period of time or a number of workouts. AliveECG is a phone app that can send an electrocardiogram instantly to a physician via email. Monitors with GPS provide an accurate estimate of distance traveled during a workout or over an entire day.

Choosing and Using Monitors

Heart rate monitors are useful if very close tracking of heart rate is important in your program. They offer several advantages:

- They are accurate, and they reduce the risk of mistakes when checking your own pulse. (Note: Chest-strap monitors are considered more accurate than strapless models. If you use a monitor built into gym equipment, its accuracy will depend on how well the device is maintained.)
- They are easy to use, although a sophisticated, multifunction monitor may take some time to master.
- They do the monitoring for you, so you don't have to worry about checking your own pulse.

When shopping for a heart rate, fitness tracker, phone app, or exercise GPS monitor, do your homework. Quality, reliability, and warranties vary. Ask personal trainers in your area for their recommendations, and look for product reviews in consumer magazines or online.

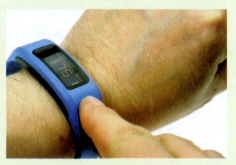

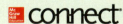

Heart rates are usually assessed in beats per minute (bpm). But counting your pulse for an entire minute isn't practical when you're exercising. And because heart rate slows rapidly when you stop exercising, a full minute's worth of counting can give inaccurate results. It's best to do a shorter count—15 seconds—and then multiply the result by 4 to get your heart rate in beats per minute. (You can also use a heart rate monitor to check your pulse. See the box "Fitness Trackers, Heart Rate Monitors, and GPS Devices" for more information.)

Interpreting Your Score

After you've completed one or more of the assessment tests, use the table under "Rating Your Cardiovascular Fitness" in Lab 3.1 to determine your current level of cardiorespiratory fitness. As you interpret your score, remember that field tests of cardiorespiratory fitness are not precise scientific measurements and have up to a 10–15% margin of error.

You can use the assessment tests to monitor the progress of your fitness program by retesting yourself from time to time. Always compare scores for the *same* test: Your scores on different tests may vary considerably because of differences in skill and motivation and quirks in the tests themselves.

DEVELOPING A CARDIORESPIRATORY ENDURANCE PROGRAM

Cardiorespiratory endurance exercises are best for developing the type of fitness associated with good health, so they should serve as the focus of your exercise program. To create a successful endurance exercise program, follow these guidelines:

- Set realistic goals.
- Set your starting frequency, intensity, and duration of exercise at appropriate levels.
- Choose suitable activities.
- Warm up and cool down.
- Adjust your program as your fitness improves.

Setting Goals

You can use the results of cardiorespiratory fitness assessment tests to set a specific oxygen consumption goal for your cardiorespiratory endurance program. Your goal should be high enough to ensure a healthy cardiorespiratory system, but not so high that it will be impossible to achieve. Scores in the fair and good ranges for maximal oxygen consumption suggest good fitness; scores in the excellent and superior ranges indicate a high standard of physical performance.

Through endurance training, an individual may be able to improve maximal oxygen consumption ($\dot{V}O_{2max}$) by about 10–30%. The amount of improvement possible depends on genetics, age, health status, and initial fitness level. People who start at a very low fitness level can improve by a greater percentage than elite athletes because the latter are already at a much higher fitness level, one that may approach their genetic physical limits. If you are tracking $\dot{V}O_{2max}$ by using the field tests described in this chapter, you may be able to increase your score by more than 30% due to improvements in other physical factors, such as muscle power, which can affect your performance on the tests.

Another physical factor you can track to monitor progress is resting heart rate—your heart rate at complete rest, measured in the morning before you get out of bed and move around. Resting heart rate may decrease by as much as 10–15 beats per minute

in response to endurance training. Changes in resting heart rate may be noticeable after only about four–six weeks of training.

You may want to set other types of goals for your fitness program. For example, if you walk, jog, or cycle as part of your fitness program, you may want to set a time or distance goal—working up to walking 5 miles in one session, completing a 4-mile run in 28 minutes, or cycling a total of 35 miles per week. A more modest goal might be to achieve the recommendation of the U.S. Department of Health and Human Services and American College of Sports Medicine (ACSM) of 150 minutes per week of moderate-intensity physical activity. Although it's best to base your program on "SMART" goals (those that are **s**pecific, **m**easurable, **a**ttainable, **r**ealistic, and **t**ime frame-specific), you may also want to set more qualitative goals, such as becoming more energetic, sleeping better, and improving the fit of your clothes.

Applying the FITT Equation

As described in Chapter 2, you can use the acronym FITT to set key parameters of your fitness program: Frequency, Intensity, Time (duration), and Type of activity.

Frequency of Training Accumulating at least 150 minutes per week of moderate-intensity physical activity (or at least 75 minutes per week of vigorous physical activity) is enough to promote health. Most experts recommend that people exercise three to five days per week to build cardiorespiratory endurance. Training more than five days per week can lead to injury and isn't necessary for the typical person on an exercise program designed to promote wellness. It is safe to do moderate-intensity activity such as walking and gardening every day. Training fewer than three days per week makes it difficult to improve your fitness (unless exercise intensity is very high) or to lose weight through exercise. Remember, however, that some exercise is better than none.

Intensity of Training Intensity is the most important factor for increasing aerobic fitness. You must exercise intensely

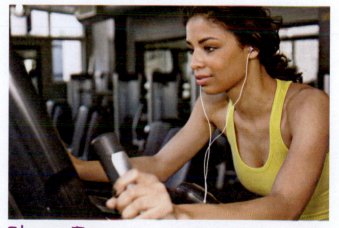

Fitness Tip Listen to fast-paced music for a better workout! In a recent study, students rode a stationary bike while listening to music at different tempos. The subjects rode harder when listening to faster music and performed less exercise in response to slower music.

enough to stress your body so that fitness improves. Four methods of monitoring exercise intensity are described in the following sections; choose the method that works best for you. Be sure to make adjustments in your intensity levels for environmental or individual factors. For example, on a hot and humid day or on your first day back to your program after an illness, you should decrease your intensity level.

TARGET HEART RATE ZONE   One of the best ways to monitor the intensity of cardiorespiratory endurance exercise is to measure your heart rate (calculated in beats per minute). It isn't necessary to exercise at your maximum heart rate to improve maximal oxygen consumption. Fitness adaptations occur at lower heart rates with a much lower risk of injury.

According to the American College of Sports Medicine, your **target heart rate zone**—a range of rates at which you should exercise to experience cardiorespiratory benefits—is between 65% and 90% of your maximum heart rate. To calculate your target heart rate zone, follow these steps:

1. Estimate your maximum heart rate (MHR) by subtracting your age from 220, or have it measured precisely by undergoing an exercise stress test in a doctor's office, hospital, or sports medicine lab. (*Note:* The formula to estimate MHR carries an error of about ±10–15 beats per minute and can be very inaccurate for some people, particularly older adults and young children. If your exercise heart rate seems inaccurate—that is, exercise within your target zone seems either too easy or too difficult—then use the perceived exertion method described in the next section, or have your maximum heart rate measured precisely.) You can get a reasonable estimate of maximal heart rate by exercising at maximal intensities on a stationary bike, treadmill, or elliptical trainer that has a built-in heart rate monitor. This method is not recommended unless you are physically fit and accustomed to intense exercise.

2. Multiply your MHR by 65% and 90% to calculate your target heart rate zone. Very unfit people should use 55% of MHR for their training threshold.

For example, a 19-year-old would calculate her target heart rate zone as follows:

$$\text{MHR} = 220 - 19 = 201 \text{ bpm}$$

$$65\% \text{ training intensity} = 0.65 \times 201 = 131 \text{ bpm}$$

$$90\% \text{ training intensity} = 0.90 \times 201 = 181 \text{ bpm}$$

target heart rate zone   The range of heart rates that should be reached and maintained during cardiorespiratory endurance exercise to obtain optimal training effects.

heart rate reserve   The difference between maximum heart rate and resting heart rate; used in one method for calculating target heart rate zone.

MET   A unit of measure that represents the body's resting metabolic rate—that is, the energy requirement of the body at rest.

TERMS

To gain fitness benefits, the young woman in our example would have to exercise at an intensity that raises her heart rate to between 131 and 181 bpm.

An alternative method for calculating target heart rate zone uses **heart rate reserve**, the difference between maximum heart rate and resting heart rate. Using this method, target heart rate is equal to resting heart rate plus between 50% (40% for very unfit people) and 85% of heart rate reserve. Although some people (particularly those with very low levels of fitness) will obtain more accurate results using this more complex method, both methods provide reasonable estimates of an appropriate target heart rate zone. Lab 3.2 gives formulas for both methods of calculating target heart rate.

If you have been sedentary, start by exercising at the lower end of your target heart rate zone (65% of maximum heart rate or 50% of heart rate reserve) for at least four–six weeks. Exercising closer to the top of the range can cause fast and significant gains in maximal oxygen consumption, but you may increase your risk of injury and overtraining. You *can* achieve significant health benefits by exercising at the bottom of your target zone, so don't feel pressure to exercise at an unnecessarily intense level. If you exercise at a lower intensity, you can increase the duration or frequency of training to obtain as much benefit to your health, as long as you are above the 65% training threshold. For people with a very low initial level of fitness, a lower training intensity of 55–64% of maximum heart rate or 40–49% of heart rate reserve may be sufficient to achieve improvements in maximal oxygen consumption, especially at the start of an exercise program. Intensities of 70–85% of maximum heart rate are appropriate for average individuals.

By monitoring your heart rate, you will always know if you are working hard enough to improve, not hard enough, or too hard. As your program progresses and your fitness improves, you will need to jog, cycle, or walk faster to reach your target heart rate zone. To monitor your heart rate during exercise, count your pulse while you're still moving or immediately after you stop exercising. Count beats for 15 seconds, then multiply that number by 4 to see if your heart rate is in your target zone. Table 3.2 shows target heart rate ranges and 15-second counts based on the maximum heart rate formula.

METS   One way scientists describe fitness is in terms of the capacity to increase metabolism (energy usage level) above rest. Scientists use METs to measure the metabolic cost of an exercise. One **MET** represents the body's resting metabolic rate—that is, the energy or calorie requirement of the body at rest. Exercise intensity is expressed in multiples of resting metabolic rate. For example, an exercise intensity of 2 METs is twice the resting metabolic rate.

METs are used to describe exercise intensities for occupational activities and exercise programs. Exercise intensities of less than 3–4 METs are considered low. Household chores and most industrial jobs fall into this category. Exercise at these intensities does not improve fitness for most people, but it will improve fitness for people with low physical capacities. Activities that increase metabolism by 6–8 METs are classified as moderate-intensity exercises and are suitable for most people beginning an

Table 3.2 — Target Heart Rate Zone and 15-Second Counts

AGE (years)	TARGET HEART RATE ZONE (bpm)*	15-SECOND COUNT (beats)
20–24	127–180	32–45
25–29	124–176	31–44
30–34	121–171	30–43
35–39	118–167	30–42
40–44	114–162	29–41
45–49	111–158	28–40
50–54	108–153	27–38
55–59	105–149	26–37
60–64	101–144	25–36
65+	97–140	24–35

*Target heart rates lower than those shown here are appropriate for individuals with a very low initial level of fitness. Ranges are based on the following formula: target heart rate = 0.65 to 0.90 of maximum heart rate, assuming maximum heart rate = 220 − age.

Table 3.3 — Approximate MET and Caloric Costs of Selected Activities for a 154-Pound Person

ACTIVITY	METs	CALORIC EXPENDITURE PER MINUTE
Rest	1	1.2
Light housework	2–4	2.4–4.8
Bowling	2–4	2.5–5
Walking	2–7	2.5–8.5
Archery	3–4	3.7–5
Dancing	3–7	3.7–8.5
Hiking	3–7	3.7–8.5
Horseback riding	3–8	3.7–10
Cycling	3–8	3.7–10
Basketball (recreational)	3–9	3.7–11
Swimming	4–8	5–10
Tennis	4–9	5–11
Fishing (fly, stream)	5–6	6–7.5
In-line skating	5–8	6–10
Skiing (downhill)	5–8	6–10
Rock climbing	5–10	6–12
Scuba diving	5–10	6–12
Skiing (cross-country)	6–12	7.5–15
Jogging	8–12	10–15

NOTE: Intensity varies greatly with effort, skill, and motivation.

SOURCE: Adapted from American College of Sports Medicine. 2013. *ACSM's Guidelines for Exercise Testing and Prescription*, 9th ed. Philadelphia: Wolters Kluwer/Lippincott Williams & Wilkins Health.

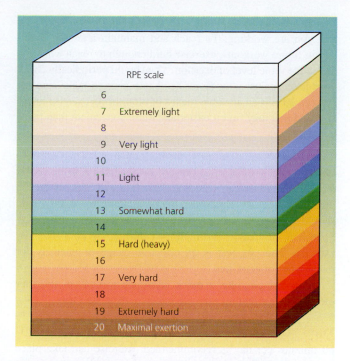

FIGURE 3.5 **Ratings of perceived exertion (RPE).** Experienced exercisers may use this subjective scale to estimate how near they are to their target heart rate zone.
SOURCE: Pick, H. L., ed. 1978. *Psychology from Research to Practice.* Kluwer Academic/Plenum Publishing Corporation. With kind permission of Springer Science and Business Media and the author.

METs are intended to be only an approximation of exercise intensity. Skill, body weight, body fat, and environment affect the accuracy of METs. As a practical matter, however, we can disregard these limitations. METs are a good way to express exercise intensity because this system is easy for people to remember and apply.

RATINGS OF PERCEIVED EXERTION Another way to monitor intensity is to monitor your perceived level of exertion. Repeated pulse counting during exercise can become a nuisance if it interferes with the activity. As your exercise program progresses, you will probably become familiar with the amount of exertion required to raise your heart rate to target levels. In other words, you will know how you feel when you have exercised intensely enough. If this is the case, you can use the scale of **ratings of perceived exertion (RPE)** shown in Figure 3.5 to monitor the intensity of your exercise session without checking your pulse.

To use the RPE scale, select a rating that corresponds to your subjective perception of how hard you are exercising when you are training in your target heart rate zone. If your target zone is about 135–155 bpm, exercise intensely enough to raise your heart rate to that level, and then associate a rating—for example,

> **ratings of perceived exertion (RPE)** **TERMS** A system of monitoring exercise intensity by assigning a number to the subjective perception of target intensity.

exercise program. Vigorous exercise increases metabolic rate by more than 10 METs. Fast running or cycling, as well as intense play in sports like racquetball, can place people in this category. Table 3.3 lists the MET ratings for various activities.

"somewhat hard" or "hard" (14 or 15)—with how hard you feel you are working. To reach and maintain a similar intensity in future workouts, exercise hard enough to reach what you feel is the same level of exertion. You should periodically check your RPE against your target heart rate zone to make sure it's correct. RPE is an accurate means of monitoring exercise intensity, and you may find it easier and more convenient than pulse counting.

TALK TEST Another easy method of monitoring exercise exertion—in particular, to prevent overly intense exercise—is the talk test. Although your breathing rate will increase during moderate-intensity cardiorespiratory endurance exercise, you should not work out so intensely that you cannot communicate. Speech is limited to short phrases during vigorous-intensity exercise. The talk test is an effective gauge of intensity for many types of activities.

Table 3.4 provides a quick reference to each of the four methods of estimating exercise intensity discussed here.

Time (Duration) of Training A total duration of 20–60 minutes per day is recommended; exercise can take place in a single session or in multiple sessions lasting 10 or more minutes. The total duration of exercise depends on its intensity. To improve cardiorespiratory endurance during a low- to moderate-intensity activity such as walking or slow swimming, you should exercise for 30–60 minutes. For high-intensity exercise performed at the top of your target heart rate zone, a duration of 20 minutes is sufficient.

Some studies have shown that 5–10 minutes of extremely intense exercise (greater than 90% of maximal oxygen consumption) improves cardiorespiratory endurance. However, training at high intensity, particularly during high-impact activities, increases the risk of injury. Also, if you experience discomfort in high-intensity exercise, you are more likely to discontinue your exercise program. Longer-duration, low- to moderate-intensity activities generally result in more gradual gains in maximal oxygen consumption. In planning your program, start with less vigorous activities and gradually increase intensity.

Type of Activity Cardiorespiratory endurance exercises include activities that involve the rhythmic use of large-muscle groups for an extended period of time, such as jogging, walking, cycling, aerobic dancing and other forms of group exercise, cross-country skiing, and swimming. Start-and-stop sports, such as tennis and racquetball, also qualify if you have enough skill to play continuously and intensely enough to raise your heart rate to target levels. Other important considerations are access to facilities, expense, equipment, and the time required to achieve an adequate skill level and workout.

Warming Up and Cooling Down

As we saw in Chapter 2, it's important to warm up before every session of cardiorespiratory endurance exercise and to cool down afterward. Because the body's muscles work better when their temperature is slightly above resting level, warming up enhances performance and decreases the chance of injury. It gives the body time to redirect blood to active muscles and the heart time to adapt to increased demands. Warming up also helps spread protective fluid throughout the joints, preventing injury to their surfaces.

A warm-up session should include low-intensity, whole-body movements similar to those in the activity that will follow, such as walking slowly before beginning a brisk walk. An active warm-up of 5–10 minutes is adequate for most types of exercise. However, warm-up time will depend on your level of fitness, experience, and individual preferences.

What about stretching as part of a warm-up? Performing *static* stretches—those in which you move a joint to the end of the range of motion and hold the position—as part of your pre-exercise warm-up has not been found to prevent injury and has little or no effect on post-exercise muscle soreness. Static stretching before exercise may also adversely affect strength, power, balance, reaction time, and movement time. (Stretching may interfere with muscle and joint receptors that are used in the performance of sport and movement skills.) For these reasons, it is often recommended that static stretches be performed at the end of your workout, after your cool-down but while your muscles are still warm and your joints are lubricated. On the flip side, *dynamic* stretches—those involving continuous movement of joints through a range of motion—can be an appropriate part of a warm-up. Slow and controlled movements such as walking lunges, heel kicks, and arm circles can raise muscle temperature while moving joints through their range of motion. (See Chapter 5 for a detailed discussion of stretching and flexibility exercises.)

Cooling down after exercise is important for returning the body to a nonexercising state. A cool-down helps maintain blood flow to the heart and brain and redirects blood from working muscles to other areas of the body. This helps prevent a large drop in blood pressure, dizziness, and other potential cardiovascular complications. A cool-down, consisting of 5–10 minutes of reduced activity, should follow every workout to allow heart rate, breathing, and circulation to return to normal. Decrease the intensity of exercise gradually during your cool-down. For example, following a running workout, begin your cool-down by jogging at half speed for 30 seconds to a minute; then do several minutes of walking, reducing your speed slowly. A good rule of thumb is to cool down at least until your heart rate drops below 100 beats per minute.

The general pattern of a safe and successful workout for cardiorespiratory fitness is illustrated in Figure 3.6.

Table 3.4	Estimating Exercise Intensity	
METHOD	MODERATE INTENSITY	VIGOROUS INTENSITY
Percentage of maximum heart rate	55–69%	70–90%
Heart rate reserve	40–59%	60–85%
Rating of perceived exertion	12–13 (somewhat hard)	14–16 (hard)
Talk test	Speech with some difficulty	Speech limited to short phrases

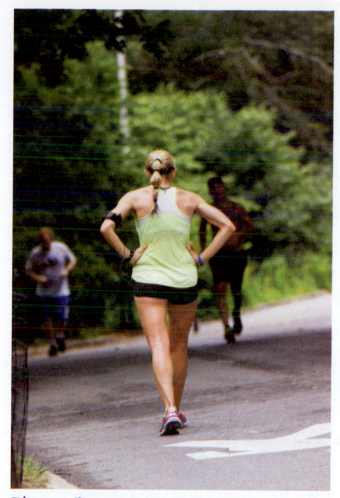

Fitness Tip Make warming up and cooling down a part of your exercise routine. Starting an exercise activity with a low-intensity version and slowing down gradually at the end helps your body adapt to being more active, protects from certain injuries, and may make the health benefits of exercise last longer.

Building Cardiorespiratory Fitness

Building fitness is as much an art as a science. Your fitness improves when you overload your body. However, you must increase the intensity, frequency, and duration of exercise carefully to avoid injury and overtraining.

General Program Progression For the initial stage of your program, which may last anywhere from three to six weeks, exercise at the low end of your target heart rate zone. Begin with a frequency of three–four days per week, and choose a duration appropriate for your fitness level: 12–15 minutes if you are very unfit, 20 minutes if you are sedentary but otherwise healthy, and 30–40 minutes if you are an experienced exerciser. Use this stage of your program to allow both your body and your schedule to adjust to your new exercise routine. When you can exercise at the upper levels of frequency (four–five days per week) and duration (30–40 minutes) without excessive fatigue or muscle soreness, you are ready to progress.

The next phase of your program is the improvement stage, lasting from four to six months. During this phase, slowly and

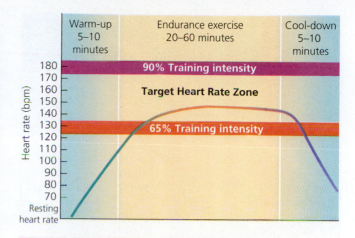

Frequency: 3–5 days per week

Intensity: 55/65–90% of maximum heart rate, 40/50–85% of heart rate reserve plus resting heart rate, or an RPE rating of about 12–18 (lower intensities—55–64% of maximum heart rate and 40–49% of heart rate reserve—are applicable to people who are quite unfit; for average individuals, intensities of 70–85% of maximum heart rate are appropriate)

Time (duration): 20–60 minutes (one session or multiple sessions lasting 10 or more minutes)

Type of activity: Cardiorespiratory endurance exercises, such as walking, jogging, biking, swimming, cross-country skiing, and rope skipping

FIGURE 3.6 The FITT principle for a cardiorespiratory endurance workout. Longer-duration exercise at lower intensities can often be as beneficial for promoting health as shorter-duration, high-intensity exercise.

gradually increase the amount of overload until you reach your target level of fitness (see the sample training progression in Table 3.5). Take care not to increase overload too quickly. It is usually best to avoid increasing both intensity and duration during the same session or increasing all three training variables (intensity, duration, and frequency) in one week. Increasing duration in increments of 5–10 minutes every two–three weeks is usually appropriate. Signs that you are increasing overload too quickly include muscle aches and pains, lack of usual interest in exercise, extreme fatigue, and inability to complete a workout. Keep an exercise log or training diary to monitor your workouts and progress.

Interval Training You will not improve your fitness indefinitely. The more fit you become, the harder you must work to improve. Few exercise techniques are more effective at improving fitness rapidly than *high-intensity interval training (HIIT)*—a series of very brief, high-intensity exercise sessions interspersed with short rest periods. The four components of interval training are distance, repetition, intensity, and rest, defined as follows:

- *Distance* refers to either the distance or the time of the exercise interval.
- *Repetition* is the number of times the exercise is repeated.

Table 3.5 — Sample Progression for an Endurance Program

STAGE/WEEK	FREQUENCY (days/week)	INTENSITY* (beats/minute)	TIME (duration in minutes)
Initial stage			
1	3	120–130	15–20
2	3	120–130	20–25
3	4	130–145	20–25
4	4	130–145	25–30
Improvement stage			
5–7	3–4	145–160	25–30
8–10	3–4	145–160	30–35
11–13	3–4	150–165	30–35
14–16	4–5	150–165	30–35
17–20	4–5	160–180	35–40
21–24	4–5	160–180	35–40
Maintenance stage			
25+	3–5	160–180	20–60

*The target heart rates shown here are based on calculations for a healthy 20-year-old with a resting heart rate of 60 beats per minute; the program progresses from an initial target heart rate of 50% to a maintenance range of 70–85% of heart rate reserve.

SOURCE: Adapted from American College of Sports Medicine. 2013. *ACSM's Guidelines for Exercise Testing and Prescription*, 9th ed. Philadelphia: Wolters Kluwer/Lippincott Williams & Wilkins Health. Reprinted with permission from the publisher.

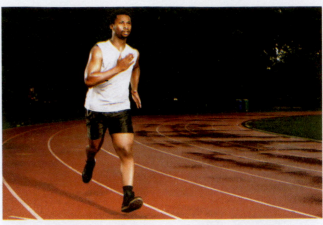

Fitness Tip High-intensity interval training can be an effective technique for boosting fitness. For a runner, HIIT might be half a dozen 200-meter sprints one to three times a week. If you decide to try HIIT, be sure start slowly, progress gradually, and listen to your body to avoid injury.

- *Intensity* is the speed at which the exercise is performed.
- *Rest* is the time spent recovering between exercises.

You can use interval training in your favorite aerobic exercises. In fact, the type of exercise you select is not important as long as you exercise at a high intensity and rest from 3 to 5 minutes between repetitions. HIIT training can even be used to help develop sports skills. For example, a runner might do 4 to 8 repetitions of 200-meter sprints at near-maximum effort. A tennis player might practice volleys against a wall as fast as possible for 4 to 8 repetitions lasting 30 seconds each. A swimmer might swim 4 to 8 repetitions of 50 meters at 100% effort.

If you add HIIT to your exercise program, do not practice interval training more than three days per week. Intervals are exhausting and easily lead to injury. Let your body tell you how many days you can tolerate. If you become overly tired after doing interval training three days per week, cut back to two days. If you feel good, try increasing the intensity or number of intervals (but not the number of days per week) and see what happens. As with any kind of exercise program, begin HIIT training slowly and progress conservatively. Although HIIT training produces substantial fitness improvements, it is best to integrate it into your total exercise program.

PROS Canadian researchers found that six sessions of high-intensity interval training on a stationary bike increased muscle oxidative capacity by 38%, muscle glycogen by 20%, and cycle endurance capacity by 100%. The subjects made these amazing improvements by exercising only 15 minutes over a period of two weeks. Each workout consisted of 4 to 7 repetitions of high-intensity exercise (each repetition consisted of 30 seconds at near maximum effort) on a stationary bike. Follow-up studies showed that practicing HIIT one to three times per week improved endurance and aerobic capacity just as well as training five times per week for 60 minutes for six weeks. These studies (and more than 50 others) showed the value of high-intensity training for building aerobic capacity and endurance.

CONS High-intensity interval training appears to be safe and effective in the short term, but there are concerns about the long-term safety and effectiveness of this type of training, so consider the following issues:

- High-intensity training could be dangerous for some people. A physician might be reluctant to give certain patients the green light for this type of exercise.
- Always warm up with several minutes of low-intensity exercise before practicing HIIT. High-intensity exercise without a warm-up can cause cardiac arrhythmias (abnormal heart rhythms), even in healthy people.
- HIIT might trigger overuse injuries in unfit people. For this reason, it is essential to start gradually, especially for someone at a low level of fitness. Exercise at submaximal intensities for at least four to six weeks before starting high-intensity interval training. Cut back on interval training or rest if you feel overly fatigued or develop overly sore joints or muscles.

Other types of high-intensity training may combine intervals with other types of exercises and training techniques; see the box "High-Intensity Conditioning Programs."

Maintaining Cardiorespiratory Fitness

There are limits to the level of fitness you can achieve, and if you increase intensity and duration indefinitely, you are likely

In recent years, high-intensity power-based "extreme" conditioning programs, such as CrossFit, Gym Jones, and Insanity, have grown in popularity. The programs typically incorporate a range of activity types and may include high-intensity aerobic exercise, interval training, free-weight exercises, and gymnastics moves. The programs may be geared toward developing whole-body fitness, limiting workout time by utilizing short but high-intensity sessions, and/or adding a competitive aspect to fitness training.

CrossFit is a popular example of a high-intensity program that emphasizes use of broad and constantly changing training stimuli. It includes activities designed to develop not only cardiorespiratory endurance but also strength, power, speed, coordination, ability, balance, and accuracy. Workouts are short and intense but should be tailored to an individual's current fitness level and age. They may include aerobic activities such as running and rope skipping, plus whole-body strength training activities such as power lifts, plyometrics, sled pulls, and kettlebell exercises.

The sample workouts below provide a flavor of this type of high-intensity training.

Sample Workouts

Complete three circuits (series) of the activities, but do not exceed 20–30 minutes for the workout. Break the exercises into sets if you cannot complete all the repetitions (e.g., 20 pull-ups). Record your time. Train as hard and as fast as you can while maintaining good technique. Select a weight that allows you to complete the reps in the sets. (Principles of resistance exercise are described in Chapter 4.) Change the exercises with every workout.

Workout 1

40 push-ups

10 standing long jumps

40 squats with hands on your hips

20 dumbbell or kettlebell swings

Skip rope rapidly for three minutes

Rest three minutes; repeat circuit 2 more times

Workout 2

20 pull-ups

20 dumbbell thrusters (front squat with barbell or dumbbells, then immediately perform an overhead press)

20 overhead squats

10 kettlebell snatches (10 for each arm)

2 minutes spinning on bike while standing, maximum intensity

Rest 3 minutes; repeat circuit 2 more times

Cautions and Guidelines

High-intensity training programs have their critics, who point to the increased risk of severe injury and lack of concern for the principle of specificity (training the way you want your body to adapt) with this type of training. Good technique is essential: The emphasis on speed and intensity can make it difficult to achieve good technique, but performing high-speed free-weight exercises such as cleans and squats improperly can lead to severe injury.

Performing high-speed, high-repetition sit-ups or squats often pushes muscles and joints to failure, causing severe knee or back injury or muscle destruction (rhabdomyolysis or "rhabdo"). Until recently, physicians encountered rhabdo only after extreme trauma from automobile accidents. These days, rhabdo may becoming more common because of the popularity of "feel the burn" high-intensity training programs. Biomechanical studies suggest that high-speed sit-ups and squats can damage the spine. The benefits of high levels of fitness are counterbalanced by the risk of injury.

In spite of the potential risks of high-intensity training, it can be a suitable option for fit individuals who enjoy and are motivated by varied, high-intensity workouts that require little time or equipment. If you are considering this type of training, consider the following:

- Follow general guidelines for medical clearance for exercise (see Chapter 2).
- Use good form and appropriate safety equipment for all exercises and activities; do not sacrifice form for speed, number of repetitions, or any other goal.
- Drink plenty of water and avoid exercise in hot and humid environments.
- Don't push yourself beyond the limits of your strength or conditioning level. Monitor yourself for signs of overtraining (unusual fatigue or muscle soreness), injuries, and rhabdomyolysis (severe muscle pain or weakness; dark, red, or cola-colored urine).
- Get advice from a qualified professional; when choosing a class, fitness facility, or trainer, follow the guidelines presented in Chapter 2.

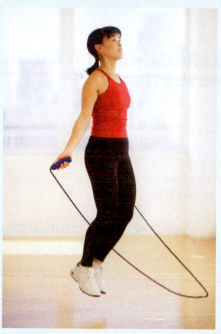

SOURCES: Smith, M. M., A. J. Sommer, B. E. Starkoff, and S. T. Devor. 2013. CrossFit-based high intensity power training improves maximal aerobic fitness and body composition. *Journal of Strength Conditioning Research.* 27(11): 3159–3172; Heinrich, K. M. 2014. High-intensity compared to moderate-intensity training for exercise initiation, enjoyment, adherence, and intentions: an intervention study. *BMC Public Health* 14: 789. Bergeron N. F., et al. 2011. *CHAMP/ACSM Executive Summary: High-Intensity Training Workshop.* (http://hprc-online.org/physical-fitness/training-exercise/exercise/guidelines/champ-acsm-high-intensity-training-conference). Skelly, L. E., et al. 2014. High-intensity interval exercise induces 24-h energy expenditure similar to traditional endurance exercise despite reduced time commitment. *Applied Physiology Nutrition Metabolism* 39(7): 845–848.

to become injured or overtrained. After an improvement stage of four–six months, you may reach your goal of an acceptable level of fitness. You can then maintain fitness by continuing to exercise at the same intensity at least three nonconsecutive days every week. If you stop exercising, you lose your gains in fitness fairly rapidly. If you take time off for any reason, start your program again at a lower level and rebuild your fitness in a slow and systematic way.

When you reach the maintenance stage, you may want to set new goals for your program and make some adjustments to maintain your motivation. For example, you might set a new goal of participating in a local 5K race. Or you might add new buddies to your program, or mix up your exercise sessions by working out in a new setting. Adding variety to your program can be a helpful strategy. Engaging in multiple types of endurance activities, an approach known as **cross-training**, can help boost enjoyment and prevent some types of injuries. For example, someone who has been jogging five days a week may change her program so she jogs three days a week, plays tennis one day a week, and goes for a bike ride one day a week.

While all these activities build endurance, alternating between them reduces the strain on specific joints and muscles. Varying your activities also offers new physical and mental challenges that can keep your fitness program fresh and fun.

EXERCISE SAFETY AND INJURY PREVENTION

Exercising safely and preventing injuries are two important challenges for people who engage in cardiorespiratory endurance exercise. This section provides basic safety guidelines that can be applied to a variety of fitness activities. Chapters 4 and 5 include additional advice specific to strength training and flexibility training.

Hot Weather and Heat Stress

Human beings require a relatively constant body temperature to survive. A change of just a few degrees in body temperature can quickly lead to distress and even death. If you lose too much water or if your body temperature gets too high, you may suffer from heat stress. Problems associated with heat stress include dehydration, heat cramps, heat exhaustion, and heatstroke.

When it is hot, exercise safety depends on the body's ability to dissipate heat and maintain blood flow to active muscles. The body releases heat from exercise through the evaporation of sweat. This process cools the skin and the blood circulating near the body's surface. Sweating is an efficient process as long as the air is relatively dry. As humidity increases, however, the sweating mechanism becomes less efficient because extra moisture in the air inhibits the evaporation of sweat from the skin. This is why it takes longer to cool down in humid weather than in dry weather.

You can avoid significant heat stress by staying fit, avoiding overly intense or prolonged exercise for which you are not prepared, drinking adequate fluids before and during exercise, and wearing clothes that allow heat to dissipate.

Dehydration Your body needs water to carry out many chemical reactions and to regulate body temperature. Sweating during exercise depletes your body's water supply and can lead to **dehydration**, excessive loss of body fluids, if fluids aren't replaced. Although dehydration is most common in hot weather, it can occur even in comfortable temperatures if fluid intake is insufficient.

Dehydration increases body temperature and decreases sweat rate, plasma volume, cardiac output, maximal oxygen consumption, exercise capacity, muscular strength, and stores of liver glycogen. You may begin to feel thirsty when you have a fluid deficit greater than about 1% of total body weight.

Drinking fluids before and during exercise is important to prevent dehydration and enhance performance. As a general rule, drink 16–20 ounces (about 2 cups) of fluid four hours before exercise, and 8–12 ounces 15 minutes immediately before exercise. During exercise lasting less than 60 minutes, drink 3–8 ounces of water every 15–20 minutes. Consume a sports drink with electrolytes every 15–20 minutes when exercising longer than 60 minutes.

Don't drink more than one quart of water per hour. Very rarely, active people consume too much water and develop *hyponatremia (water intoxication),* a condition that can cause lung congestion, muscle weakness, nervous system problems, and even death. Following the guidelines presented here can help prevent this condition.

To determine if you're drinking enough fluid, weigh yourself before and after an exercise session; any weight loss is due to fluid loss that needs to be replaced. Urine color is a good marker of hydration (see Figure 3.7). A dark color means that you might be dehydrated. Diet and supplements can affect urine color, which affects the accuracy of the test.

Bring a water bottle when you exercise so you can replace your fluids while they're being depleted. For exercise sessions lasting less than 60 minutes, cool water is an excellent fluid

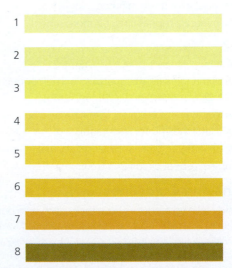

FIGURE 3.7 Urine chart to assess hydration. A large amount of light-colored urine means you are well hydrated. The darker the color, the more dehydrated you are. Vitamins and some foods can make urine darker.

SOURCE: American College of Sports Medicine. 2011. Selecting and Effectively Using Hydration for Fitness. Indianapolis, IN: American College of Sports Medicine.

replacement. For longer workouts, choose sports drinks containing water and small amounts of electrolytes (sodium, potassium, and magnesium) and simple carbohydrates ("sugar," usually in the form of sucrose, glucose, lactate, or glucose polymers). Electrolytes, which are lost from the body in sweat, are important because they help regulate the balance of fluids in body cells and the bloodstream. The carbohydrates in typical sports drinks are rapidly digestible, which enables them to help maintain blood glucose levels. Choose a beverage with no more than eight grams of simple carbohydrate per 100 milliliters of fluid. Nonfat milk and chocolate milk, for those who can tolerate dairy products, are excellent fluid replacement beverages because they promote long-term hydration. See Chapter 8 for more on diet and fluid recommendations for active people.

Heat Cramps Involuntary cramping and spasms in the muscle groups used during exercise are sometimes called **heat cramps**. Although depletion of sodium and potassium from the muscles is involved with the problem, the primary cause of cramps is muscle fatigue. Children are particularly susceptible to heat cramps, but the condition can also occur in adults, even those who are fit. The best treatment for heat cramps is a combination of gentle stretching, replacement of fluid and electrolytes, and rest.

Heat Exhaustion Symptoms of **heat exhaustion** include the following:

- Rapid, weak pulse
- Low blood pressure
- Headache
- Faintness, weakness, dizziness
- Profuse sweating
- Pale face
- Psychological disorientation (in some cases)
- Normal or slightly elevated core body temperature

Heat exhaustion occurs when an insufficient amount of blood returns to the heart because so much of the body's blood volume is being directed to working muscles (for exercise) and to the skin (for cooling). Treatment for heat exhaustion includes resting in a cool area, removing excess clothing, applying cool or damp towels to the body, and drinking fluids. An affected individual should rest for the remainder of the day and drink plenty of fluids for the next 24 hours.

Heatstroke **Heatstroke** is a major medical emergency resulting from the failure of the brain's temperature regulatory center. The body does not sweat enough, and body temperature rises dramatically to extremely dangerous levels. In addition to high body temperature, symptoms can include the following:

- Hot, flushed skin (dry or sweaty), red face
- Chills, shivering
- Very high or very low blood pressure
- Confusion, erratic behavior
- Convulsions, loss of consciousness

A heatstroke victim should be cooled as rapidly as possible and immediately transported to a hospital. To lower body temperature, get out of the heat, remove excess clothing, drink cold fluids, and apply cool or damp towels to the body or immerse the body in cold water. People experiencing heatstroke during exercise may still be sweating.

Cold Weather

In extremely cold conditions, problems can occur if a person's body temperature drops or if particular parts of the body are exposed. If the body's ability to warm itself through shivering or exercise can't keep pace with heat loss, the core body temperature begins to drop. This condition, known as **hypothermia**, depresses the central nervous system, resulting in sleepiness and a lower metabolic rate. As metabolic rate drops, body temperature declines even further, and coma and death can result. The risk of hypothermia is particularly severe in cold water.

Frostbite—the freezing of body tissues—is another potential danger of exercise in extremely cold conditions. Frostbite most commonly occurs in exposed body parts like earlobes, fingers, and the nose. It can cause permanent circulatory damage; its symptoms are numbness, pale color, and lack of sensation to cold in the affected areas. Hypothermia and frostbite both require immediate medical treatment.

To exercise safely in cold conditions, don't stay out in very cold temperatures for too long. Take both the temperature and the wind into account when planning your exercise session. Frostbite is possible within 30 minutes in calm conditions when the temperature is colder than −5°F, or in windy conditions (30 mph or more) if the temperature is below 10°F. **Wind chill** values that reflect a combination of the temperature and the wind speed are available as part of a local weather forecast and from the National Weather Service (http://www.weather.gov).

Appropriate clothing provides insulation and helps trap warm air next to the skin. Dress in layers so you can remove them as you warm up and can put them back on if you get cold. A substantial amount of heat loss comes from the head and

cross-training Alternating activities to improve components of fitness.

TERMS

dehydration Excessive loss of body fluids.

heat cramps Sudden muscle spasms and pain associated with intense exercise in hot weather.

heat exhaustion Heat illness resulting from exertion in hot weather.

heatstroke A severe and often fatal heat illness characterized by significantly elevated core body temperature.

hypothermia Low body temperature due to exposure to cold conditions.

frostbite Freezing of body tissues characterized by pallor, numbness, and a loss of cold sensation.

wind chill A measure of how cold it feels based on the rate of heat loss from exposed skin caused by cold and wind.

neck, so keep these areas covered. In subfreezing temperatures, protect the areas of your body most susceptible to frostbite—fingers, toes, ears, nose, and cheeks—with warm socks, mittens or gloves, and a cap, hood, or ski mask. Wear clothing that breathes and will wick moisture away from your skin to avoid being cooled or overheated by trapped perspiration. Many types of comfortable, lightweight clothing that provide good insulation are available. It's also important in cold conditions to warm up thoroughly and to drink plenty of fluids.

Poor Air Quality

Air pollution can decrease exercise performance and negatively affect health, particularly if you smoke or have respiratory problems such as asthma, bronchitis, or emphysema. The effects of smog are worse during exercise than at rest because air enters the lungs faster. Polluted air may also contain carbon monoxide, which displaces oxygen in the blood and reduces the amount of oxygen available to working muscles. One study found that exercise in polluted air could decrease lung function to the same extent as heavy smoking. Another study found that training in a polluted environment counteracted the normally beneficial effects of exercise on the brain. Symptoms of exercising in poor air quality include eye and throat irritations, difficulty breathing, and possibly headache and malaise.

Do not exercise outdoors during a smog alert or if air quality is very poor. If you have any type of cardiorespiratory difficulty, you should take particular care to avoid exertion outdoors in poor air quality. You can avoid some smog and air pollution by exercising in indoor facilities, in parks, near water (riverbanks, lakeshores, and ocean beaches), or in residential areas with less traffic. Air quality is also usually better in the early morning and late evening, before and after the commute hours.

Exercise Injuries

Most injuries are annoying rather than serious or permanent. However, an injury that isn't cared for properly can escalate into a chronic problem, sometimes serious enough to permanently curtail the activity. It's important to learn how to deal with injuries so they don't derail your fitness program. Strategies for the care of common exercise injuries and discomforts appear in Table 3.6; some general guidelines are given in the following sections.

When to Call a Physician Some injuries require medical attention. Consult a physician for the following:

- Head and eye injuries
- Possible ligament injuries

Table 3.6	Care of Common Exercise Injuries and Discomforts

INJURY	SYMPTOMS	TREATMENT
Blister	Accumulation of fluid in one spot under the skin	Don't pop or drain it unless it interferes too much with your daily activities. If it does pop, clean the area with antiseptic and cover with a bandage. Do not remove the skin covering the blister.
Bruise (contusion)	Pain, swelling, and discoloration	R-I-C-E: rest, ice, compression, elevation.
Fracture and/or dislocation	Pain, swelling, tenderness, loss of function, and deformity	Seek medical attention, immobilize the affected area, and apply cold.
Joint sprain	Pain, tenderness, swelling, discoloration, and loss of function	R-I-C-E; apply heat when swelling has disappeared. Stretch and strengthen affected area.
Muscle cramp	Painful, spasmodic muscle contractions	Gently stretch for 15–30 seconds at a time and/or massage the cramped area. Drink fluids and increase dietary salt intake if exercising in hot weather.
Muscle soreness or stiffness	Pain and tenderness in the affected muscle	Stretch the affected muscle gently; exercise at a low intensity; apply heat. Nonsteroidal anti-inflammatory drugs, such as ibuprofen, help some people.
Muscle strain	Pain, tenderness, swelling, and loss of strength in the affected muscle	R-I-C-E; apply heat when swelling has disappeared. Stretch and strengthen the affected area.
Plantar fasciitis	Pain and tenderness in the connective tissue on the bottom of the foot	Apply ice, take nonsteroidal anti-inflammatory drugs, and stretch. Wear night splints when sleeping.
Shin splint	Pain and tenderness on the front of the lower leg; sometimes also pain in the calf muscle	Rest; apply ice to the affected area several times a day and before exercise; wrap with tape for support. Stretch and strengthen muscles in the lower legs. Purchase good-quality footwear and run on soft surfaces.
Side stitch	Pain on the side of the abdomen	Stretch the arm on the affected side as high as possible; if that doesn't help, try bending forward while tightening the abdominal muscles.
Tendinitis	Pain, swelling, and tenderness of the affected area	R-I-C-E; apply heat when swelling has disappeared. Stretch and strengthen the affected area.

- Reduce the initial inflammation using the R-I-C-E principle (see text).

- After 36–48 hours, apply heat *if the swelling has disappeared completely*. Immerse the affected area in warm water or apply warm compresses, a hot water bottle, or a heating pad. As soon as you feel comfortable, begin moving the affected joints slowly. If you feel pain, or if the injured area begins to swell again, reduce the amount of movement. Continue gently stretching and moving the affected area until you have regained normal range of motion.

- Gradually begin exercising the injured area to build strength and endurance. Depending on the type of injury, weight training, walking, and resistance training can all be effective.

- Gradually reintroduce the stress of an activity until you can return to full intensity. Don't progress too rapidly or you'll re-injure yourself. Before returning to full exercise participation, you should have a full range of motion in your joints, normal strength and balance among your muscles, normal coordinated patterns of movement (with no injury compensation movements, such as limping), and little or no pain.

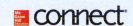

- Broken bones
- Internal disorders: chest pain, fainting, elevated body temperature, intolerance to hot weather

Also seek medical attention for ostensibly minor injuries that do not get better within a reasonable amount of time. You may need to modify your exercise program for a few weeks to allow an injury to heal.

Managing Minor Exercise Injuries For minor cuts and scrapes, stop the bleeding and clean the wound. Treat injuries to soft tissue (muscles and joints) with the R-I-C-E principle: rest, ice, compression, and elevation.

- *Rest:* Stop using the injured area as soon as you experience pain. Avoid any activity that causes pain.

- *Ice:* Apply ice to the injured area to reduce swelling and alleviate pain. Apply ice immediately for 10–20 minutes, and repeat every few hours as needed for pain. Let the injured part return to normal temperature between icings, and do not apply ice to one area for more than 20 minutes. An easy method for applying ice is to freeze water in a paper cup, peel some of the paper away, and rub the exposed ice on the injured area. If the injured area is large, you can surround it with several bags of crushed ice or ice cubes, or bags of frozen vegetables. Place a thin towel between the bag and your skin. If you use a cold gel pack, limit application time to 10 minutes. Some experts recommend regular icing for up to about 6 hours after an injury, while others suggest continuing as long as swelling persists.

- *Compression:* Wrap the injured area firmly with an elastic or compression bandage between icings. If the area starts throbbing or begins to change color, the bandage may be wrapped too tightly. Do not sleep with the wrap on.

- *Elevation:* Raise the injured area above heart level to decrease the blood supply and reduce swelling. When lying down use pillows, books, or a low chair or stool to raise the injured area.

The day after the injury, some experts recommend also taking an over-the-counter medication, such as aspirin, ibuprofen, or naproxen, to decrease inflammation. To rehabilitate your body, follow the steps listed in the box "Rehabilitation Following a Minor Athletic Injury."

Preventing Injuries The best method for dealing with exercise injuries is to prevent them. If you choose activities for your program carefully and follow the training guidelines described here and in Chapter 2, you should be able to avoid most types of injuries. Important guidelines for preventing athletic injuries include the following:

- Train regularly and stay in condition.
- Gradually increase the intensity, duration, or frequency of your workouts.
- Avoid or minimize high-impact activities such as running; alternate them with low-impact activities such as swimming or cycling.
- Get proper rest between exercise sessions.
- Drink plenty of fluids.
- Warm up thoroughly before you exercise and cool down afterward.
- Achieve and maintain a normal range of motion in your joints.
- Use proper body mechanics when lifting objects or executing sports skills.
- Don't exercise when you are ill or overtrained.
- Use proper equipment, particularly shoes, and choose an appropriate exercise surface. If you exercise on a grass field, soft track, or wooden floor, you are less likely to be injured than on concrete or a hard track. (For information on athletic shoes, see the box "Choosing Exercise Footwear.")
- Don't return to your normal exercise program until any athletic injuries have healed. Restart your program at a lower intensity and gradually increase the amount of overload.

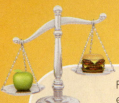

CRITICAL CONSUMER
Choosing Exercise Footwear

Footwear is perhaps the most important item of equipment for almost any activity. Shoes protect and support your feet and improve your traction. When you jump or run, you place as much as six times more force on your feet than when you stand still. Shoes can help cushion against the stress that this additional force places on your lower legs, thereby preventing injuries. Some athletic shoes are also designed to help prevent ankle rollover, another common source of injury.

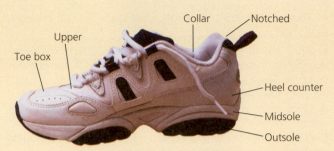

General Guidelines

When choosing athletic shoes, first consider the activity you've chosen for your exercise program. Shoes appropriate for different activities have very different characteristics.

Foot type is another important consideration. If your feet tend to roll inward excessively, you may need shoes with additional stability features on the inner side of the shoe to counteract this movement. If your feet tend to roll outward excessively, you may need highly flexible and cushioned shoes that promote foot motion. Most women will get a better fit if they choose shoes specifically designed for women's feet rather than downsized versions of men's shoes.

Successful Shopping

For successful shoe shopping, keep the following strategies in mind:

- Shop late in the day or, ideally, following a workout. Your foot size increases over the course of the day and after exercise.

- Wear socks like those you plan to wear during exercise.

- Try on both shoes and wear them for 10 or more minutes. Try walking on a noncarpeted surface. Approximate the movements of your activity: walk, jog, run, jump, and so on.

- Check the fit and style carefully:

  - Is the toe box roomy enough? Your toes will spread out when your foot hits the ground or when you push off. There should be at least one thumb's width of space from the longest toe to the end of the toe box.

  - Do the shoes have enough cushioning? Do your feet feel supported when you bounce up and down? Try bouncing on your toes and on your heels.

- Do your heels fit snugly into the shoe? Do they stay put when you walk, or do they slide up?

- Are the arches of your feet right on top of the shoes' arch supports?

- Do the shoes feel stable when you twist and turn on the balls of your feet? Try twisting from side to side while standing on one foot.

- Do you feel any pressure points?

- If you exercise at dawn or dusk, choose shoes with reflective sections for added visibility and safety.

- Replace athletic shoes about every three months or 300–500 miles of jogging or walking.

Barefoot Shoes or Minimalist Footwear

Two-thirds of runners experience an injury every year. Humans have evolved to run, so some scientists blame running shoes for the high injury rate. Most runners strike heel first when using heavily padded running shoes. Barefoot runners strike the ground with their forefoot (at least they're supposed to), which better uses the shock absorbing capacity of the skeleton. Some researchers speculate that using "minimalist" footwear allows people to run more naturally, which should cut down on the injury rate. Other research suggests that traditional running shoes provide a physiological advantage that makes running easier. We need more research to determine whether barefoot running is safe and viable or just the latest running fad.

TIPS FOR TODAY AND THE FUTURE

Regular, moderate exercise, even in short bouts spread through the day, can improve cardiorespiratory fitness.

RIGHT NOW YOU CAN
- Assess your cardiorespiratory fitness by using one of the methods discussed in this chapter and in Lab 3.1.
- Do a short bout of endurance exercise, such as 10–15 minutes of walking, jogging, or cycling.

- If you have physical activity planned for later in the day, drink some fluids now to make sure you are fully hydrated for your workout.
- Consider the exercise equipment, including shoes, you currently have on hand. If you need new equipment, start researching your options to get the best equipment you can afford.

IN THE FUTURE YOU CAN
- Graduate to a different, more challenging fitness assessment as your cardiorespiratory fitness improves.
- Vary the exercises in your cardiorespiratory endurance training to keep yourself challenged and motivated.

Touring the Cardiorespiratory System

The Cardiorespiratory System

The Heart and Lungs

Atherosclerosis: The Process of Cardiovascular Disease

Diabetes: A Disorder of Metabolism

GOALS OF THE TOUR

1. **The Cardiorespiratory System.** You will be able to identify the parts of the cardiorespiratory system and the pattern of blood flow through the body.

2. **The Heart and Lungs.** You will be able to identify the chambers of the heart and describe the flow of blood through the right side of the heart to the lungs (pulmonary circulation) and through the left side of the heart to the body (systemic circulation).

3. **Atherosclerosis.** You will be able to explain the process of cardiovascular disease and compare and contrast the outcomes affecting the heart and the brain.

4. **Diabetes.** You will be able to describe how the body uses digested food for energy and growth and how this process is disrupted when a person has diabetes.

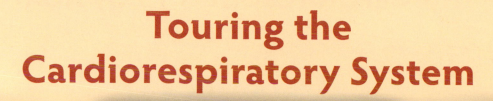

The Cardiorespiratory System

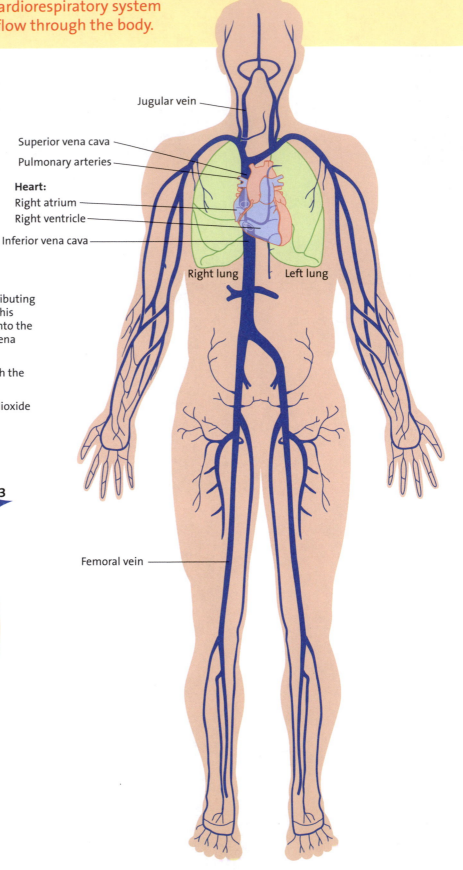

Jugular vein

Superior vena cava

Pulmonary arteries

Heart:

Right atrium

Right ventricle

Inferior vena cava

Right lung   Left lung

Femoral vein

Return of deoxygenated blood to the heart

1. Blood travels through the body, distributing oxygen and picking up carbon dioxide. This waste-laden, oxygen-poor blood flows into the right side of the heart via the superior vena cava and the inferior vena cava.

2. From there, blood is pumped through the pulmonary arteries into the lungs.

3. In the lungs, blood discards carbon dioxide and picks up oxygen.

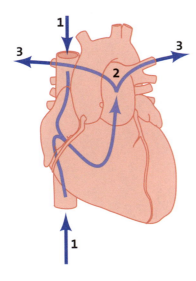

The Heart and Lungs

Identify the chambers of the heart and describe the flow of blood through the right side of the heart to the lungs (pulmonary circulation) and through the left side of the heart to the body (systemic circulation).

2

Blood is supplied to the heart muscle by the right and left coronary arteries, which branch off the aorta.

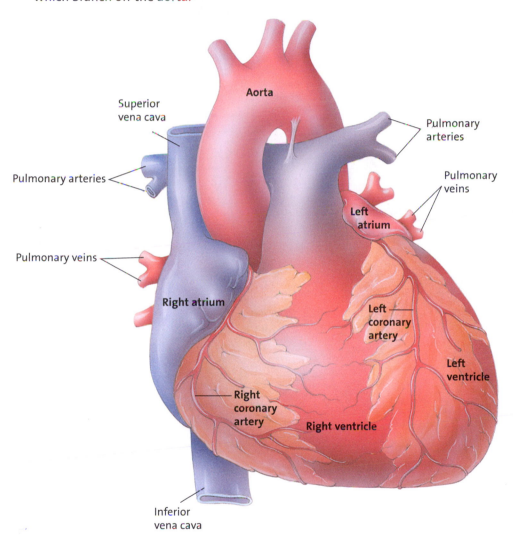

Superior vena cava

Aorta

Pulmonary arteries

Pulmonary arteries

Pulmonary veins

Left atrium

Pulmonary veins

Right atrium

Left coronary artery

Left ventricle

Right coronary artery

Right ventricle

Inferior vena cava

Atherosclerosis: The Process of Cardiovascular Disease

3 Explain the process of cardiovascular disease and compare and contrast the outcomes affecting the heart and the brain.

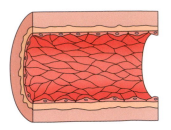

1. A healthy artery allows blood to flow through freely.

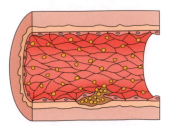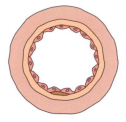

2. Plaque buildup begins when endothelial cells lining the arteries are damaged by smoking, high blood pressure, oxidized LDL cholesterol, and other causes. Excess cholesterol particles collect beneath these cells.

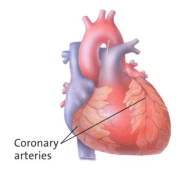

Coronary arteries

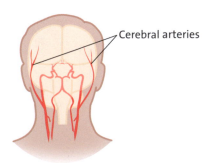

Cerebral arteries

Diabetes: A Disorder of Metabolism

Describe how the body uses digested food for energy and growth and how this process is disrupted when a person has diabetes.

Normal metabolism

1. When a meal is consumed, food is broken down into nutrients that the body can use to produce energy and build and nourish cells. Carbohydrates are broken down into glucose, which is the body's primary source of energy.

2. When glucose enters the bloodstream, the pancreas secretes the hormone insulin, which allows glucose to enter body cells.

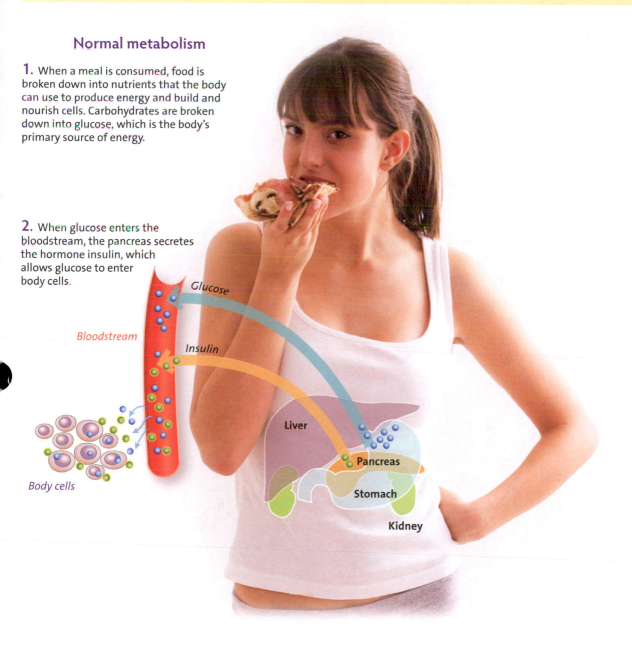

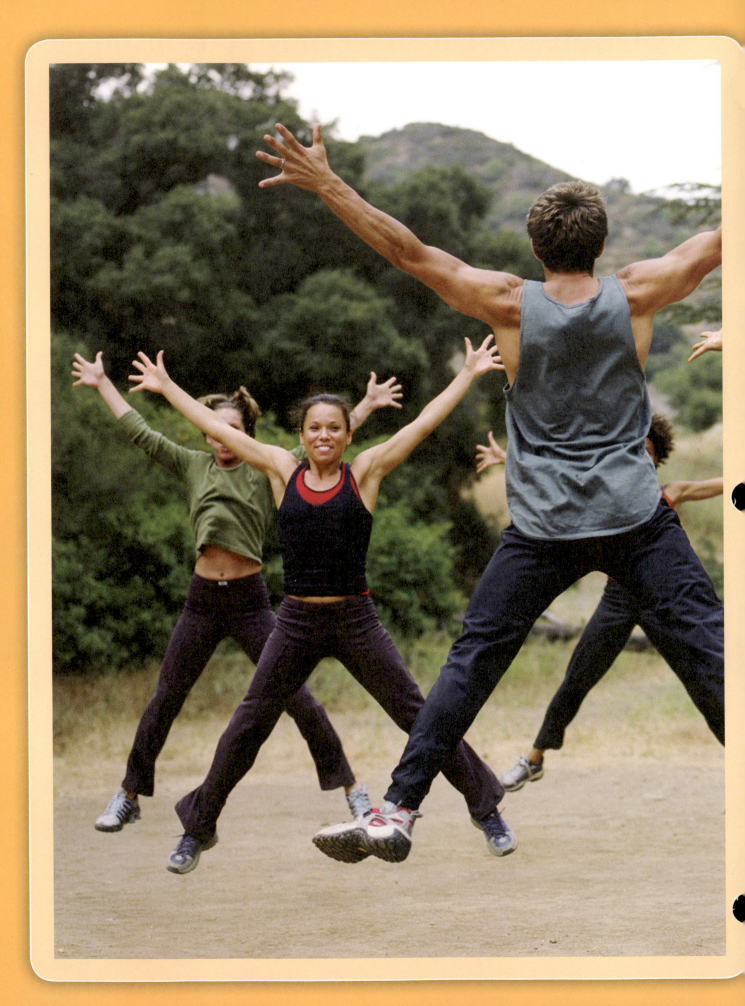

COMMON QUESTIONS ANSWERED

Q **Do I need a special diet for my endurance exercise program?**

A No. For most people, a nutritionally balanced diet contains all the energy and nutrients needed to sustain an exercise program. Don't waste your money on unnecessary supplements. (Chapter 8 provides detailed information about putting together a healthy diet.)

Q **How can I measure how far I walk or run?**

A The simplest way to measure distance is with a GPS-based phone app, which measures your distance, speed, and change in elevation. You can also use a pedometer, which counts your steps. Although stride length varies among individuals, 2000 steps typically equals about one mile, and 10,000 steps equals about five miles. To track your distance and your progress using a pedometer, follow the guidelines in Lab 2.3.

Q **How can I avoid being so sore when I start an exercise program?**

A Post-exercise muscle soreness is caused by muscle injury followed by muscle inflammation. Muscles get stronger and larger in response to muscle tension and injury. However, excessive injury can delay progress. The best approach is to begin conservatively with low-volume, low-intensity workouts, and gradually increase the severity of the exercise sessions. If you are currently sedentary, begin with 5 to 10 minutes of exercise and gradually increase the distance and speed you walk, run, cycle, or swim.

Q **Is it OK to do cardiorespiratory endurance exercise while menstruating?**

A Yes. There is no evidence that exercise during menstruation is unhealthy or that it has negative effects on performance. If you have headaches, backaches, and abdominal pain during menstruation, you may not feel like exercising. For some women, exercise helps relieve these symptoms. Listen to your body and exercise at whatever intensity is comfortable for you.

Q **Will high altitude affect my ability to exercise?**

A At high altitude (above 1500 meters, or about 4900 feet), there is less oxygen available in the air than at lower altitude. High altitude doesn't affect anaerobic exercise, such as stretching and weight lifting, but it does affect aerobic activities—that is, any type of cardiovascular endurance exercise—because the heart and lungs have to work harder, even when the body is at rest, to deliver enough oxygen to body cells. The increased cardiovascular strain of exercise at high altitude reduces endurance. To play it safe when at high altitude, avoid heavy exercise—at least for the first few days—and drink plenty of water. And don't expect to reach your normal lower-altitude exercise capacity.

SUMMARY

- The cardiorespiratory system consists of the heart, blood vessels, and respiratory system; it picks up and transports oxygen, nutrients, and waste products.

- The body takes chemical energy from food and uses it to produce ATP and fuel cellular activities. ATP is stored in the body's cells as the basic form of energy.

- During exercise, the body supplies ATP and fuels cellular activities by combining three energy systems: immediate, for short periods of activity; nonoxidative (anaerobic), for intense activity; and oxidative (aerobic), for prolonged activity. Which energy system predominates depends on the duration and intensity of the activity.

- Cardiorespiratory endurance exercise improves cardiorespiratory functioning and cellular metabolism; it reduces the risk of chronic diseases such as heart disease, cancer, type 2 diabetes, obesity, and osteoporosis; and it improves immune function and psychological and emotional well-being.

- Cardiorespiratory fitness is measured by determining how well the cardiorespiratory system transports and uses oxygen. The upper limit of this measure, called maximal oxygen consumption, or VO_{2max} can be measured precisely in a laboratory, or it can be estimated reasonably well through self-assessment tests.

- To create a successful exercise program, set realistic goals, choose suitable activities, begin slowly, and always warm up and cool down. As fitness improves, exercise more often, longer, and/or harder.

- Intensity of training can be measured through target heart rate zone, METs, ratings of perceived exertion, or the talk test.

- With careful attention to fluid intake, clothing, duration of exercise, and exercise intensity, endurance training can be safe in hot and cold weather conditions.

- Serious injuries require medical attention. Application of the R-I-C-E principle (rest, ice, compression, elevation) is appropriate for treating many types of muscle or joint injuries.

FOR FURTHER EXPLORATION

American Academy of Orthopaedic Surgeons: Sports and Exercise. Provides fact sheets on many fitness and sports topics, including how to begin a program, how to choose equipment, and how to prevent and treat many types of injuries.

http://orthoinfo.aaos.org/menus/sports.cfm

American Cancer Society: Eat Healthy and Get Active. Provides tools for managing an exercise program and discusses the links between cancer and lifestyle, including the importance of physical activity in preventing some cancers.

http://www.cancer.org/healthy/eathealthygetactive/

American Heart Association: Exercise and Fitness. Provides information on cardiovascular health and disease, including the role of exercise in maintaining heart health and exercise tips for people of all ages.

http://www.heart.org/HEARTORG/GettingHealthy/PhysicalActivity/
Physical-Activity_UCM_001080_SubHomePage.jsp

Centers for Disease Control and Prevention: Physical Activity for Everyone. Explains the latest government recommendations on exercise and physical activity and provides strategies for getting the appropriate type and amount of exercise.

http://www.cdc.gov/physicalactivity/

CrossFit Journal. A fitness, health, and lifestyle publication dedicated to the improvement of athletic performance, with new articles published daily and an archive of articles, videos, and audio files covering exercise technique, nutrition, injuries and rehab, equipment, coaching, and more.

http://journal.crossfit.com/

President's Challenge Adult Fitness Test: Aerobics. Provides step-by-step instructions for taking and interpreting standard tests of aerobic fitness.

http://www.adultfitnesstest.org

Runner's World Online. Contains a wide variety of information about running, including tips for beginning runners, advice about training, and a shoe buyer's guide.

http://www.runnersworld.com

Weight-control Information Network: Walking. An online fact sheet that explains the benefits of walking for exercise, tips for starting a walking program, and techniques for getting the most from walking workouts.

http://win.niddk.nih.gov

Women's Sports Foundation. Provides information and links about training and about many specific sports activities.

http://www.womenssportsfoundation.org

SELECTED BIBLIOGRAPHY

American College of Sports Medicine. 2009. *ACSM's Resource Manual for Guidelines for Exercise Testing and Prescription,* 6th ed. Philadelphia: Lippincott Williams and Wilkins.

American College of Sports Medicine. 2012. *ACSM's Health/Fitness Facility Standards and Guidelines,* 4th ed. Champaign, Ill: Human Kinetics.

American College of Sports Medicine. 2013. *ACSM's Guidelines for Exercise Testing and Prescription,* 9th ed. Philadelphia: Wolters Kluwer/Lippincott Williams & Wilkins Health.

Andrews, J. R., and D. Yaeger. 2013. *Any Given Monday: Sports Injuries and How to Prevent Them for Athletes, Parents, and Coaches—Based on My Life in Sports Medicine.* New York: Scribner.

Arem, H., et al. 2015. Leisure time physical activity and mortality: A detailed pooled analysis of the dose-response relationship. *Journal American Medical Association Internal Medicine.* Published online April 6, 2015.

Bacon, A. P., et al. 2013. $\dot{V}O_{2max}$ trainability and high intensity interval training in humans: a meta-analysis. *PLoS One* 8(9): e73182.

Bouchard, C., et al. 2012. Adverse metabolic response to regular exercise: is it a rare or common occurrence? *PLoS One* 7(5): e37887.

Brooks, G. A., et al. 2005. *Exercise Physiology: Human Bioenergetics and Its Applications,* 4th ed. New York: McGraw-Hill.

Centers for Disease Control and Prevention. 2010. *Promoting Physical Activity: A Guide for Community Action,* 2nd ed. Champaign, Ill.: Human Kinetics.

Curlik, D. M., and T. J. Shors. 2013. Training your brain: Do mental and physical (MAP) training enhance cognition through the process of neurogenesis in the hippocampus? *Neuropharmacology* 64 (1): 506–514.

Denadai, B. S., et al. 2006. Interval training at 95% and 100% of the velocity at $\dot{V}O_{2max}$: Effects on aerobic physiological indexes and running performance. *Applied Physiology, Nutrition, and Metabolism* 31(6): 737–743.

Denis, G. V. and M. S. Obin. 2013. Metabolically healthy obesity: origins and implications. *Molecular Aspects of Medicine* 34(1): 59–70.

Doral, M. N., and J. Karlsson. 2015. *Sports Injuries: Prevention, Diagnosis, Treatment and Rehabilitation.* New York: Springer.

Edwards, S. 2012. *Zoning: Fitness in a Blink.* Sacramento, Calif.: Zoning.

Falcone, P. H., et al. 2015. Caloric expenditure of aerobic, resistance, or combined high-intensity interval training using a hydraulic resistance system in healthy men. *Journal of Strength Conditioning Research* 29(3): 779–785.

Franz, J. R., C. M. Wierzbinski, and R. Kram. 2012. Metabolic cost of running barefoot versus shod: is lighter better? *Medicine and Science in Sports and Exercise* 44(8): 1519–1525.

Garber, C. E., et al. 2011. Quantity and quality of exercise for developing and maintaining cardiorespiratory, musculoskeletal, and neuromotor fitness in apparently healthy adults: Guidance for prescribing exercise. *Medicine and Science in Sport and Exercise* 43(7):1334–1359.

Gebel, K., et al. 2015. Effect of moderate to vigorous physical activity on all-cause mortality in middle-aged and older Australians. *Journal American Medical Association Internal Medicine.* Published online April 6, 2015.

Gonzales, M. M., et al. 2013. Aerobic fitness and the brain: increased N-acetyl-aspartate and choline concentrations in endurance-trained middle-aged adults. *Brain Topography* 26(1): 126–134.

Griffin, J. 2015. *Nutrition for Cyclists.* Ramsbury, UK: Crowood Press.

Hanssen, H., et al. 2015. Acute effects of interval versus continuous endurance training on pulse wave reflection in healthy young men. *Atherosclerosis* 238(2): 399–406.

Hardee, J. P., et al. 2014. The effect of resistance exercise on all-cause mortality in cancer survivors. *Mayo Clinic Proceedings* 89(8): 1108–1115.

Hawkins, J. D., and S. Hawkins. 2013. *Walking for Fun and Fitness.* Independence, Ky: Cengage Learning.

Howley, E., and D. Thompson. 2012. *Fitness Professional's Handbook.* 6th ed. Champaign, Ill.: Human Kinetics.

Larsen, S., et al. 2015. The effect of high-intensity training on mitochondrial fat oxidation in skeletal muscle and subcutaneous adipose tissue. *Scandinavian Journal of Medicine and Science in Sports* 25(1): e59–69.

Lucas, S. J., et al. 2015. High-intensity interval exercise and cerebrovascular health: curiosity, cause, and consequence. *Journal of Cerebral Blood Flow and Metabolism.* Published online April 1, 2015.

MacIntosh, B. J., et al. 2014. Impact of a single bout of aerobic exercise on regional brain perfusion and activation responses in healthy young adults. *PLoS One* 9(1): e85163.

McDougall, C. 2012. *Born to Run: A Hidden Tribe, Superathletes, and the Greatest Race the World Has Never Seen.* New York: Knopf.

Meeusen, R. 2014. Exercise, nutrition and the brain. *Sports Medicine* 44 Suppl 1: S47–56.

Metzl, J., and C. Kowalchik. 2015. *Dr. Jordan Metzl's Running Strong: The Sports Doctor's Complete Guide to Staying Healthy and Injury-Free for Life.* New York: Rodale.

Mozaffarian, D., et al. 2015. *Heart Disease and Stroke Statistics—2015 Update.* Circulation 131 (4): e29–e322.

Muller, J., et al. 2015. Acute effects of submaximal endurance training on arterial stiffness in healthy middle- and long-distance runners. *Journal of Clinical Hypertension* 17(5): 371–374.

Nagamatsu, L. S., et al. 2014. Exercise is medicine, for the body and the brain. *British Journal of Sports Medicine* 48(12): 943–944.

Nieman, D. C. 2010. *Exercise Testing and Prescription: A Health-Related Approach,* 7th ed. New York: McGraw-Hill.

Physical Activity Guidelines Advisory Committee. 2008. *Physical Activity Guidelines Advisory Committee Report, 2008.* Washington, D.C.: U.S. Department of Health and Human Services.

Puterman, E., et al. 2015. Determinants of telomere attrition over 1 year in healthy older women: stress and health behaviors matter. *Molecular Psychiatry* 20(4): 529–535.

Ramos, J. S., et al. 2015. The impact of high-intensity interval training versus moderate-intensity continuous training on vascular function: a systematic review and meta-analysis. *Sports Medicine* 45(5): 679–692.

Ruiz, J. R., et al. 2011. Strenuous endurance exercise improves life expectancy: It's in our genes. *British Journal of Sports Medicine* 45(3): 159–161.

Schnohr, P., et al. 2015. Dose of jogging and long-term mortality: The Copenhagen City Heart Study. *Journal of the American College of Cardiology* 65(5): 411–419.

Schnohr, P., J. L. Marott, P. Lange, and G. B. Jensen. 2013. Longevity in male and female joggers: The Copenhagen City heart study. *American Journal of Epidemiology,* 177(7): 683–689.

Snigdha, S., et al. 2014. Exercise enhances memory consolidation in the aging brain. *Frontiers of Aging Neuroscience* 6: 3.

Tyndall, A. V., et al. 2013. The brain-in-motion study: effect of a 6-month aerobic exercise intervention on cerebrovascular regulation and cognitive function in older adults. *BMC Geriatrics* 13(1): 21.

U.S. Department of Health and Human Services. 2008. *Physical Activity Guidelines for Americans.* Washington, D.C.: U.S. Department of Health and Human Services.

Vardar Yagli, N., et al. 2015. Do yoga and aerobic exercise training have impact on functional capacity, fatigue, peripheral muscle strength, and quality of life in breast cancer survivors? *Integrative Cancer Therapies* 14(2): 125–132.

Vincent, G., et al. 2015. Changes in mitochondrial function and mitochondria associated protein expression in response to 2 weeks of high intensity interval training. *Frontiers in Physiology* 6: 51.

Voss, M. W., et al. 2013. Neurobiological markers of exercise-related brain plasticity in older adults. *Brain Behavior Immunity* 28 (supplement): 90–99.

Weston, M., et al. 2014. Effects of low-volume high-intensity interval training (HIIT) on fitness in adults: a meta-analysis of controlled and non-controlled trials. *Sports Medicine* 44(7): 1005–1017.

Yeo, W. K., et al. 2011. Fat adaptation in well-trained athletes: effects on cell metabolism. *Applied Physiology Nutrition Metabolism* 36(1): 12–22.

Zwetsloot, K. A., et al. 2014. High-intensity interval training induces a modest systemic inflammatory response in active, young men. *Journal of Inflammation Research* 7: 9–17.

Name _____ Section _____ Date _____

LAB 3.1   Assessing Your Current Level of Cardiorespiratory Endurance

The conditions for exercise safety given in Chapter 2 apply to all fitness assessment tests. Talk to a physician if needed, and if you experience any unusual symptoms while taking a test, stop exercising and discuss your condition with your instructor. Additional cautions and prerequisites for the five test options presented in this lab are described below.

1-Mile Walk Test	Recommended for anyone who meets the criteria for safe exercise. This test can be used by people who cannot perform other tests because of low fitness level or injury.
3-Minute Step Test	If you suffer from joint problems in your ankles, knees, or hips or are significantly overweight, check with your physician before taking this test. People with balance problems or for whom a fall would be particularly dangerous, including older adults and pregnant women, should use special caution or avoid this test.
1.5-Mile Run-Walk Test	Recommended for people who are healthy and at least moderately active. If you have been sedentary, you should participate in a 4- to 8-week walk-run program before taking the test. Don't take this test in extremely hot or cold weather or if you aren't used to exercising under those conditions.
Beep Test	Recommended for fit individuals; the test is highly strenuous and requires the ability to jog, run, and sprint. Don't take this test unless you can complete at least 10 sets of 50-meter sprints.
12-Minute Swim Test	Recommended for relatively strong swimmers who are confident in the water; if needed, ask a qualified swimming instructor to evaluate your swimming ability before attempting this test.

Choose one of the tests based on your fitness level and available facilities. For best results, don't exercise strenuously or consume caffeine the day of the test, and don't smoke or eat a heavy meal within about three hours of the test.

The 1-Mile Walk Test

Equipment

1. A track or course that provides a measurement of 1 mile
2. A stopwatch, clock, or watch with a second hand
3. A weight scale

Preparation

Measure your body weight (in pounds) before taking the test.
Body weight: _____ lbs

Instructions

1. Warm up before taking the test. Do some walking, easy jogging, or calisthenics.
2. Cover the 1-mile course as quickly as possible. Walk at a pace that is brisk but comfortable. You must raise your heart rate above 120 beats per minute (bpm).
3. As soon as you complete the distance, note your time and take your pulse for 15 seconds.
   Walking time: _____ min _____ sec
   15-second pulse count: _____ beats
4. Cool down after the test by walking slowly for several minutes.

Determining Maximal Oxygen Consumption

1. Convert your 15-second pulse count into a value for exercise heart rate by multiplying it by 4.
   Exercise heart rate: _____ × 4 = _____ bpm
2. Convert your walking time from minutes and seconds to a decimal figure. For example, a time of 14 minutes and 45 seconds would be 14 + (45/60), or 14.75 minutes.
   Walking time: _____ min + (_____ sec ÷ 60 sec/min) = _____ min
3. Insert values for your age, gender, weight, walking time, and exercise heart rate in the following equation, where
   W = your weight (in pounds)
   A = your age (in years)

G = your gender (male = 1; female = 0)

T = your time to complete the 1-mile course (in minutes)

H = your exercise heart rate (in beats per minute)

$\dot{V}O_{2max}$ = 132.853 − (0.0769 × W) − (0.3877 × A) + (6.315 × G) − (3.2649 × T) − (0.1565 × H) = _____ ml/kg/min (maximum oxygen consumption measured in milliliters of oxygen used per minute per kilogram of body weight)

For example, a 20-year-old, 190-pound male with a time of 14.75 minutes and an exercise heart rate of 152 bpm would calculate maximal oxygen consumption as follows:

$\dot{V}O_{2max}$ = 132.853 − (0.0769 × 190) − (0.3877 × 20) + (6.315 × 1) − (3.2649 × 14.75) − (0.1565 × 152) = 45 ml/kg/min

$\dot{V}O_{2max}$ = **132.853 − (0.0769 ×** _____ **) − (0.3877 ×** _____ **) + (6.315 ×** _____ **)**
  weight (lb)   age (years)   gender

− (3.2649 × _____ **) − (0.1565 ×** _____ **) =** _____ **ml/kg/min**
  walking time (min)   exercise heart rate (bpm)

4. Copy this value for $\dot{V}O_{2max}$ into the appropriate place in the chart on page 90.

The 3-Minute Step Test

Equipment

1. A step, bench, or bleacher step that is 16.25 inches from ground level

2. A stopwatch, clock, or watch with a second hand

3. A metronome

Preparation

Practice stepping up onto and down from the step before you begin the test. Each step has four beats: up-up-down-down. Males should perform the test with the metronome set for a rate of 96 beats per minute, or 24 steps per minute. Females should set the metronome at 88 beats per minute, or 22 steps per minute.

Instructions

1. Warm up before taking the test. Do some walking or easy jogging.

2. Set the metronome at the proper rate. Your instructor or a partner can call out starting and stopping times; otherwise, have a clock or watch within easy viewing during the test.

3. Begin the test and continue to step at the correct pace for three minutes.

4. Stop after three minutes. Remain standing and count your pulse for the 15-second period from 5 to 20 seconds into recovery.
   15-second pulse count: _____ beats

5. Cool down after the test by walking slowly for several minutes.

Determining Maximal Oxygen Consumption

1. Convert your 15-second pulse count to a value for recovery heart rate by multiplying by 4.
   Recovery heart rate: _____ × 4 = _____ **bpm**
                 15-sec pulse count

2. Insert your recovery heart rate in the equation below, where

   H = recovery heart rate (in beats per minute)

   Males: $\dot{V}O_{2max}$ = 111.33 − (0.42 × H)

   Females: $\dot{V}O_{2max}$ = 65.81 − (0.18470 × H)

   For example, a man with a recovery heart rate of 162 bpm would calculate maximal oxygen consumption as follows:

   $\dot{V}O_{2max}$ = 111.33 − (0.42 × 162) = 43 ml/kg/min

   Males: $\dot{V}O_{2max}$ = 111.33 − (0.42 × _____ **) =** _____ **ml/kg/min**
                      recovery heart rate (bpm)

   Females: $\dot{V}O_{2max}$ = 65.81 − (0.1847 × _____ **) =** _____ **ml/kg/min**
                      recovery heart rate (bpm)

3. Copy this value for $\dot{V}O_{2max}$ into the appropriate place in the chart on page 90.

The 1.5-Mile Run-Walk Test

Equipment

1. A running track or course that is flat and provides exact measurements of up to 1.5 miles

2. A stopwatch, clock, or watch with a second hand

Preparation

You may want to practice pacing yourself prior to taking the test to avoid going too fast at the start and becoming prematurely fatigued. Allow yourself a day or two to recover from your practice run before taking the test.

Instructions

1. Warm up before taking the test. Do some walking or easy jogging.

2. Try to cover the distance as fast as possible without overexerting yourself. If possible, monitor your own time, or have someone call out your time at various intervals of the test to determine whether your pace is correct.

3. Record the amount of time, in minutes and seconds, it takes you to complete the 1.5-mile distance.
   Running-walking time: _____ min _____ sec

4. Cool down after the test by walking or jogging slowly for about five minutes.

Determining Maximal Oxygen Consumption

1. Convert your running time from minutes and seconds to a decimal figure. For example, a time of 14 minutes and 25 seconds would be 14 + (25/60), or 14.4 minutes.
   Running-walking time: _____ min + (_____ sec ÷ 60 sec/min) = _____ min

2. Insert your running time into the equation below, where

   T = running time (in minutes)

   $\dot{V}O_{2max} = (483 \div T) + 3.5$

   For example, a person who completes 1.5 miles in 14.4 minutes would calculate maximal oxygen consumption as follows:

   $\dot{V}O_{2max} = (483 \div 14.4) + 3.5 = 37 \ ml/kg/min$

   $\dot{V}O_{2max} = (483 \div \underline{\hspace{3cm}}) + 3.5 = \underline{\hspace{3cm}} \textbf{ ml/kg/min}$

   run-walk time (min)

3. Copy this value for $\dot{V}O_{2max}$ into the appropriate place in the chart on page 90.

The Beep Test

This is also called the Multi-Stage Fitness Test, Pacer Test, Yo Yo test, or 20-Meter Shuttle Run Test.

Description

The Beep Test involves running a series of 20-meter shuttles at a specified pace. The pace gets faster each minute as you go to another level. For example, the series begins at a speed of 8.5 kilometers per hour and then increases by 0.5 kilometers per hour with each advancing level. The MP3 audio recording or phone app signals the end of a shuttle with a single beep and the start of the next level with three beeps. The object of the test is to keep up with the beeps as long as possible.

Facilities and Equipment

1. Running track, open field, or gymnasium

2. Two cones or field markers set 20 meters (21 yards, 32 inches) apart (use four cones if testing a large group)

3. Beep Test app or MP3 recording of beeps (widely available free on the Internet—e.g., http://www.beeptestacademy.com; free Beep Test apps are also available for the iPhone and Android smart phones)

4. Method of playing Beep Test: MP3 player with speaker, smart phone with speaker, iPad with speaker. You could run this test by yourself if you have an MP3 player with earphones.

Preparation

Don't take this test until you are prepared. A good technique is to run intervals on a track or playing field. For example, run 50 meters, rest 30 seconds, repeat. Gradually, increase the speed and number of repetitions until you can complete at least 10 sets of 50-meter sprints.

Instructions

The Beep Test is a popular assessment of cardiovascular endurance levels and maximal oxygen consumption.

1. Set up the audio alert system for the test (MP3 player with speaker, or personal MP3 player, or smart phone with headphones).

2. Run back and forth between two cones or field markers placed 20 meters apart, keeping pace with an audio beep that plays during the test. The test is arranged in levels. The beeps get faster with each increasing stage. A single beep will sound at the end of the time for each shuttle. A triple beep sounds at the end of each level. The triple beep is a signal that the pace will get faster. Do not stop when you hear the triple beat; continue running toward the other field marker or cone.

LABORATORY ACTIVITIES

3. The test ends when you can't keep pace with the beeps for two consecutive shuttles.
4. Note your level and the total number of shuttles you completed. Record your maximal oxygen consumption and enter it on the chart labeled "Rating Your Cardiovascular Fitness."

Videos of the test are widely available on the Internet.

Level	Speed (miles per hour)	Minutes per mile	Total Shuttles	Predicted $\dot{V}O_{2max}$ (milliliters oxygen per kilogram body weight)
1	5.3	11.4	2	16.6
1	5.3	11.4	4	17.5
1	5.3	11.4	6	18.5
2	5.6	10.7	8	20.0
2	5.6	10.7	10	20.9
2	5.6	10.7	12	21.8
2	5.6	10.7	14	22.6
3	5.9	10.2	16	23.4
3	5.9	10.2	18	24.3
3	5.9	10.2	20	25.1
3	5.9	10.2	22	26.0
4	6.2	9.7	24	26.8
4	6.2	9.7	26	27.6
4	6.2	9.7	28	28.3
4	6.2	9.7	31	29.5
5	6.5	9.2	33	30.2
5	6.5	9.2	35	31.0
5	6.5	9.2	37	31.8
5	6.5	9.2	40	32.9
6	6.8	8.8	42	33.6
6	6.8	8.8	44	34.3
6	6.8	8.8	46	35.0
6	6.8	8.8	48	35.7
6	6.8	8.8	50	36.4
7	7.2	8.4	52	37.1
7	7.2	8.4	54	37.8
7	7.2	8.4	56	38.5
7	7.2	8.4	58	39.2
7	7.2	8.4	60	39.9
8	7.5	8.0	62	40.5
8	7.5	8.0	64	41.1
8	7.5	8.0	66	41.8
8	7.5	8.0	68	42.4
8	7.5	8.0	71	43.3
9	7.8	7.7	73	43.9
9	7.8	7.7	75	44.5
9	7.8	7.7	76	45.2
9	7.8	7.7	78	45.8
9	7.8	7.7	81	46.8
10	8.1	7.4	83	47.4
10	8.1	7.4	85	48.0
10	8.1	7.4	87	48.7
10	8.1	7.4	89	49.3
10	8.1	7.4	92	50.2

Level	Speed (miles per hour)	Minutes per mile	Total Shuttles	Predicted $\dot{V}O_{2max}$ (milliliters oxygen per kilogram body weight)
11	8.4	7.2	94	50.8
11	8.4	7.2	96	51.4
11	8.4	7.2	98	51.9
11	8.4	7.2	100	52.5
11	8.4	7.2	102	53.1
11	8.4	7.2	104	53.7
12	8.7	6.9	106	54.3
12	8.7	6.9	108	54.8
12	8.7	6.9	110	55.4
12	8.7	6.9	112	56.0
12	8.7	6.9	114	56.5
12	8.7	6.9	116	57.1
13	9.0	6.7	118	57.6
13	9.0	6.7	120	58.2
13	9.0	6.7	122	58.7
13	9.0	6.7	124	59.3
13	9.0	6.7	126	59.8
13	9.0	6.7	129	60.6
14	9.3	6.4	131	61.1
14	9.3	6.4	133	61.7
14	9.3	6.4	135	62.2
14	9.3	6.4	137	62.7
14	9.3	6.4	139	63.2
14	9.3	6.4	142	64.0
15	9.6	6.2	144	64.6
15	9.6	6.2	146	65.1
15	9.6	6.2	148	65.6
15	9.6	6.2	150	66.2
15	9.6	6.2	152	66.7
15	9.6	6.2	154	67.5
16	9.9	6.0	156	68.0
16	9.9	6.0	158	68.5
16	9.9	6.0	160	69.0
16	9.9	6.0	162	69.5
16	9.9	6.0	164	69.9
16	9.9	6.0	166	70.5
16	9.9	6.0	168	70.9
17	10.3	5.9	170	71.4
17	10.3	5.9	172	71.9
17	10.3	5.9	174	72.4
17	10.3	5.9	176	72.9
17	10.3	5.9	178	73.4
17	10.3	5.9	180	73.9
17	10.3	5.9	182	74.4
18	10.6	5.7	184	74.8
18	10.6	5.7	186	75.3
18	10.6	5.7	188	75.8
18	10.6	5.7	190	76.2
18	10.6	5.7	192	76.7
18	10.6	5.7	194	77.2
18	10.6	5.7	197	77.9

Level	Speed (miles per hour)	Minutes per mile	Total Shuttles	Predicted $\dot{V}O_{2max}$ (milliliters oxygen per kilogram body weight)
19	10.9	5.5	199	78.3
19	10.9	5.5	201	78.8
19	10.9	5.5	203	79.2
19	10.9	5.5	205	79.7
19	10.9	5.5	207	80.2
19	10.9	5.5	209	80.6
19	10.9	5.5	212	81.3
20	11.2	5.4	214	81.8
20	11.2	5.4	216	82.2
20	11.2	5.4	218	82.6
20	11.2	5.4	220	83.0
20	11.2	5.4	222	83.5
20	11.2	5.4	224	83.9
20	11.2	5.4	226	84.8

Record your score. Copy this value for $\dot{V}O_{2max}$ into the appropriate place in the chart below:

Highest level: _____

Total shuttles run: _____

Predicted $\dot{V}O_{2max}$: _____

SOURCE: Adapted from Ramsbottom, R., J. Brewer, and C. Williams. 1988. A progressive shuttle run test to estimate maximal oxygen uptake. *British Journal of Sports Medicine* 22(4): 141–144.

Rating Your Cardiovascular Fitness

Record your $\dot{V}O_{2max}$ score(s) and the corresponding fitness rating from the table below.

Women	Very Poor	Poor	Fair	Good	Excellent	Superior
Age: 18–29	Below 31.6	31.6–35.4	35.5–39.4	39.5–43.9	44.0–50.1	Above 50.1
30–39	Below 29.9	29.9–33.7	33.8–36.7	36.8–40.9	41.0–46.8	Above 46.8
40–49	Below 28.0	28.0–31.5	31.6–35.0	35.1–38.8	38.9–45.1	Above 45.1
50–59	Below 25.5	25.5–28.6	28.7–31.3	31.4–35.1	35.2–39.8	Above 39.8
60–69	Below 23.7	23.7–26.5	26.6–29.0	29.1–32.2	32.3–36.8	Above 36.8
Men						
Age: 18–29	Below 38.1	38.1–42.1	42.2–45.6	45.7–51.0	51.1–56.1	Above 56.1
30–39	Below 36.7	36.7–40.9	41.0–44.3	44.4–48.8	48.9–54.2	Above 54.2
40–49	Below 34.6	34.6–38.3	38.4–42.3	42.4–46.7	46.8–52.8	Above 52.8
50–59	Below 31.1	31.1–35.1	35.2–38.2	38.3–43.2	43.3–49.6	Above 49.6
60–69	Below 27.4	27.4–31.3	31.4–34.9	35.0–39.4	39.5–46.0	Above 46.0

SOURCE: Ratings based on norms from The Cooper Institute of Aerobic Research, Dallas, Tex.; from *The Physical Fitness Specialist Manual,* Revised 2002. Used with permission.

	$\dot{V}O_{2max}$	Cardiovascular Fitness Rating
1-Mile Walk Test		
3-Minute Step Test		
1.5-M Run-Walk Test		
Beep Test		

The 12-Minute Swim Test

If you enjoy swimming and prefer to build a cardiorespiratory training program around this type of exercise, you can assess your cardiorespiratory endurance by taking the 12-Minute Swim Test. You will receive a rating based on the distance you can swim in 12 minutes. A complete fitness program based on swimming is presented in Chapter 7.

Note, however, that this test is appropriate only for relatively strong swimmers who are confident in the water. If you are unsure about your swimming ability, this test may not be appropriate for you. If necessary, ask your school's swim coach or a qualified swimming instructor to evaluate your ability in the water before attempting this test.

Equipment

1. A swimming pool that provides measurements in yards
2. A wall clock that is clearly visible from the pool, or someone with a watch who can time you

Preparation

You may want to practice pacing yourself before taking the test to avoid going too fast at the start and becoming prematurely fatigued. Allow yourself a day or two to recover from your practice swim before taking the test.

Instructions

1. Warm up before taking the test. Do some walking or light jogging before getting in the pool. Once in the water, swim a lap or two at an easy pace to make sure your muscles are warm and you are comfortable.
2. Try to cover the distance as fast as possible without overexerting yourself. If possible, monitor your own time, or have someone call out your time at various intervals of the test to determine whether your pace is correct.
3. Record the distance, in yards, that you were able to cover during the 12-minute period.
4. Cool down after the test by swimming a lap or two at an easy pace.
5. Use the following chart to gauge your level of cardiorespiratory fitness.

DISTANCE IN YARDS

Women	Needs Work	Better	Fair	Good	Excellent
Age: 13–19	Below 500	500–599	600–699	700–799	Above 800
20–29	Below 400	400–499	500–599	600–699	Above 700
30–39	Below 350	350–449	450–549	550–649	Above 650
40–49	Below 300	300–399	400–499	500–599	Above 600
50–59	Below 250	250–349	350–449	450–549	Above 550
60 and over	Below 250	250–299	300–399	400–499	Above 500
Men					
Age: 13–19	Below 400	400–499	500–599	600–699	Above 700
20–29	Below 300	300–399	400–499	500–599	Above 600
30–39	Below 250	250–349	350–449	450–549	Above 550
40–49	Below 200	200–299	300–399	400–499	Above 500
50–59	Below 150	150–249	250–349	350–449	Above 450
60 and over	Below 150	150–199	200–299	300–399	Above 400

100 yards = 91 meters

SOURCE: Cooper, K. H. 1982. *The Aerobics Program for Total Well-Being.* New York: Bantam Books.

Record your fitness rating:

	Cardiovascular Fitness Rating
12-Minute Swim Test	

LABORATORY ACTIVITIES

Using Your Results

How did you score? Does your rating for cardiovascular fitness surprise you? Are you satisfied with your current rating?

If you're not satisfied, set a realistic goal for improvement: _____

_____

Are you satisfied with your current level of cardiovascular fitness as evidenced in your daily life—your ability to walk, run, bicycle, climb stairs, do yard work, or engage in recreational activities?

If you're not satisfied, set some realistic goals for improvement, such as completing a 5K run or 25-mile bike ride: _____

_____

What should you do next? Enter the results of this lab in the Preprogram Assessment column in Appendix C. If you've set goals for improvement, begin planning your cardiorespiratory endurance exercise program by completing the plan in Lab 3.2. After several weeks of your program, complete this lab again, and enter the results in the Postprogram Assessment column of Appendix C. How do the results compare? (Remember, it's best to compare $\dot{V}O_{2max}$ scores for the same test.)

SOURCES: Brooks, G. A., and T. D. Fahey. 1987. *Fundamentals of Human Performance.* New York: Macmillan; Kline, G. M., et al. 1987. Estimation of $\dot{V}O_{2max}$ from a one-mile track walk, gender, age, and body weight. *Medicine and Science in Sports and Exercise* 19(3): 253–259; McArdle, W. D., F. I. Katch, and V. L. Katch. 2010. *Exercise Physiology: Nutrition, Energy, and Human Performance.* Philadelphia: Lea and Febiger, 243–246.

Name _____ Section _____ Date _____

LAB 3.2 Developing an Exercise Program for Cardiorespiratory Endurance

1. *Goals.* List goals for your cardiorespiratory endurance exercise program. Your goals can be specific or general, short or long term. In the first section, include specific, measurable goals that you can use to track the progress of your fitness program. These goals might be things like raising your cardiorespiratory fitness rating from fair to good or swimming laps for 30 minutes without resting. In the second section, include long-term and more qualitative goals, such as improving self-confidence and reducing your risk for chronic disease.

   Specific Goals: Current Status   Final Goals

   _____   _____

   _____   _____

   _____   _____

   Other goals: _____

   _____

2. *Type of Activities.* Choose one or more endurance activities for your program. These can include any activity that uses large-muscle groups, can be maintained continuously, and is rhythmic and aerobic in nature. Examples include walking, jogging, cycling, ebike cycling, group exercise such as aerobic dance, rowing, rope skipping, stair-climbing, cross-country skiing, swimming, skating, and endurance game activities such as soccer and tennis. Choose activities that are both convenient and enjoyable. Fill in the activity names on the program plan.

3. *Frequency.* On the program plan, fill in how often you plan to participate in each activity; the ACSM recommends participating in cardiorespiratory endurance exercise three–five days per week.

Program Plan

Type of Activity	Frequency (check ✓)							Intensity (bpm or RPE)	Time (min)
	M	T	W	TH	F	SA	SU		

4. *Intensity.* Determine your exercise intensity using one of the following methods, and enter it on the program plan. Begin your program at a lower intensity and slowly increase intensity as your fitness improves, so select a range of intensities for your program.

   a. Target heart rate zone: Calculate target heart rate zone in beats per minute and then calculate the corresponding 15-second exercise count by dividing the total count by 6. For example, the 15-second exercise counts corresponding to a target heart rate zone of 122–180 bpm would be 20–30 beats.

   Maximum heart rate: 200 − _____ = _____ bpm
                                         age (years)

   ### Maximum Heart Rate Method

   65% training intensity = _____ bpm × 0.65 = _____ bpm
                                maximum heart rate

   90% training intensity = _____ bpm × 0.90 = _____ bpm
                                maximum heart rate

   Target heart rate zone = _____ **to** _____ **bpm**   **15-second count =** _____ **to** _____

LABORATORY ACTIVITIES

Heart Rate Reserve Method

Resting heart rate: _____ bpm (taken after 10 minutes of complete rest)

Heart rate reserve = _____ bpm − _____ bpm = _____ bpm
                         maximum heart rate   resting heart rate

50% training intensity = (_____ bpm × 0.50) + _____ bpm = _____ bpm
                              heart rate reserve   resting heart rate

85% training intensity = (_____ bpm × 0.85) + _____ bpm = _____ bpm
                              heart rate reserve   resting heart rate

Target heart rate zone = _____ to _____ bpm

15-second count = _____ to _____

b. Ratings of perceived exertion (RPE): If you prefer, determine an RPE value that corresponds to your target heart rate range (see p. 71–72 and Figure 3.5).

5. *Time (Duration).* A total time of 20–60 minutes per exercise session is recommended; your duration of exercise will vary with intensity. For developing cardiorespiratory endurance, higher-intensity activities can be performed for a shorter duration; lower intensities require a longer duration. Enter a duration (or a range of duration) on the program plan.

6. *Monitoring Your Program.* Complete a log like the one below to monitor your program and track your progress. Note the date on top, and fill in the intensity and time (duration) for each workout. If you prefer, you can also track other variables such as distance. For example, if your cardiorespiratory endurance program includes walking and swimming, you may want to track miles walked and yards swum in addition to the duration of each exercise session.

Activity/Date												
1	Intensity											
	Time											
	Distance											
2	Intensity											
	Time											
	Distance											
3	Intensity											
	Time											
	Distance											
4	Intensity											
	Time											
	Distance											

7. *Making Progress.* Follow the guidelines in the chapter and in Table 3.5 and Figure 3.6 to slowly increase the amount of overload in your program. Continue keeping a log, and periodically evaluate your progress.

Progress Checkup: Week _____ of program

Goals: Original Status   Current Status

_____   _____

_____   _____

_____   _____

List each activity in your program and describe how satisfied you are with the activity and with your overall progress. List any problems you've encountered or any unexpected costs or benefits of your fitness program so far.

Muscular Strength and Endurance

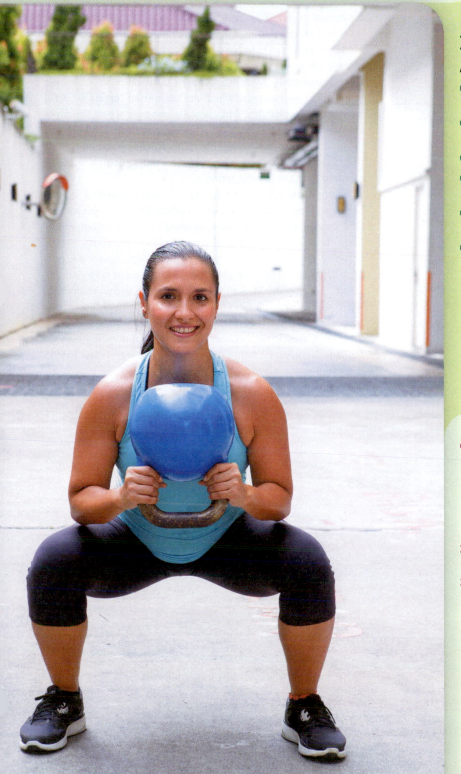

LOOKING AHEAD...

After reading this chapter, you should be able to

- Describe the basic physiology of muscles and explain how strength training affects muscles.

- Define muscular strength and endurance, and describe how they relate to wellness.

- Assess muscular strength and endurance.

- Apply the FITT principle to create a safe and successful strength training program.

- Describe the effects of supplements and drugs that are marketed to active people and athletes.

- Explain how to safely perform common strength training exercises using body weight, free weights, and weight machines.

TEST YOUR KNOWLEDGE

1. For women, weight training typically results in which of the following?
   a. bulky muscles
   b. significant increases in body weight
   c. improved body image

2. To maximize strength gains, it is a good idea to hold your breath as you lift a weight. True or false?

3. Regular strength training is associated with which of the following benefits?
   a. denser bones
   b. reduced risk of heart disease
   c. improved body composition
   d. fewer injuries
   e. improved metabolic health
   f. Increased longevity

See answers on the next page.

Muscles make up more than 40% of your body mass. You depend on them for movement, and, because of their mass, they are the sites of a large portion of the energy reactions (metabolism) that take place in your body. Strong, well-developed muscles help you perform daily activities with greater ease, protect you from injury, and enhance your well-being in other ways.

As described in Chapter 2, muscular strength is the amount of force a muscle can produce with a single maximum effort; muscular endurance is the ability to hold or repeat a muscular contraction for a long time. This chapter explains the benefits of *strength training* (also called *resistance training* or *weight training*) and describes methods of assessing muscular strength and endurance. It then explains the basics of strength training and provides guidelines for setting up your own training program. The musculoskeletal system is depicted on pages T4-2 and T4-3 of the color transparency insert "Touring the Musculoskeletal System" in this chapter. You can refer to this illustration as you set up your program.

BASIC MUSCLE PHYSIOLOGY AND THE EFFECTS OF STRENGTH TRAINING

Muscles move the body and enable it to exert force. When a muscle contracts (shortens), it moves a bone by pulling on the tendon that attaches the muscle to the bone.

Muscle Fibers

Muscles consist of individual muscle cells, or **muscle fibers**, connected in bundles called fascicles (Figure 4.1). A single muscle is made up of many bundles of muscle fibers and is covered by layers of connective tissue that hold the fibers together. Muscle fibers, in turn, are made up of smaller protein structures called **myofibrils**. Myofibrils consist of a series of contractile units called *sarcomeres,* which are composed largely of actin and myosin molecules. Muscle cells contract when the myosin molecules glide across the actin molecules in a ratchet-like movement. Each muscle cell has many **nuclei** containing genes that direct the production of enzymes and structural proteins required for muscle contraction.

Strength training increases the size and number of myofibrils, resulting in larger individual muscle fibers. Larger muscle fibers mean a larger and stronger muscle. The development of large muscle fibers is called **hypertrophy**; inactivity causes **atrophy**, the reversal of this process. For a depiction of the process of hypertrophy, see page T4-4 of the color transparency insert "Touring the Musculoskeletal System" in this chapter. In some species, muscles can increase in size through a separate process called **hyperplasia**, which involves an increase in the *number* of muscle fibers rather than the *size* of muscle fibers. In humans, hyperplasia is not thought to play a significant role in determining muscle size.

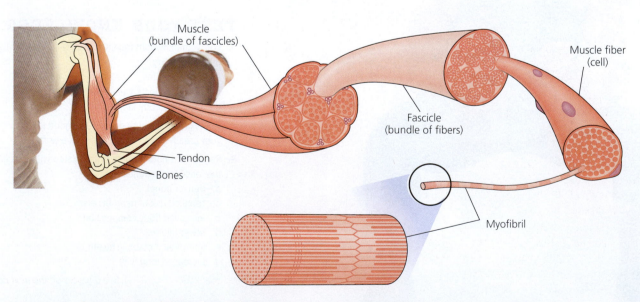

FIGURE 4.1 Components of skeletal muscle tissue.

Muscle fibers are classified as slow-twitch or fast-twitch fibers according to their strength, speed of contraction, and energy source. (See Chapter 3 for more on energy systems.)

- **Slow-twitch muscle fibers** are relatively fatigue resistant, but they don't contract as rapidly or strongly as fast-twitch fibers. The principal energy system that fuels slow-twitch fibers is aerobic (oxidative). Slow-twitch muscle fibers are typically reddish in color.
- **Fast-twitch muscle fibers** contract more rapidly and forcefully than slow-twitch fibers but fatigue more quickly. Although oxygen is important in the energy system that fuels fast-twitch fibers, they rely more on anaerobic (nonoxidative) metabolism than do slow-twitch fibers. Fast-twitch muscle fibers are typically whitish in color (e.g., white meat versus dark meat in a turkey).

Most muscles contain both slow-twitch and fast-twitch fibers. The proportion of the types of fibers varies significantly among different muscles and different individuals, and that proportion is largely fixed at birth, although fibers can contract faster or slower following a period of training or a period of inactivity. The type of fiber that acts during a particular activity depends on the type of work required. Endurance activities like jogging tend to use slow-twitch fibers, whereas strength and **power** activities like sprinting, use fast-twitch fibers. Strength training can increase the size and strength of both fast-twitch and slow-twitch fibers, although fast-twitch fibers are preferentially increased.

Motor Units

To exert force, a muscle recruits one or more motor units to contract. A **motor unit** is made up of a nerve connected to a number of muscle fibers. The number of muscle fibers in a motor unit varies from two to hundreds. Small motor units contain slow-twitch fibers, whereas large motor units contain fast-twitch fibers. When a motor unit calls on its fibers to contract, all fibers contract to their full capacity. The number of motor units recruited depends on the amount of strength required: When you pick up a small weight, you use fewer and smaller motor units than when picking up a large weight.

Strength training improves the body's ability to recruit motor units—a phenomenon called **muscle learning**—which increases strength even before muscle size increases. The physiological changes and benefits that result from strength training are summarized in Table 4.1; see the box "Gender Differences in Muscular Strength" for additional information on hormonal and nervous system influences on muscle tissue.

As a person ages, motor nerves can become disconnected from the portion of muscle they control. By age 70, 15% of the motor nerves in most people are no longer connected to muscle tissue. Aging and inactivity also cause muscles to become slower and therefore less able to perform quick, powerful movements. Strength training helps maintain motor nerve connections and the quickness of muscles.

Osteoporosis (bone loss) is common in people over age 55, particularly postmenopausal women. Osteoporosis leads to fractures that can be life-threatening. Hormonal changes from aging account for much of the bone loss that occurs, but lack of bone mass due to inactivity and a poor diet are contributing factors. Strength training can lessen bone loss even if it is taken up later in life; if practiced regularly, strength training may even build bone mass in postmenopausal women and older men. Increased muscle strength can also help prevent falls, which are a major cause of injury in people with osteoporosis (see the box "Benefits of Muscular Strength and Endurance").

Metabolic and Heart Health

Strength training helps prevent and manage both cardiovascular disease (CVD) and diabetes by doing the following:

- Improving glucose metabolism
- Increasing maximal oxygen consumption
- Reducing blood pressure
- Increasing HDL cholesterol and reducing LDL cholesterol (in some people)
- Improving blood vessel health

Stronger muscles reduce the demand on the heart during ordinary daily activities such as lifting and carrying objects. The benefits of resistance exercise to the heart are so great that the American Heart Association recommends strength training two to three days per week for healthy adults and many low-risk cardiac patients. Resistance training may not be appropriate for people with some types of heart disease.

---

muscle fiber   A single muscle cell, usually classified according to strength, speed of contraction, and energy source. **TERMS**

myofibrils   Protein structures that make up muscle fibers.

nucleus   A cell structure containing DNA and genes that direct the production of proteins; plural, *nuclei*.

hypertrophy   An increase in the size of muscle fibers, usually stimulated by muscular overload, as occurs during strength training.

atrophy   A decrease in the size of muscle fibers, usually attributable to inactivity.

hyperplasia   An increase in the number of muscle fibers.

slow-twitch muscle fibers   Red muscle fibers that are fatigue resistant but have a slow contraction speed and a lower capacity for tension; usually recruited for endurance activities.

fast-twitch muscle fibers   White muscle fibers that contract rapidly and forcefully but fatigue quickly; usually recruited for actions requiring strength, power, or speed.

power   The ability to exert force rapidly.

motor unit   A motor nerve (one that initiates movement) connected to one or more muscle fibers.

muscle learning   The improvement in the body's ability to recruit motor units, brought about through strength training.

Table 4.1 — Physiological Changes and Benefits from Strength Training

CHANGE	BENEFITS
Increased muscle mass* and strength	Increased muscular strength
	Improved body composition
	Higher rate of metabolism
	Improved capacity to regulate fuel use with aging
	Toned, healthy-looking muscles
	Increased longevity
	Improved quality of life
Increased utilization of motor units during muscle contractions	Increased muscular strength and power
Improved coordination of motor units	Increased muscular strength and power
Increased strength of tendons, ligaments, and bones	Lower risk of injury to these tissues
Increased storage of fuel in muscles	Increased resistance to muscle fatigue
Increased size of fast-twitch muscle fibers (from a high-resistance program)	Increased muscular strength and power
Increased size of slow-twitch muscle fibers (from a high-repetition program)	Increased muscular endurance
Increased blood supply to muscles (from a high-repetition program) and improved blood vessel health	Increased delivery of oxygen and nutrients Faster elimination of wastes
Biochemical improvements (for example, increased sensitivity to insulin)	Enhanced metabolic health and, possibly, increased life span
Improved blood fat levels	Reduced risk of heart disease
Increased muscle endurance	Enhanced ability to exercise for long periods and maintain good body posture

*Due to genetic and hormonal differences, men will build more muscle mass than women, but both men and women make about the same percentage gains in strength through a good program.

ASSESSING MUSCULAR STRENGTH AND ENDURANCE

Muscular strength is usually assessed by measuring the maximum amount of weight a person can lift in a single effort. This single maximum effort is called a **repetition maximum (RM)**. You can assess the strength of your major muscle groups by taking the one–repetition maximum (1 RM) test for the bench press and by taking functional leg strength tests. You can measure 1 RM directly or estimate it by doing multiple repetitions with a submaximal (lighter) weight. It is best to train for several weeks before attempting a direct 1 RM test; after you have a baseline value, you can retest after 6–12 weeks to check your progress. See Lab 4.1 for guidelines on taking these tests. For more accurate results, avoid strenuous weight training for 48 hours beforehand.

Muscular endurance is usually assessed by counting the maximum number of **repetitions** of an exercise a person can do (such as in push-ups or kettlebell snatches) or the maximum amount of time a person can hold a muscular contraction (such as in the flexed-arm hang). You can test the muscular endurance of major muscle groups in your body by taking the curl-up test, the push-up test, the core muscle plank test (Chapter 5), and the squat endurance test. See Lab 4.2 for complete instructions on taking these assessment tests.

CREATING A SUCCESSFUL STRENGTH TRAINING PROGRAM

When the muscles are stressed by a greater load than they are used to, they adapt and improve their function. The type of adaptation that occurs depends on the type of stress applied.

Static versus Dynamic Strength Training Exercises

Strength training exercises are generally classified as static or dynamic. Each involves a different way of using and strengthening muscles.

TERMS

repetition maximum (RM) The maximum amount of resistance that can be moved a specified number of times. 1-RM is the maximum amount of weight that can be lifted one time; 5-RM is the maximum amount of weight that can be lifted five times.

repetitions The number of times an exercise is performed during one set.

tendon A tough band of fibrous tissue that connects a muscle to a bone or other body part and transmits the force exerted by the muscle.

ligament A tough band of tissue that connects the ends of bones to other bones or supports organs in place.

cartilage Tough, resilient tissue that acts as a cushion between the bones in a joint.

testosterone The principal male hormone, responsible for the development of secondary sex characteristics and important in increasing muscle size.

Enhanced muscular strength and endurance can lead to improvements in the areas of performance, injury prevention, body composition, self-image, lifetime muscle and bone health, and metabolic health. Most important, greater muscular strength and endurance reduce the risk of premature death. Stronger people—particularly men—have a lower death rate due to all causes, including cardiovascular disease and cancer. The link between strength and death rate is independent of age, physical activity, smoking, alcohol intake, body composition, and family history of cardiovascular disease.

Improved Performance of Physical Activities

A person with a moderate to high level of muscular strength and endurance can perform everyday tasks—such as climbing stairs and carrying groceries—with ease. Increased strength can enhance enjoyment of recreational sports by making it possible to achieve high levels of performance and to handle advanced techniques. Strength training also results in modest improvements in maximal oxygen consumption. People with poor muscle strength tire more easily and are less effective in both everyday and recreational activities.

Injury Prevention

Increased muscular strength and endurance help protect you from injury in two key ways:

- By enabling you to maintain good posture. Good muscle strength and endurance help stabilize the spine, which protects against back and neck injuries.

- By encouraging proper body mechanics during everyday activities such as walking and lifting.

Good muscle strength and, particularly, endurance in the abdomen, hips, lower back, and legs maintain the spine in proper alignment and help prevent low-back pain, which afflicts more than 85% of Americans at some time in their lives. (Prevention of low-back pain is discussed in Chapter 5.)

Training for muscular strength and endurance also makes the **tendons**, **ligaments**, and **cartilage** cells stronger and less susceptible to injury. Resistance exercise prevents injuries best when the training program is gradual and progressive and builds all the major muscle groups.

Improved Body Composition

Healthy body composition means that the body has a high proportion of fat-free mass and a relatively small proportion of fat. Strength training improves body composition by increasing muscle mass, thereby tipping the body composition ratio toward fat-free mass and away from fat.

Building muscle mass through strength training also helps with losing fat because metabolic rate is related to muscle mass: The greater your muscle mass, the higher your metabolic rate. A high metabolic rate means that a nutritionally sound diet coupled with regular exercise will not lead to an increase in body fat. Strength training can boost resting metabolic rate by up to 15%, depending on how hard you train.

Resistance exercise also increases muscle temperature, which in turn slightly increases the rate at which you burn calories over the hours following a weight training session.

Enhanced Self-Image and Quality of Life

Strength training leads to an enhanced self-image in both men and women by providing stronger, firmer muscles and a toned, healthy-looking body. Women tend to lose inches, increase strength, and develop greater muscle definition. Men tend to build larger, stronger muscles. The larger muscles in men combine with high levels of the hormone **testosterone** for a strong tissue-building effect; see the box "Gender Differences in Muscular Strength."

Because strength training involves measurable objectives (pounds lifted, repetitions accomplished), a person can easily recognize improved performance, leading to greater self-confidence and self-esteem. Strength training also improves quality of life by increasing energy, preventing injuries, and making daily activities easier and more enjoyable.

Improved Muscle and Bone Health with Aging

Research has shown that good muscular strength helps people live healthier lives. A lifelong program of regular strength training prevents muscle and nerve degeneration that can compromise the quality of life and increase the risk of hip fractures and other potentially life-threatening injuries.

In the general population, people begin to lose muscle mass after age 30, a condition called *sarcopenia*. At first they may notice that they cannot play sports as well as they could in high school. After more years of inactivity and strength loss, people may have trouble performing even the simple movements of daily life, such as walking up a flight of stairs or doing yard work. By age 75, about 25% of men and 75% of women cannot lift more than 10 pounds overhead. Although aging contributes to decreased strength, inactivity causes most of the loss. Poor strength makes it much more likely that a person will be injured during everyday activities.

Increased Longevity

Strength training helps you live longer. A number of studies have associated greater muscular strength with lower rates of death from all causes, including cancer and cardiovascular disease. A study of more than 9,000 men showed that compared to men with the lowest levels of muscular strength, stronger men were 1.5 times less likely to die from all causes; 1.6 times less likely to die from cardiovascular disease; and 1.25 times less likely to die from cancer. The results were particularly striking in men age 60 and older with low levels of muscular strength, who were more than four times more likely to die from cancer than similar-age men with greater muscular strength.

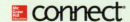

Men are generally stronger than women because they typically have larger bodies and a larger proportion of their total body mass is made up of muscle. But when strength is expressed per unit of cross-sectional area of muscle tissue, men are only 1–2% stronger than women in the upper body and about equal to women in the lower body. Because of the larger proportion of muscle tissue in the upper male body, men can more easily build upper-body strength than women can. Individual muscle fibers are larger in men, but the metabolism of cells within those fibers is the same in both sexes.

Two factors that help explain these disparities are testosterone levels and the speed of nervous control of muscle. Testosterone promotes the growth of muscle tissue in both males and females, but testosterone levels are 5–10 times higher in men than in women, allowing men to have larger muscles. Also, because the male nervous system can activate muscles faster, men tend to have more power.

Women are often concerned that they will develop large muscles from strength

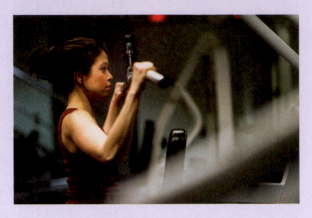

training. Because of hormonal differences, however, most women do not develop big muscles unless they train intensely over many years or take anabolic steroids. Women do gain muscle and improve body composition through strength training, but they don't develop bulky muscles or gain significant amounts of weight. A study of average women who weight trained two–three days per week for eight weeks found that they gained about 1.75 pounds of muscle and lost about 3.5 pounds of fat. Losing muscle over time is a much greater health concern for women than small gains in muscle weight, especially because any gains in muscle weight are typically more than offset by loss of fat weight. Both men and women lose muscle mass and power as they age, but because men start out with more muscle and don't lose power as quickly, older women tend to have greater impairment of muscle function than older men. This may partially account for the higher incidence of life-threatening falls in older women.

The bottom line is that both men and women can increase strength through strength training. Women may not be able to lift as much weight as men, but pound for pound of muscle, they have nearly the same capacity to gain strength as men.

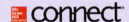

Static Exercise Also called **isometric** exercise, **static exercise** causes a muscle contraction without changing the length of the muscle or the angle in the joint on which the muscle acts (Figure 4.2A). In isometrics, the muscle contracts, but there is no movement. To perform an isometric exercise, a person can use an immovable object like a wall to provide resistance, or simply tighten a muscle while remaining still (for example, tightening the abdominal muscles while sitting at a desk). The spine extension and the side bridge, shown on page 112, are both isometric exercises.

Static exercises are particularly important for developing stiff core or torso muscles that support the spine and provide a firm foundation for whole body motions. During almost all movements some muscles contract statically to support the skeleton so other muscles can contract dynamically. For example, when you throw something, hit a ball, or ski, the core muscles in the abdomen and back stabilize the spine. This stability allows more powerful contractions in the lower- and upper-body muscles. The core muscles also contract statically during dynamic exercises, such as squats, lunges, and overhead presses.

Static exercises are useful in strengthening muscles after an injury or surgery, when movement of the affected joint could delay healing. Isometrics are also used to overcome weak points in an individual's range of motion. Statically strengthening a muscle at its weakest point will allow more weight to be lifted with that muscle during dynamic exercise. Certain types of calisthenics and Pilates exercises (described in more detail later in the chapter) also involve static contractions. For maximum strength gains, hold the isometric contraction maximally for six seconds; do 2–10 repetitions.

Dynamic Exercise Also called **isotonic** exercise, **dynamic exercise** causes a muscle contraction and a change in the length of the muscle and the angle of the joint (Figure 4.2 B,C). Dynamic exercises are the most popular type of exercises for increasing muscle strength and seem to be most valuable for developing strength that can be transferred to other forms of physical activity. They can be performed with weight machines, free weights, or a person's own body weight (as in curl-ups or push-ups).

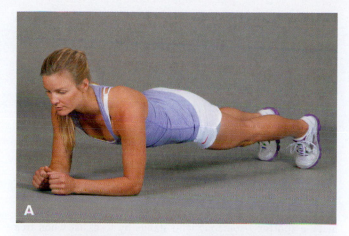

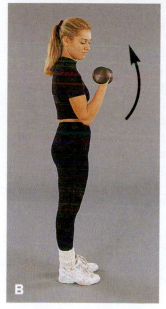
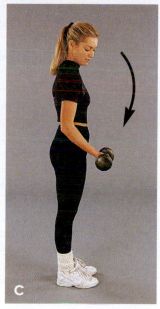

FIGURE 4.2 A static (isometric) exercise such as a plank (A) involves muscle contraction without movement; the position is held. A dynamic exercise such as a biceps curl involves muscle contraction with a change in the length of the muscle and angle of the joint. Dynamic muscle contractions can be concentric (B), in which the muscle shortens as it contracts, or eccentric (C), in which the muscle lengthens as it contracts.

There are two kinds of dynamic muscle contractions:

- A **concentric muscle contraction** (also called a *miometric contraction*) occurs when the muscle applies enough force to overcome resistance and shortens as it contracts.
- An **eccentric muscle contraction** (also called a *pliometric contraction*) occurs when the resistance is greater than the force applied by the muscle and the muscle lengthens as it contracts.

For example, in an arm curl, the biceps muscle works concentrically as the weight is raised toward the shoulder and eccentrically as the weight is lowered.

CONSTANT AND VARIABLE RESISTANCE Two of the most common dynamic exercise techniques are constant resistance exercise and variable resistance exercise. Both exercises are extremely effective for building muscular strength and endurance.

- **Constant resistance exercise** uses a constant load (weight) throughout a joint's full range of motion. Training with free weights is a form of constant resistance exercise. A problem with this technique is that, because of differences in leverage, there are points in a joint's range of motion where the muscle controlling the movement is stronger and points where it is weaker. The weakest point in the range limits the amount of weight a person can lift.
- In **variable resistance exercise**, the load is changed to provide maximum load throughout the entire range of motion. This form of exercise uses machines that place more stress on muscles at the end of the range of motion, where a person has better leverage and can exert more force. Use elastic bands and chains with free weights to add variable resistance to the exercises.

OTHER DYNAMIC EXERCISE TECHNIQUES Athletes use four other kinds of isotonic techniques, primarily for training and rehabilitation.

- **Eccentric (pliometric) loading** places a load on a muscle as it lengthens. The muscle contracts eccentrically to control the weight. Eccentric loading is practiced during most types of resistance training. For example, you are performing an eccentric movement as you lower the weight to your chest during a bench press in preparation for the active movement. You can also perform exercises designed specifically to overload muscle eccentrically, a technique called *negatives*.
- **Plyometrics** is the sudden eccentric loading and stretching of muscles followed by a forceful concentric

contraction—a movement that scientists call the stretch-shortening cycle. An example would be the action of the lower-body muscles when jumping from a bench to the ground and then jumping back onto the bench. This type of exercise helps develop explosive strength; it also helps build and maintain bone density.

- In **speed loading** you move a weight as rapidly as possible in an attempt to approach the speeds used in movements like throwing a softball or sprinting. In the bench press, for example, speed loading might involve doing 5 repetitions as fast as possible using a weight that is half the maximum load you can lift. You can gauge your progress by timing how fast you can perform the repetitions.

Training with a **kettlebell**—an iron ball with a handle—is a type of speed loading. Kettlebell training is highly ballistic, meaning that many exercises involve fast, pendulum-type motions, extreme decelerations, and high-speed eccentric muscle contractions. Kettlebell swings require dynamic concentric muscle contractions during the upward phase of the exercise followed by high-speed eccentric contractions to control the movement when returning to the starting position.

- **Isokinetic exercise** involves exerting force at a constant speed against an equal force exerted by a special strength training machine. The isokinetic machine provides variable resistance at different points in the joint's range of motion, matching the effort applied by the individual while keeping the speed of the movement constant. Isokinetic exercises are excellent for building strength and endurance.

Comparing Static and Dynamic Exercise Static exercises require no equipment, so they can be done virtually anywhere. They build strength rapidly and are useful for rehabilitating injured joints and stabilizing joints in the shoulder and spine. On the other hand, they have to be performed at several different angles for each joint to improve strength throughout its entire range of motion. Dynamic exercises can be performed without equipment (calisthenics) or with equipment (weight training). Not only are they excellent for building muscular strength and endurance, but they also tend to build strength through a joint's full range of motion. Most people develop muscular strength and endurance using dynamic

exercises. Ultimately, however, the type of exercise a person chooses depends on individual goals, preferences, and access to equipment.

Weight Machines, Free Weights, and Body Weight Exercises

Muscles get stronger when made to work against resistance. Resistance can be provided by free weights, body weight, or exercise machines. Many people prefer machines because they are safe, convenient, and easy to use. You just set the resistance, sit down at the machine, and start working. Machines make it easy to isolate and work specific muscles. You don't need a **spotter**—someone who stands by to assist when free weights are used—and you don't have to worry about dropping a weight on yourself. Many machines provide support for the back.

Free weights, such as barbells and kettlebells, require more care, balance, and coordination to use than machines, but they strengthen your body in ways that are more adaptable to real life. They are also more popular with athletes for developing functional strength for sports, especially sports that require a great deal of strength. Free weights are widely available, inexpensive, and convenient for home use.

Exercises that use body weight, elastic bands, rocks, or soup cans as resistance enable you to do workouts at home. You can purchase elastic bands at sporting good stores or any home improvement or hardware store. A basic principle of resistant exercise is to "train movements and not muscles." This means that you can overload the body in everyday movements like sitting and standing from a chair, climbing a fence, getting out of a swimming pool without a ladder, and standing after lying on the ground.

Other Training Methods and Types of Equipment

You don't need a fitness center or expensive equipment to strength train. If you prefer to train at home or like low-cost alternatives, consider the following options.

Resistance Bands Resistance or exercise bands are elastic strips or tubes of rubber material that are inexpensive, lightweight, and portable. They are available in a variety of styles and levels of resistance. Some are sold with instructional guides or DVDs, and classes may be offered at fitness centers. Many free-weight exercises can be adapted for resistance bands. For example, you can do biceps curls by standing on the center of the band and holding one end of the band in each hand; the band provides resistance when you stretch it to perform the curl.

Exercise (Stability) Balls The exercise or stability ball is an extra-large inflatable ball. It was originally developed for use in physical therapy but has become a popular piece of exercise equipment for use in the home or gym. It can be used to work the entire body, but it is particularly effective for working the core stabilizing muscles in the abdomen, chest, and

---

TERMS

speed loading Moving a load as rapidly as possible.

kettlebell A large iron weight with a connected handle; used for ballistic weight training exercises such as swings and one-arm snatches.

isokinetic exercise A type of dynamic exercise that provides variable resistance to a movement, so the movement occurs at a constant speed no matter how much effort is exerted.

spotter A person who assists with a weight training exercise done with free weights.

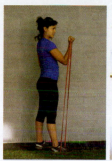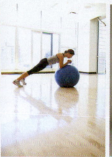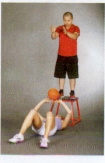

Fitness Tip There are many options for resistance training available, many at little cost. Try different types of equipment and exercises to add variety to your program and stimulate strength development.

back—muscles that are important for preventing back problems. The ball's instability forces the exerciser to use the stability muscles to balance the body, even when just sitting on the ball. The "stir the pot" exercise—a plank position with elbows resting on the ball, which is then moved in small circles—is an example of a core-building exercise that uses the stability ball.

There are many ways to incorporate a stability ball into a typical workout. For example, you can perform crunches or curl-ups while lying on a ball instead of on the floor. Lying facedown across a ball provides different leverage points for pushups. A variety of resistance training exercises can be performed on a stability ball, but experts recommend using dumbbells rather than barbells when lifting weights on a ball.

When selecting a ball, make sure your thighs are parallel to the ground when you sit on it; if you are a beginner or have back problems, choose a larger ball so your thighs are at an angle, with hips higher than knees. Beginners should use caution until they feel comfortable with the movements and take care to avoid poor form due to fatigue (Table 4.2).

Vibration Training Vibration training consists of doing basic exercises, such as squats, push-ups, lunges, and modified pull-ups, on a vibrating platform. Vibration is transferred to whichever part of the body is in contact with the vibrating plate or handlebars. Vibration activates stretch receptors in the muscles, which triggers thousands of small reflex muscle

contractions. Most studies have found that vibration training caused little or no additional effects above weight training alone.

Pilates Pilates (*pil LAH teez*) was developed by German gymnast and boxer Joseph Pilates early in the 20th century. Pilates focuses on strengthening and stretching the core muscles in the back, abdomen, and buttocks to create a solid base of support for whole-body movement; the emphasis is on concentration, control, movement flow, and breathing. Pilates often makes use of specially designed resistance training devices, although some classes feature just mat or floor work. Mat exercises can be done at home, but because there are hundreds of Pilates exercises, some of them strenuous, it is best to begin with some qualified instruction.

Medicine Balls, Suspension Training, Stones, and Carrying Exercises Almost anything that provides resistance to movement will develop strength. Rubber medicine balls weighing up to 50 pounds can be used for a variety of functional movements, such as squats and overhead throws. Suspension training (e.g., TRX system) uses body weight as the resistance in exercises using ropes or cords attached to a hook, bar, door jam, or sturdy tree branch. You can train with a stone found in your backyard or local riverbank in performing exercises such as squats, presses, and carries. Walking while carrying dumbbells, farmer's bars, or heavy stones is an easy and effective way to develop whole-body strength. Carrying exercises are particularly useful for building the core muscles.

Power-Based Conditioning Programs This type of training combines aerobics, weight training, gymnastics, and high-intensity interval training. Programs such as CrossFit and GymJones employ different exercises every day. More traditional circuit training methods often use the same exercises set up in series. (See the box "High-Intensity Conditioning Programs" in Chapter 3.)

Applying the FITT Principle: Selecting Exercises and Putting Together a Program

A complete weight training program works all the major muscle groups. It usually takes about 8–10 different exercises to

Table 4.2	The Pros and Cons of Stability Balls
PROS	CONS
Stability balls activate muscle and nerve groups that might not otherwise get involved in a particular exercise.	Muscle activation when training on unstable surfaces is less effective than traditional training for building strength in muscle groups responsible for a movement or in trunk-stabilizing muscle groups.
Some exercises, such as the stir the pot exercise, can enhance the stability of supporting joints throughout the body.	Some exercises (such as curl-ups) can be more stressful to certain joints and muscles and promote back or shoulder pain in susceptible people.
Stability balls can be useful for some older adults because they require balance and can enhance overall stability.	Falling off an unstable surface, especially while holding weights, can cause serious injury.
Stability balls add variety and challenge to a workout	

Want to get stronger? Then you need to focus on developing your skills at least as much as you focus on lifting more weight. Improving skill is the best way to increase strength during movements such as hitting a tennis ball or baseball, performing a bench press, driving a golf ball, skiing down a slope, or carrying a bag of groceries up a flight of stairs. In the world of weight training, skill means lifting weights with proper form; the better your form, the better your results.

The brain develops precise neural pathways as you learn a skill. As you improve, the pathways conduct nervous impulses faster and more precisely until the movement almost becomes reflexive. The best way to learn a skill is through focused practice that involves identifying mistakes, correcting them, and practicing the refined movement many times. However, simply practicing the skill is not enough if you want to improve and perform more powerful movements. You must perform the movements correctly instead of practicing mistakes or poor form over and over again.

Here's where technology can help. Watch videos of people performing weight training movements correctly. You may be able to borrow videos from your instructor, purchase low-cost training videos through magazines and sporting goods stores, or find them on the Internet. If you watch training videos online, however, make sure they were produced by an authoritative source on weight training. Otherwise, you may be learning someone else's mistakes.

Film your movements using a phone camera or inexpensive video camera. Compare your movements with those of a more skilled person performing them correctly. Make a note of movement patterns that need work and try to change your technique to make it more mechanically correct. Share your videos with your instructor or a certified personal trainer, who can help you identify poor form and teach you ways to correct your form. Smart phone apps such as Coaches' Eye, Hudl Technique and Dartfish allow you to analyze movements in slow motion, compare movements side by side, and share your videos with others.

---

get a complete full-body workout. Use the FITT principle—frequency, intensity, time, and type—to set the parameters of your program.

Frequency of Exercise For general fitness, the American College of Sports Medicine (ACSM) recommends a frequency of at least two nonconsecutive days per week for weight training. Allow your muscles at least one day of rest between workouts; if you train too often, your muscles won't be able to work with enough intensity to improve their fitness, and soreness and injury are more likely to result. If you enjoy weight training and want to train more often, try working different muscle groups on alternate days—a training plan called a *split routine*. For example, work your arms and upper body one day, work your lower body the next day, and then return to upper-body exercises on the third day.

Intensity of Exercise: Amount of Resistance The amount of weight (resistance) you lift in weight training exercises is equivalent to intensity in cardiorespiratory endurance training. It determines how your body will adapt to weight training and how quickly these adaptations will occur.

Choose weights based on your current level of muscular fitness and your fitness goals. Choose a weight heavy enough to fatigue your muscles but light enough for you to complete the repetitions with good form. (For tips on perfecting your form, see the box "Improving Your Technique with Video.") To build strength rapidly, you should lift weights as heavy as 80% of your maximum capacity (1 RM). If you're more interested in building endurance, choose a lighter weight (perhaps 40–60% of 1 RM), and do more repetitions. New research has found that you can stimulate muscle hypertrophy using only 30–50% of maximum capacity if you stress the muscles adequately.

For example, if your maximum capacity for the leg press is 160 pounds, you might lift 130 pounds to build strength and 80 pounds in more repetitions to build endurance. For a general fitness program to develop both muscular strength and endurance, choose a weight in the middle of this range, perhaps 70% of 1 RM. Or you can create a program that includes both higher-intensity exercise (80% of 1 RM for 8–10 repetitions) and lower-intensity exercise (60% of 1 RM for 15–20 repetitions); this routine will develop both fast-twitch and slow-twitch muscle fibers.

Because it can be tedious and time-consuming to continually reassess your maximum capacity for each exercise, you might find it easier to choose a weight based on the number of repetitions of an exercise you can perform with a given resistance.

Time of Exercise: Repetitions and Sets To improve fitness, you must do enough repetitions of each exercise to fatigue your muscles. The number of repetitions needed to cause fatigue depends on the amount of resistance: The heavier the weight, the fewer repetitions to reach fatigue. In general, a heavy weight and a low number of repetitions (1–5) build strength and overload primarily fast-twitch fibers, whereas a light weight and a high number of repetitions (15–20) build endurance and overload primarily slow-twitch fibers.

For a general fitness program to build both strength and endurance, try to do about 8–12 repetitions of each exercise; a few exercises, such as abdominal crunches and calf raises, may require more. To avoid injury, older (approximately age 50–60 and above) and frailer people should perform more repetitions (10–15) using a lighter weight.

In weight training, a **set** refers to a group of repetitions of an exercise followed by a rest period. To develop strength and endurance for general fitness, you can make gains doing a single set of each exercise, provided you use enough resistance to fatigue your muscles. (You should just barely be able to complete the 8–12 repetitions—using good form—for each exercise.) Doing more than one set of each exercise will increase strength development; most serious weight trainers do at least three sets of each exercise (see the section "More Advanced Strength Training Programs" for guidelines on more advanced programs).

If you perform more than one set of an exercise, you need to rest long enough between sets to allow your muscles to work with enough intensity to increase fitness. The length of the rest interval depends on the amount of resistance. In a program to develop a combination of strength and endurance for wellness, a rest period of one–three minutes between sets is appropriate. If you are lifting heavier loads to build strength, rest three–five minutes between sets. You can save time in your workouts by alternating sets of different exercises. One muscle group can rest between sets while you work on another group.

Overtraining—doing more exercise than your body can recover from—can occur in response to heavy resistance training. Possible signs of overtraining include lack of progress or decreased performance, chronic fatigue, decreased coordination, and chronic muscle soreness. The best remedy for overtraining is rest; add more days of recovery between workouts. With extra rest, chances are you'll be refreshed and ready to train again. Adding variety to your program, as discussed later in the chapter, can also help you avoid overtraining with resistance exercise.

Type or Mode of Exercise For overall fitness, you need to include exercises for your neck, upper back, shoulders, arms, chest, abdomen, lower back, thighs, buttocks, and calves—about 8–10 exercises in all. If you are also training for a particular sport, include exercises to strengthen the muscles important for optimal performance *and* the muscles most likely to be injured. Weight training exercises for general fitness are presented later in this chapter.

BALANCE EXERCISES FOR OPPOSING MUSCLE GROUPS It is important to balance exercises between antagonistic muscle groups. When a muscle contracts, the opposing muscle must relax. Whenever you do an exercise that moves a joint in one direction, also select an exercise that works the joint in the opposite direction. For example, if you do knee extensions to develop the muscles on the front of your thighs, also do leg curls to develop the antagonistic muscles on the back of your thighs.

SETTING ORDER OF EXERCISES The order of exercises can also be important. Do exercises for large-muscle groups or for more than one joint before you do exercises that use small-muscle groups or single joints. This allows for more effective overload of the larger, more powerful muscle groups. Small-muscle groups fatigue more easily than larger ones, and small-muscle fatigue limits your capacity to overload large-muscle groups. For example, lateral raises, which work the shoulder muscles, should be performed after bench presses, which work the chest and arms in addition to the shoulders. If you fatigue your shoulder muscles by doing lateral raises first, you won't be able to lift as much weight and effectively fatigue all the key muscle groups used during the bench press.

Warm-up 5–10 minutes	Strength training exercises for major muscle groups (8–10 exercises)		Cool-down 5–10 minutes
	Sample program		
	Exercise	*Muscle group(s) developed*	
	Bench press	Chest, shoulders, triceps	
	Pull-ups	Lats, biceps	
	Shoulder press	Shoulders, trapezius, triceps	
	Upright rowing	Deltoids, trapezius	
	Biceps curls	Biceps	
	Lateral raises	Shoulders	
	Squats	Gluteals, quadriceps	
	Heel raises	Calves	
	Abdominal curls	Abdominals	
	Spine extensions	Low- and mid-back spine extensors	
	Side bridges	Obliques, quadratus lumborum	
Start			*Stop*

Frequency: 2–3 nonconsecutive days per week

Intensity/Resistance: Weights heavy enough to cause muscle fatigue when exercises are performed with good form for the selected number of repetitions

Time: Repetitions: 8–12 of each exercise (10–15 with a lower weight for people over age 50–60); **Sets:** 1 (doing more than 1 set per exercise may result in faster and greater strength gains); rest 1–2 minutes between exercises.

Type of activity: 8–10 strength training exercises that focus on major muscle groups

FIGURE 4.3 The FITT principle for a strength training workout.

Also, order exercises so you work opposing muscle groups in sequence, one after the other. For example, follow biceps curls, which work the biceps, with triceps extensions, which exercise the triceps—the antagonistic muscle to the biceps.

The Warm-Up and Cool-Down

As with cardiorespiratory endurance exercise, you should warm up before every weight training session and cool down afterward (Figure 4.3). You should do both a general warm-up—several minutes of walking or easy jogging and a warm-up for the weight training exercises you plan to perform. For example, if you plan to do one or more sets of 10 repetitions of bench presses with 125 pounds, you might do one set of 10 repetitions with 50 pounds as a warm-up. Do similar warm-up exercises for each exercise in your program.

set A group of repetitions followed by a rest period. **TERMS**

To cool down after weight training, relax for 5–10 minutes after your workout. Although this is controversial, a few studies have suggested that including a period of post-exercise stretching may help prevent muscle soreness; warmed-up muscles and joints make the cool-down period a particularly good time to work on flexibility.

Getting Started and Making Progress

The first few sessions of weight training should be devoted to learning the movements and allowing your nervous system to practice communicating with your muscles so you can develop strength effectively. To start, choose a weight that you can move easily through 8–12 repetitions, do only one set of each exercise, and rest one–two minutes between exercises. Gradually add weight and (if you want) sets to your program over the first few weeks until you are doing one to three sets of 8–12 repetitions of each exercise.

As you progress, add weight according to the "two-for-two" rule: When you can perform two additional repetitions with a given weight on two consecutive training sessions, increase the load. For example, if your target is to perform 8–10 repetitions per exercise, and you performed 12 repetitions in your previous two workouts, it would be appropriate to increase your load. If adding weight means you can do only 7 or 8 repetitions, stay with that weight until you can again complete 12 repetitions per set. If you can do only 4–6 repetitions after adding weight, or if you can't maintain good form, you've added too much and should take some off.

You can add more resistance in large-muscle exercises, such as squats and bench presses, than you can in small-muscle exercises, such as curls. For example, when you can complete 12 repetitions of squats with good form, you may be able to add 10–20 pounds of additional resistance; for curls, on the other hand, you might add only 3–5 pounds. As a general guideline, try increases of approximately 5%, which is half a pound of additional weight for each 10 pounds you are currently lifting.

You can expect to improve rapidly during the first 6–10 weeks of training—a 10–30% increase in the amount of weight lifted. Gains will then come more slowly. Your rate of improvement will depend on how hard you work and how your body responds to resistance training. Factors such as age, gender, motivation, and heredity also will affect your progress.

After you achieve the level of strength and muscularity you want, you can maintain your gains by training two–three days per week. You can monitor the progress of your program by recording the amount of resistance and the number of repetitions and sets you perform on a workout card like the one shown in Figure 4.4.

More Advanced Strength Training Programs

The program just described is sufficient to develop and maintain muscular strength and endurance for general fitness. Performing more sets and fewer repetitions with a heavier load will cause greater increases in strength. Such a program might include three to five sets of 4–6 repetitions each; the load should be heavy enough to cause fatigue with the smaller

Exercise	Wt	Sets	Reps/secs
Bench press	45	2	10
Pull-ups (assisted)	0	2	7
Shoulder press	25	2	10
Upright rowing	10	2	10
Biceps curls	15	2	8
Lateral raise	5	2	12
Squats	45	2	12
Heel raises	45	2	11
Abdominal curls	0	2	25
Spine extensions	0	2	10
Side bridge	0	2	65

Session date: March 5

FIGURE 4.4 A sample workout log for a general fitness strength training program.

number of repetitions. Rest long enough after a set (three–five minutes) to allow your muscles to recover and work intensely during the next set.

Experienced weight trainers often practice some form of cycle training, also called *periodization*, in which the exercises, number of sets and repetitions, and intensity vary within a workout and/or between workouts. For example, you might do a particular exercise more intensely during some sets or on some days than others. You might also vary the exercises you perform for particular muscle groups. For more detailed information on these more advanced training techniques, consult a certified strength coach. If you decide to adopt a more advanced training regimen, start off slowly to give your body a chance to adjust and to minimize the risk of injury.

Weight Training Safety

Injuries happen in weight training. Maximum physical effort, elaborate machinery, rapid movements, and heavy weights can

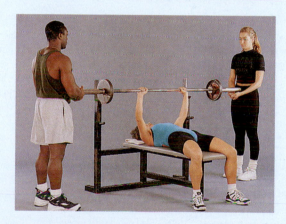

General Guidelines

- When beginning a program or trying new exercises or equipment, ask a qualified trainer or instructor to show you how to do exercises safely and correctly.

- Lift weights from a stabilized body position; keep weights as close to your body as possible.

- Protect your back by maintaining control of your spine and avoiding dangerous positions. Don't twist your body while lifting.

- Observe proper lifting techniques and good form at all times. Don't lift beyond the limits of your strength.

- Don't hold your breath while doing weight training exercises. Doing so causes a decrease in blood returning to the heart and can make you dizzy and faint. It can also increase blood pressure to dangerous levels. Exhale when exerting the greatest force, and inhale when moving the weight into position for the active phase of the lift. Breathe smoothly and steadily.

- Don't use defective equipment. Be aware of broken collars or bolts, frayed cables, broken chains, or loose cushions.

- Don't exercise if you're ill, injured, or overtrained. Do not try to work through the pain.

Free Weights

- Make sure the bar is loaded evenly on both sides and weights are secured with collars or spring clips.

- When you pick a weight up from the ground, keep your back straight and your head level. Don't bend at the waist with straight legs.

- Lift weights smoothly; don't jerk them. Control the weight through the entire range of motion.

- Do most of your lifting with your legs. Keep your hips and buttocks back. When doing standing lifts, maintain a good posture so that you protect your back. Bend at the hips, not with the spine. Feet should be shoulder-width apart, heels and balls of the feet in contact with the floor, and knees slightly bent.

- Don't bounce weights against your body during an exercise.

Spotting

- Use spotters for free-weight exercises in which the bar crosses the face or head (e.g., the bench press), is placed on the back (e.g., squats), or is racked in front of the chest (e.g., overhead press from the rack holding the weight).

- If one spotter is used, the spotter should stand behind the lifter; if two spotters are used, one spotter should stand at each end of the barbell.

- For squats with heavy resistance, use at least three spotters—one behind the lifter (hands near lifter's hips, waist, or torso) and one at each end of the bar. Squatting in a power rack will increase safety during this exercise. A power rack consists of four vertical posts with two movable horizontal bar catchers on each side.

- Spot dumbbell exercises at the forearms, as close to the weights as possible.

- For over-the-face and over-the-head lifts, the spotter should hold the bar with an alternate grip (one palm up and one palm down) inside the lifter's grip.

- Spotter and lifter should ensure good communication by agreeing on verbal signals before the exercise.

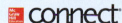

combine to make the weight room a dangerous place if proper precautions aren't taken. To help ensure that your workouts are safe and productive, follow the guidelines in the box "Safe Weight Training" and the following suggestions.

Use Proper Lifting Technique Every exercise has a proper technique that is important for obtaining maximum benefits and preventing injury. Your instructor or weight room attendant can help explain the specific techniques for different exercises and weight machines.

Perform exercises smoothly and with good form. Lift or push the weight forcefully during the active phase of the lift and then lower it with control. Perform all lifts through the full range of motion and strive to maintain a neutral spine position during each exercise.

Use Spotters and Collars with Free Weights Spotters are necessary when an exercise has potential for danger; a weight that is out of control or falls can cause a serious injury. A spotter can assist you if you cannot complete a lift or if the weight tilts. A spotter can also help you move a weight into position before a lift and provide help or additional resistance during a lift. Spotting requires practice and coordination between the lifter and the spotter(s).

Collars are devices that secure weights to a barbell or dumbbell. Although people lift weights without collars, doing so is dangerous. It is easy to lose your balance or to raise one side of the weight faster than the other. Without collars, the weights can slip off and crash to the floor. If you use spring clip collars, make sure they fit the bar tightly. Worn spring collars can slide off the bar easily.

Be Alert for Injuries Report any obvious muscle or joint injuries to your instructor or physician, and stop exercising the affected area. Training with an injured joint or muscle can lead to a more serious injury. Make sure you get the necessary first aid. Even minor injuries heal faster if you use the R-I-C-E principle of treating injuries described in Chapter 3.

Consult a physician if you have any unusual symptoms during exercise or if you're uncertain whether weight training is a proper activity for you. Weight training can aggravate conditions such as heart disease and high blood pressure. Immediately report symptoms such as headaches; dizziness; labored breathing; numbness; vision disturbances; and chest,

neck, or arm pain. As discussed in Chapter 3, pushing muscles to failure can sometimes result in rhabdomyolysis (destruction of muscle cells), which can cause serious illness or even death.

A Caution about Supplements and Drugs

Many active people use nutritional supplements and drugs in the quest for improved performance and appearance. Table 4.3 lists a selective summary of "performance aids" along with their potential side effects. While some of these substances improve performance, most are ineffective and expensive, and some are dangerous. A balanced diet should be your primary nutritional strategy.

WEIGHT TRAINING EXERCISES

A general book on fitness and wellness cannot include a detailed description of all weight training exercises. The following pages present a basic program for developing muscular strength and endurance for general fitness using body weight (no equipment), free weights, and weight machines. Photographs and

Table 4.3	Performance Aids Marketed to Weight Trainers		
SUBSTANCE	SUPPOSED EFFECTS	ACTUAL EFFECTS	SELECTED POTENTIAL SIDE EFFECTS
Adrenal androgens, such as dehydroepiandrosterone (DHEA), androstenedione	Increased testosterone, muscle mass, and strength; decreased body fat	Increased testosterone, strength, and fat-free mass; decreased fat in older subjects (more studies needed in younger people)	Gonadal suppression, prostate hypertrophy, breast development in males, masculinization in women and children; long-term effects unknown
Amino acids	Increased muscle mass	No effects if dietary protein intake is adequate; consuming before or after training may promote muscle protein synthesis (particularly leucine)	Minimal side effects; unbalanced amino acid intake can cause problems with protein metabolism
Amphetamines	Prevention of fatigue; increased confidence and training intensity	Increased arousal, wakefulness, and confidence; feeling of enhanced decision-making ability	Depression and fatigue, extreme confusion; aggressiveness, paranoia, hallucinations, restlessness, irritability, heart arrhythmia, high blood pressure, and chest pain
Anabolic steroids (steroids are controlled substances*)	Increased muscle mass, strength, power, psychological aggressiveness, and endurance	Increased strength, power, fat-free mass, and aggression; no effects on endurance	Liver damage and tumors, abnormal blood lipids, impaired reproductive health, hypertension, depressed immunity, insulin resistance, psychological disturbances, acne, breast development in males, masculinization in women and children, heart disease, thicker blood, and increased risk of cancer
Caffeine	Weight loss; improved endurance, strength, and power output; stimulant effect	Improves sports performance in low to moderate doses (three-six mg/kg body weight); improves endurance and high-intensity exercise capacity	Abnormal heart rhythm and insomnia; caffeine is addictive
Creatine monohydrate	Increased creatine phosphate levels in muscles, muscle mass, and capacity for high-intensity exercise	Increased muscle mass and performance in some types of high-intensity exercise	Minimal side effects; long-term effects unknown

SUBSTANCE	SUPPOSED EFFECTS	ACTUAL EFFECTS	SELECTED POTENTIAL SIDE EFFECTS
Diuretics	Promote loss of body fluid	Promote loss of body fluid to accentuate muscle definition; often taken with potassium supplements and very low-calorie diets	Muscle cell destruction, low blood pressure, blood chemistry abnormalities, and heart problems
Energy drinks	Increased energy, strength, power	Increased training volume; caffeine and carbohydrates are main ingredients; products are overpriced	Insomnia, increased blood pressure, heart palpitations
Erythropoietin	Enhanced performance during endurance events	Stimulated growth of red blood cells; enhanced oxygen uptake and endurance	Increased blood viscosity (thickness), can cause potentially fatal blood clots
Ginseng	Decreased effects of physical and emotional stress; increased oxygen consumption	Most well-controlled studies show no effect on performance	No serious side effects; high doses can cause high blood pressure, nervousness, and insomnia
Growth hormone (extremely expensive controlled substance*)	Increased muscle mass, strength, and power; decreased body fat	Increased muscle mass and strength; decreased fat mass; little effect on exercise performance	Elevated blood sugar, high insulin levels, and carpal tunnel syndrome; enlargement of the heart and other organs
Beta-hydroxy beta-methylbutyrate (HMB)	Increased strength and muscle mass; decreased body fat	Some studies show increased fat-free mass and decreased fat; more research needed	No reported side effects; long-term effects unknown
Insulin	Increased muscle mass	Effectiveness in stimulating muscle growth unknown	Insulin shock (characterized by extremely low blood sugar), which can lead to unconsciousness and death
"Metabolic-optimizing" meals for athletes	Increased muscle mass and energy supply; decreased body fat	No proven effects beyond those of balanced meals	No reported side effects, extremely expensive
Nitric oxide boosters (arginine, beet root)	Increased blood flow by stimulating nitric oxide production in blood vessels	Might increase endurance (beet root); little evidence that they promote muscle hypertrophy	Generally safe; could lower blood pressure in some people and make herpes infections worse
Protein, amino acids, polypeptide supplements	Increased muscle mass and growth hormone release; accelerated muscle development; decreased body fat	No effects if dietary protein intake is adequate; may promote protein synthesis if taken immediately before or after weight training	Can be dangerous for people with liver or kidney disease; substituting amino acid or polypeptide supplements for protein-rich food can cause nutrient deficiencies

*Possession of a controlled substance is illegal without a prescription, and physicians are not allowed to prescribe controlled substances for the improvement of athletic performance. In addition, the use of anabolic steroids, growth hormone, or any of several other substances listed in this table is banned for athletic competition. Some apparently safe supplements may contain substances banned for use in sport.

SOURCES: Fahey, T., et al. 2015. Sport and exercise physiology: Performance-enhancing substances—anabolic steroids, in *Sports Science and Physical Education*, ed., L. Georgescu, in *Encyclopedia of Life Support Systems (EOLSS)*, developed under the auspices of UNESCO. Oxford, UK: EOLSS Publishers; Brooks, G. A., et al. 2005. *Exercise Physiology: Human Bioenergetics and Its Applications*, 4th ed. New York: McGraw-Hill; Pasiakos, S. M., et al. 2015. The effects of protein supplements on muscle mass, strength, and aerobic and anaerobic power in healthy adults: A systematic review. *Sports Medicine.* 45(1): 111–131.

a list of the muscles being trained accompany instructions for each exercise. See pages T4-2 and T4-3 of the color transparency insert "Touring the Musculoskeletal System" in this chapter for a clear illustration of the deep and superficial muscles referenced in the exercises.

Labs 4.2 and 4.3 will help you assess your current level of muscular endurance and design your own weight training program. If you want to develop strength for a particular activity, your program should contain exercises for general fitness, exercises for the muscle groups most important for the activity, and exercises for muscle groups most often injured. Regardless of the goals of your program or the type of equipment you use, your program should be structured so that you obtain maximum results without risking injury.

EXERCISE 1

Instructions: (a) Keep your back straight and head level; stand with feet slightly more than shoulder-width apart and toes pointed slightly outward. Hold your hands out in front of you. **(b)** Squat down until your thighs are below parallel with the floor. Let your thighs move laterally (outward) so that you "squat between your legs." Hinge at your hips and don't let your back sag. This will help keep your back straight and your heels on the floor. Drive upward toward the starting position, hinging at the hips and keeping your back in a fixed position throughout the exercise.

Air Squats

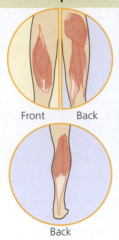

Front   Back

Back

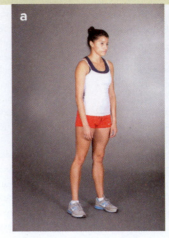

a

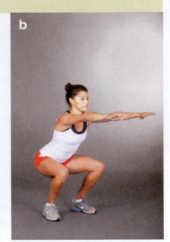

b

Muscles developed:

Quadriceps, gluteus maximus, hamstrings, gastrocnemius

EXERCISE 2

Instructions: (a) Stand with one foot about two feet in front of the other. **(b)** Lunge forward with the front leg, bending it until the thigh is parallel to the floor. The heel of the lead leg should stay on the ground. Do not shift your weight so far forward that the knee moves out past the toes. Repeat the exercise using the other leg. Keep your back and head as straight as possible and maintain control while performing the exercise.

Lunges

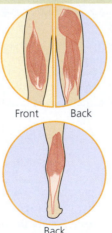

Front   Back

Back

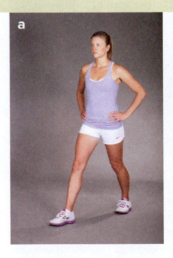

a

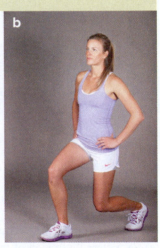

b

Muscles developed:

Quadriceps, gluteus maximus, hamstrings, gastrocnemius

Burpees with a Push-up

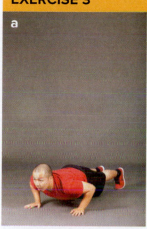
a

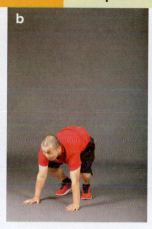
b

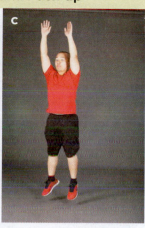
c

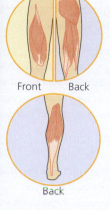
Front   Back

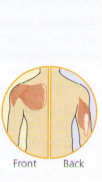
Back

Front   Back

Instructions: (a) From a standing position, squat down and place your hands on the floor; and then kick your legs behind you and land in the "up" push-up position. Do a push-up. (b) Then move your knees forward until you are in a squat position; (c) spring up as high as you can into a full jump. Repeat.

Muscles developed:
Quadriceps, gluteus maximus, hamstrings, gastrocnemius, deltoids, pectoralis major, triceps

EXERCISE 4   Curl-Up or Crunch

Instructions: (a) Lie on your back on the floor with your arms folded across your chest and your feet on the floor or on a bench. (b) Curl your trunk up, minimizing your head and shoulder movement. Lower to the starting position. Focus on using your abdominal muscles rather than the muscles in your shoulders, chest, and neck.

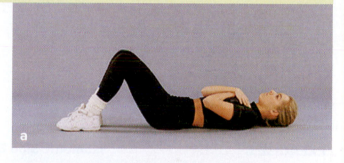
a

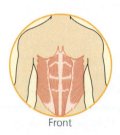
Front

Muscles developed:
Rectus abdominis, obliques

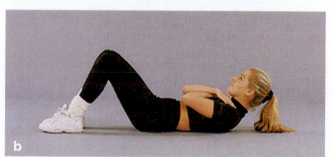
b

Instructions: Begin on all fours with your knees below your hips and your hands below your shoulders.

Unilateral spine extension:

(a) Extend your right leg to the rear and reach forward with your right arm. Keep your spine neutral and your raised arm and leg in line with your torso. Don't arch your back or let your hip or shoulder sag. Hold this position for 10–30 seconds. Repeat with your left leg and left arm.

Bilateral spine extension:

(b) Extend your left leg to the rear and reach forward with your right arm. Keep your spine neutral and your raised arm and leg in line with your torso. Don't arch your back or let your hip or shoulder sag. Hold this position for 10–30 seconds. Repeat with your right leg and left arm.

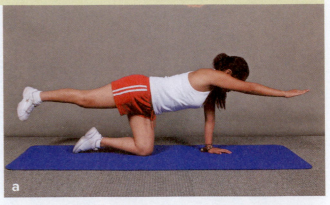

a

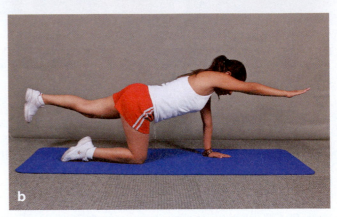

b

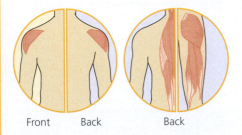

Front   Back   Back

Muscles developed: Erector spinae, gluteus maximus, hamstrings, deltoids

You can make this exercise more difficult by making box patterns with your arms and legs.

Instructions: Lie on the floor on your side with your knees bent and your top arm lying alongside your body. Lift and drive your hips forward so your weight is supported by your forearm and knee. Hold this position for 3–10 seconds, breathing normally. Repeat on the other side. Perform 3–10 repetitions on each side.

Variation: You can make the exercise more difficult by keeping your legs straight and supporting yourself with your feet and forearm (see Lab 5.3) or with your feet and hand (with elbow straight). An advanced version of this exercise that builds the core and shoulder muscles is to do a side bridge on the right side, rotate to a front plank, and then rotate to a side bridge on the left side. Hold each position for three seconds.

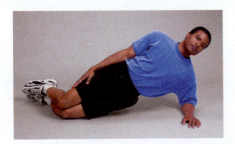

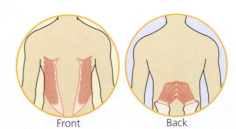

Front   Back

Muscles developed:

Obliques, quadratus lumborum

Touring the Musculoskeletal System

The Muscular System: Anterior View

The Muscular System: Posterior View

Muscle Hypertrophy: Gaining Muscle Through Strength Training

The Knee: Supporting and Maintaining Joint Stability

GOALS OF THE TOUR

5. **The Muscular System, Anterior View.** You will be able to use the illustration as a reference point for identifying the deep and superficial muscles of the front of the body in the context of understanding and performing strength training exercises.

6. **The Muscular System, Posterior View.** You will be able to use the illustration as a reference point for identifying the deep and superficial muscles of the back of the body in the context of understanding and performing strength training exercises.

7. **Muscle Hypertrophy.** You will be able to identify the components of skeletal muscle tissue and describe the process of muscle hypertrophy.

8. **The Knee.** You will be able to identify the muscles that support and stabilize the knee and describe the exercises that strengthen and stretch these muscles.

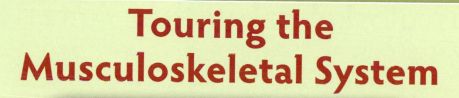

The Musculoskeletal System: Anterior View

5 Become familiar with and use the illustration as a reference point for identifying the deep and superficial muscles of the front of the body in the context of understanding and performing strength training exercises.

Deep Muscles

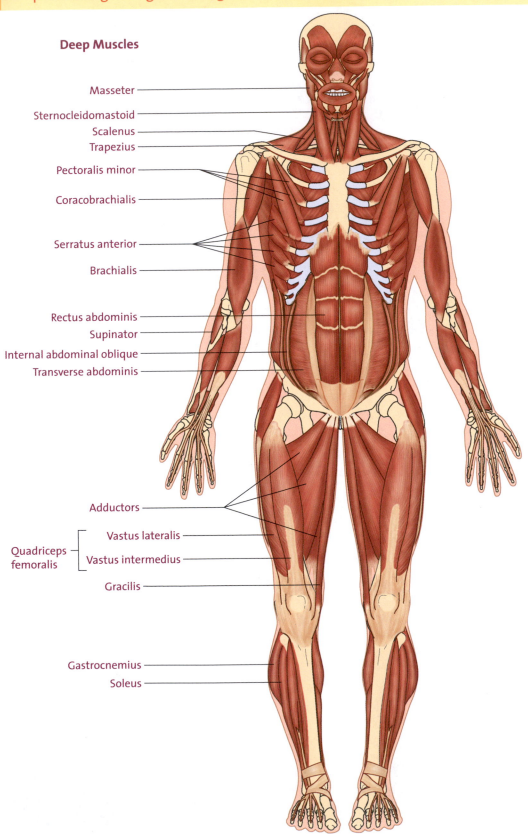

Masseter

Sternocleidomastoid

Scalenus

Trapezius

Pectoralis minor

Coracobrachialis

Serratus anterior

Brachialis

Rectus abdominis

Supinator

Internal abdominal oblique

Transverse abdominis

Adductors

Vastus lateralis

Quadriceps femoralis

Vastus intermedius

Gracilis

Gastrocnemius

Soleus

The Muscular System: Posterior View

Deep Muscles

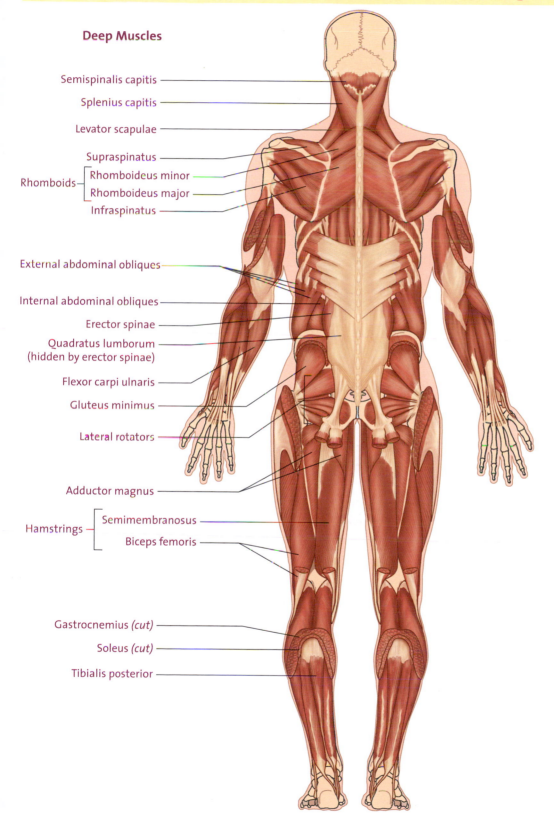

Semispinalis capitis

Splenius capitis

Levator scapulae

Supraspinatus

Rhomboids
- Rhomboideus minor
- Rhomboideus major

Infraspinatus

External abdominal obliques

Internal abdominal obliques

Erector spinae

Quadratus lumborum
(hidden by erector spinae)

Flexor carpi ulnaris

Gluteus minimus

Lateral rotators

Adductor magnus

Hamstrings
- Semimembranosus
- Biceps femoris

Gastrocnemius *(cut)*

Soleus *(cut)*

Tibialis posterior

Muscle Hypertrophy: Gaining Muscle Through Strength Training

Skeletal muscles are found throughout the body; they are attached to bones by tendons. Contraction of skeletal muscles allows the body to maintain posture and move. The number of muscle fibers a person has is set in childhood and does not change.

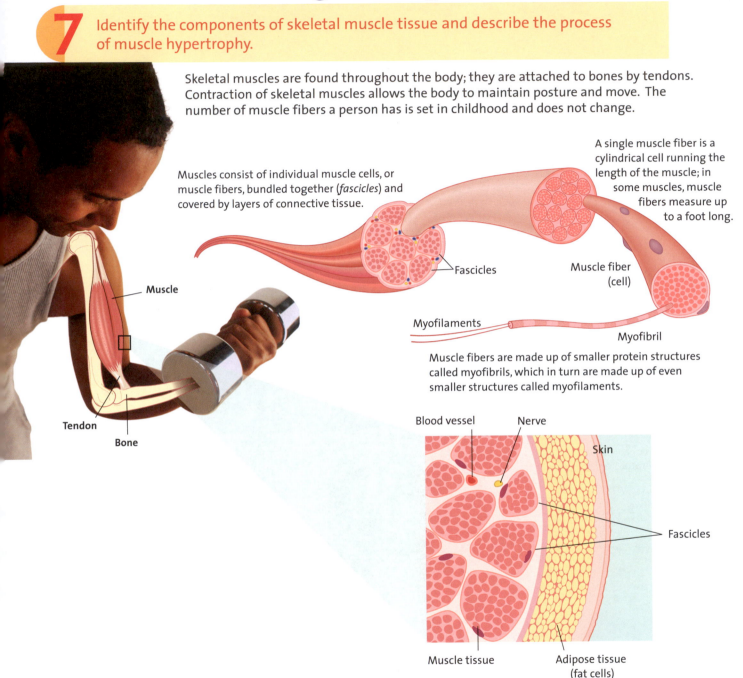

Muscles consist of individual muscle cells, or muscle fibers, bundled together (*fascicles*) and covered by layers of connective tissue.

A single muscle fiber is a cylindrical cell running the length of the muscle; in some muscles, muscle fibers measure up to a foot long.

Muscle
Tendon
Bone

Fascicles
Muscle fiber (cell)
Myofilaments
Myofibril

Muscle fibers are made up of smaller protein structures called myofibrils, which in turn are made up of even smaller structures called myofilaments.

Blood vessel
Nerve
Skin
Fascicles
Muscle tissue
Adipose tissue (fat cells)

The Knee: Supporting and Maintaining Joint Stability

Identify the muscles that support and stabilize the knee, and describe the exercises that strengthen and stretch these muscles.

8

The knee is important both for weight bearing and for locomotion. Because of the stresses and strains placed on this joint, it is often subject to injury. Powerful muscles help provide support for the joint. The development of strength, endurance, and flexibility in these muscles is essential for injury prevention and maintenance of stability of the joint.

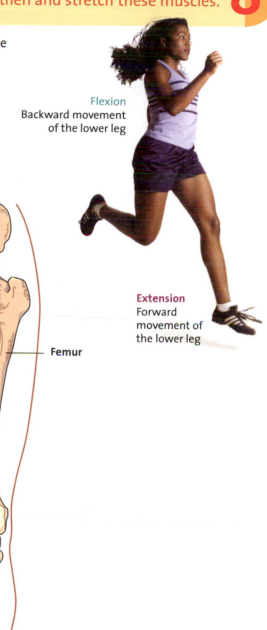

Flexion
Backward movement of the lower leg

Extension
Forward movement of the lower leg

The knee is a hinge joint operating between the femur (thigh bone) and tibia (shin bone). Its primary movements are extension and flexion.

Cartilage
Flexible connective tissue lines the ends of the bones and protects them from wear.

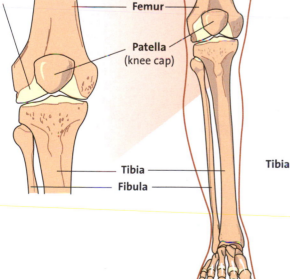

Femur

Patella
(knee cap)

Tibia

Fibula

Femur

Tibia

Anterior   **Posterior**

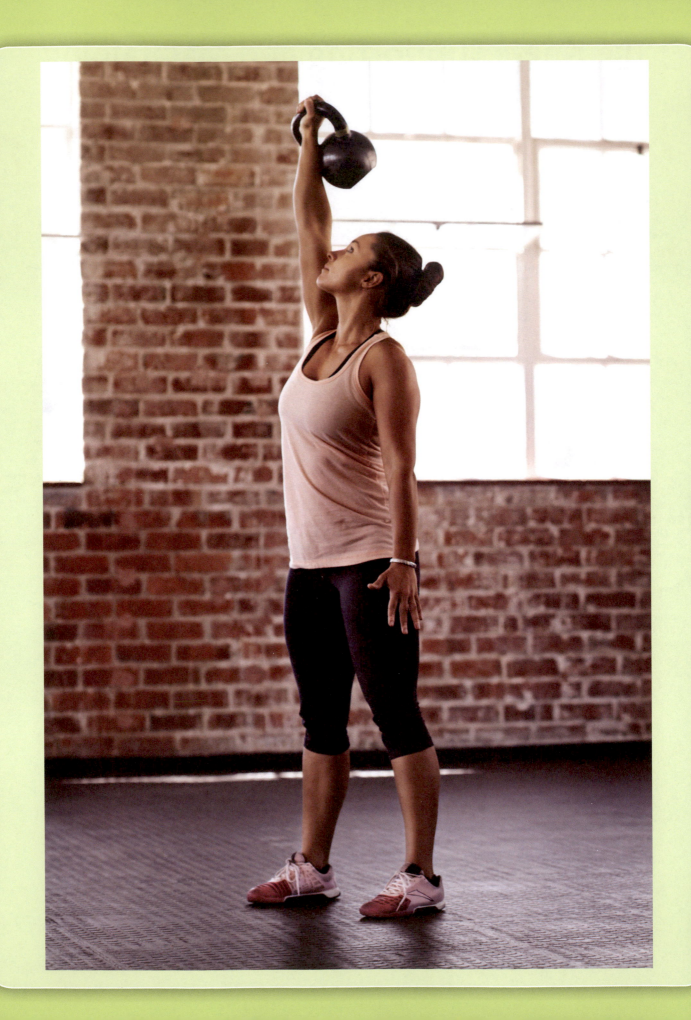

EXERCISE 7 — Thrusters

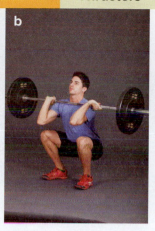
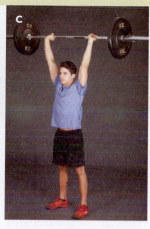
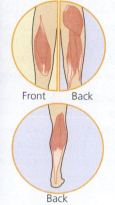
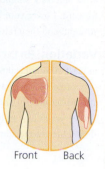

Front   Back

Back   Front   Back

Instructions: **(a)** From a standing position, hold stones, soup cans, dumbbells, or barbells (or a single rock with both hands) at chest level with palms facing outward. **(b)** Squat down until your thighs are parallel with the floor. **(c)** Immediately stand and press the objects overhead in one continuous motion. Lower the objects to the starting position and immediately repeat the exercise.

Muscles developed: Quadriceps, gluteus maximus, hamstrings, gastrocnemius, deltoids, pectoralis major, triceps

EXERCISE 8 — Overhead squats

Instructions: **(a)** Stand holding a broom handle, stones, barbell, or soup cans overhead with straight arms, feet placed slightly more than shoulder-width apart, toes pointed out slightly, head neutral, and back straight. Center your weight over your arches or slightly behind. **(b)** Squat down, keeping your weight centered over your arches, and actively flex the hips (hinge at the hips with buttocks back) until your legs break parallel. During the movement, keep your back straight, shoulders back, and chest out, and let your thighs part to the side so that you are "squatting between your legs." Try to "spread the floor" with your feet. Push up to the starting position, maximizing the use of the posterior hip and thigh muscles, and maintaining a straight back and neutral head position.

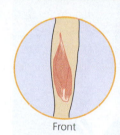

Front

Muscles developed: Quadriceps, gluteus maximus

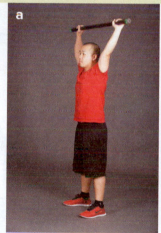
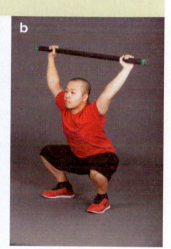

EXERCISE 9 — Front Plank

Instructions: Lying on your front with body straight, raise your body upward, supporting your weight on forearms and toes. Hold the position. Begin with 10-second holds and progress until you can hold the plank for at least two minutes. Breathe normally. Tighten your abs, glutes, and quads as you do this exercise.

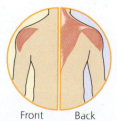
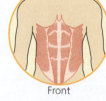

Front   Back   Front

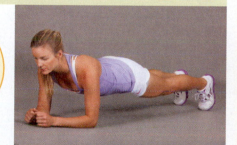

Muscles developed: Rectus abdominis, erector spinae, trapezius, rhomboids, deltoids, pectorals, gluteals

EXERCISE 10 — Push-ups

Instructions: (a) Start in the push-up position with your body weight supported by your hands and feet. Your arms and back should be straight and your fingers pointed forward. Lower your chest to the floor with your back straight, and then return to the starting position.

Variation: (b) Do modified push-ups if you can't do at least 10 regular push-ups. Start with your body weight supported by your hands and knees. Your arms and back should be straight and your fingers pointed forward. Lower your chest to the floor with your back straight, and then return to the starting position.

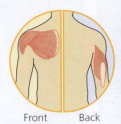

Front   Back

Muscles developed: Pectoralis muscles, triceps, deltoids

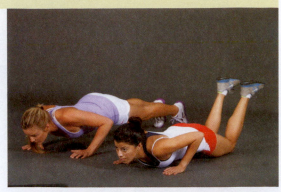

WEIGHT TRAINING EXERCISES Free Weights

EXERCISE 1 — Bench Press

Instructions: (a) Lying on a bench on your back with your feet on the floor, grasp the bar with palms upward and hands shoulder-width apart. If the weight is on a rack, move the bar carefully from the supports to a point over the middle of your chest or slightly above it (at the lower part of the sternum). **(b)** Lower the bar to your chest. Then press it in a straight line to the starting position. Don't arch your back or bounce the bar off your chest. You can also do this exercise with dumbbells or one arm at a time (unilateral training).

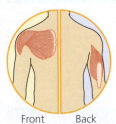

Muscles developed: Pectoralis major, triceps, deltoids

Front   Back

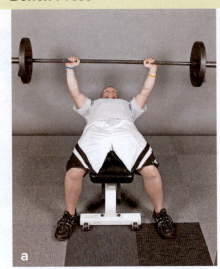

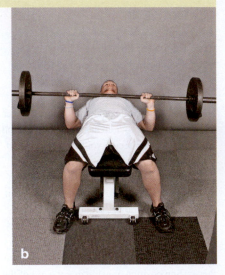

Note: *To allow an optimal view of exercise technique, a spotter does not appear in these demonstration photographs; however, spotters should be used for most exercises with free weights.*

Pull-Up

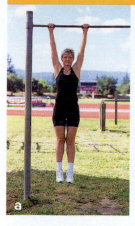

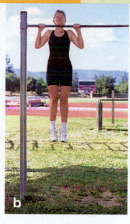

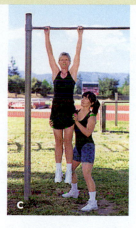

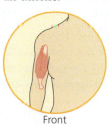

Assisted pull-up: (**c**) This is done as described for a pull-up, except that a spotter assists the person by pushing upward at the waist, hips, or legs during the exercise.

Front

Back

Instructions: (**a**) Begin by grasping the pull-up bar with both hands, palms facing forward and elbows extended fully. (**b**) Pull yourself upward until your chin goes above the bar. Then return to the starting position.

Muscles developed:

Latissimus dorsi, biceps

EXERCISE 3

Shoulder Press (Overhead or Military Press)

Instructions: This exercise can be done standing or seated, with dumbbells or a barbell. The shoulder press begins with the weight at your chest, preferably on a rack. (**a**) Grasp the weight with your palms facing away from you. (**b**) Push the weight overhead until your arms are extended. Then return to the starting position (weight at chest). Be careful not to arch your back excessively.

If you are a more advanced weight trainer, you can "clean" the weight (lift it from the floor to your chest). The clean should be attempted only after instruction from a knowledgeable coach; otherwise, it can lead to injury.

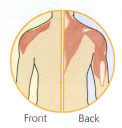

Front   Back

Muscles developed:

Deltoids, triceps, trapezius

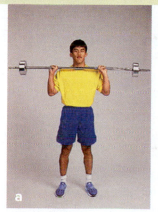

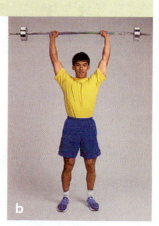

EXERCISE 4

Upright Rowing

Instructions: (**a**) From a standing position with arms extended fully, grasp a barbell with a close grip (hands about 6–12 inches apart) and palms facing the body. (**b**) Raise the bar to about the level of your collarbone, keeping your elbows above bar level at all times. Return to the starting position.

This exercise can be done using dumbbells, a weighted bar (shown), or a barbell.

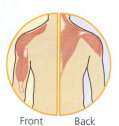

Front   Back

Muscles developed:

Trapezius, deltoids, biceps

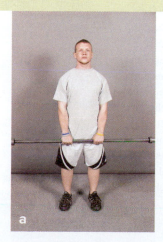

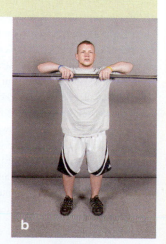

EXERCISE 5 — Biceps Curl

Instructions: (a) From a standing position, grasp the bar with your palms facing away from you and your hands shoulder-width apart. (b) Keeping your upper body rigid, flex (bend) your elbows until the bar reaches a level slightly below the collarbone. Return the bar to the starting position.

This exercise can be done using dumbbells, a curl bar (shown), or a barbell; some people find that using a curl bar places less stress on the wrists.

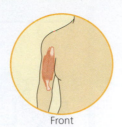

Front

Muscles developed:
Biceps, brachialis

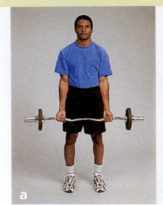

a

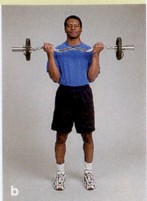

b

EXERCISE 6 — Lateral Raise

Instructions: (a) Stand with feet shoulder-width apart and a dumbbell in each hand. Hold the dumbbells in front of you and parallel to each other. (b) With elbows slightly bent, slowly lift both weights to the side until they reach shoulder level. Keep your wrists in a neutral position, in line with your forearms. Return to the starting position.

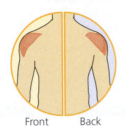

Front   Back

Muscles developed:
Deltoids

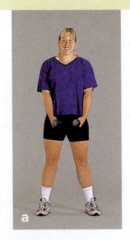

a

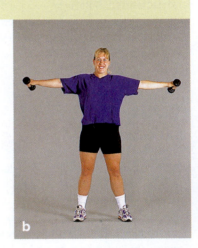

b

EXERCISE 7 — Squat

Instructions: (a) If the bar is racked, place the bar on the fleshy part of your upper back and grasp the bar at shoulder width. Keeping your back straight and head level, remove the bar from the rack and take a step back. Stand with feet slightly more than shoulder-width apart and toes pointed slightly outward. (b) Rest the bar on the back of your shoulders, holding it there with palms facing forward. (c) Keeping your head level and lower back straight and pelvis back, squat down until your thighs are below parallel with the floor. Let your thighs move laterally (outward) so that you "squat between your legs." This will help keep your back straight and keep your heels on the floor. Drive upward toward the starting position, hinging at the hips and keeping your back in a fixed position throughout the exercise.

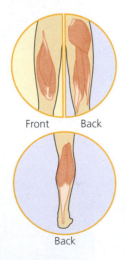

Front   Back

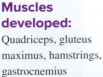

Back

Muscles developed:
Quadriceps, gluteus maximus, hamstrings, gastrocnemius

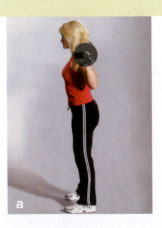

a

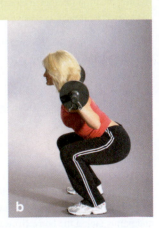

b

EXERCISE 8

Heel Raise

Instructions: Stand with feet shoulder-width apart and toes pointed straight ahead. **(a)** Rest the bar on the back of your shoulders, holding it there with palms facing forward. **(b)** Press down with your toes while lifting your heels. Return to the starting position.

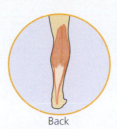

Back

Muscles developed:

Gastrocnemius, soleus

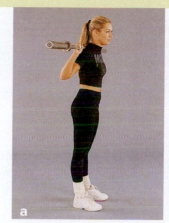

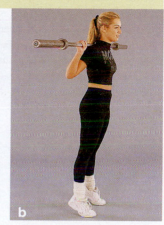

EXERCISE 9

Kettlebell Swing

Instructions: (a) Begin by holding the kettlebell in both hands with palms facing toward you, in a standing position with knees bent, feet placed slightly more than shoulder-width apart, hips flexed, back straight, chest out, and head in a neutral position. **(b)** Holding the kettlebell at knee level, swing the weight to a horizontal position by initiating the motion with the hips, thighs, and abs (tighten the quads, glutes, and ab muscles as hard as you can), keeping your arm straight and relaxed during the movement. Let the weight swing back between your legs in a "football hiking motion" and then repeat the exercise. During the movement, hinge at the hips and not at the spine.

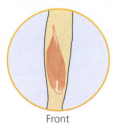

Front

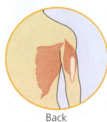

Back

Muscles developed:

Quadriceps, gluteals, latissimus dorsi

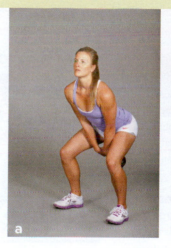

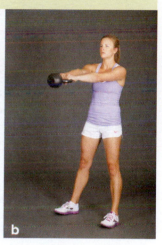

EXERCISE 10

Kettlebell One-Arm Snatch

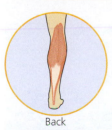

Back

Muscles developed:

Quadriceps, gluteals, latissimus dorsi, shoulder muscles

Instructions: (a) Begin by holding the kettlebell in one hand with your palm facing toward you, in a standing position with knees bent, feet placed slightly more than shoulder-width apart, hips flexed, back straight, chest out, and head in a neutral position.

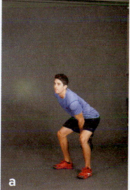

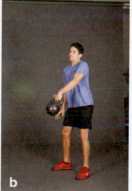

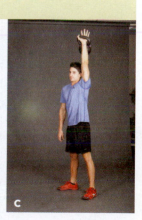

Hold the kettlebell at knee level. **(b)** Swing the weight to a horizontal position by initiating the motion with the hips, thighs, and abs (tighten the quads, glutes, and ab muscles as hard as you can), bending your arm as it approaches the chest and continuing the motion until straightening it overhead. The kettlebell should rotate from the front of your hand to the back during the motion. Use an upward punching motion at the top of the movement to prevent injuring your forearm. **(c)** Let the weight swing back between your legs in a "football hiking motion" and then repeat the exercise. During the movement, hinge at the hips and not at the spine.

EXERCISE 11 — Kettlebell or Dumbbell Carry (Suitcase Carry)

Instructions: This is an excellent exercise for building the core muscles. Pick up a dumbbell or kettlebell in one or both hands. Maintaining good posture, walk 20 to 100 yards carrying the weight. Carry 10 to several hundred pounds, depending on your fitness.

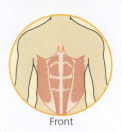

Front

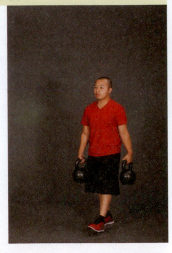

Muscles developed:
Core muscles, trapezius, leg and hip muscles

WEIGHT TRAINING EXERCISES   Weight Machines

EXERCISE 1 — Bench Press (Chest or Vertical Press) Weight Machines

Instructions: Sit or lie on the seat or bench, depending on the type of machine and the manufacturer's instructions. Your back, hips, and buttocks should be pressed against the machine pads. Place your feet on the floor or the foot supports.

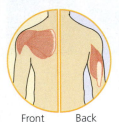

Muscles developed:
Pectoralis major, anterior deltoids, triceps

Front   Back

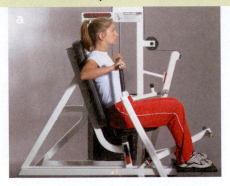

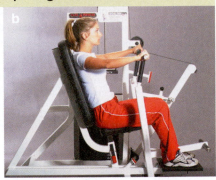

(a) Grasp the handles with your palms facing away from you; the handles should be aligned with your armpits.

(b) Push the bars until your arms are fully extended, but don't lock your elbows. Return to the starting position.

EXERCISE 2 — Lat Pull

Instructions: Begin in a seated or kneeling position, depending on the type of lat machine and the manufacturer's instructions.

Note: *This exercise focuses on the same major muscles as the assisted pull-up (Exercise 3); choose an appropriate exercise for your program based on your preferences and equipment availability.*

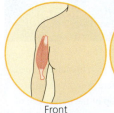

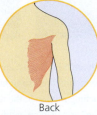

Muscles developed:
Latissimus dorsi, biceps

Front   Back

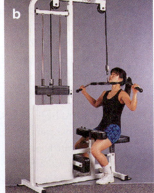

(a) Grasp the bar of the machine with arms fully extended.

(b) Slowly pull the weight down until it reaches the top of your chest. Slowly return to the starting position.

EXERCISE 3 — Assisted Pull-Up

Instructions: Set the weight according to the amount of assistance you need to complete a set of pull-ups—the heavier the weight, the more assistance provided.

(a) Stand or kneel on the assist platform, and grasp the pull-up bar with your elbows fully extended and your palms facing away.

(b) Pull up until your chin goes above the bar, and then return to the starting position.

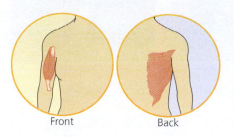

Front   Back

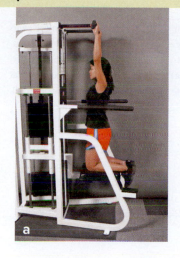

a

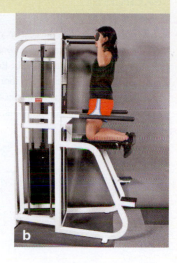

b

Muscles developed: Latissimus dorsi, biceps

EXERCISE 4 — Overhead Press (Shoulder Press)

Instructions: Adjust the seat so your feet are flat on the ground and the hand grips are slightly above your shoulders. **(a)** Sit down, facing away from the machine, and grasp the hand grips with your palms facing forward. **(b)** Press the weight upward until your arms are extended. Return to the starting position.

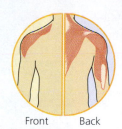

Front   Back

Muscles developed: Deltoids, trapezius, triceps

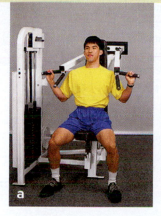

a

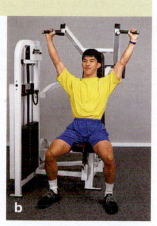

b

EXERCISE 5 — Biceps Curl

Instructions: (a) Adjust the seat so that your back is straight and your arms rest comfortably against the top and side pads. Place your arms on the support cushions and grasp the hand grips with your palms facing up. **(b)** Keeping your upper body still, flex (bend) your elbows until the hand grips almost reach your collarbone. Return to the starting position.

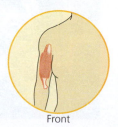

Front

Muscles developed: Biceps, brachialis

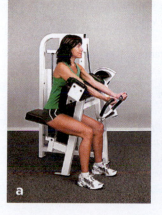

a

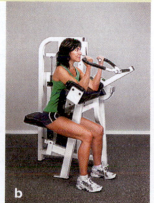

b

Pullover

Instructions: Adjust the seat so your shoulders are aligned with the cams. Push down on the foot pads with your feet to bring the bar forward until you can place your elbows on the pads. Rest your hands lightly on the bar. If possible, place your feet flat on the floor. **(a)** To get into the starting position, let your arms go backward as far as possible. **(b)** Pull your elbows forward until the bar almost touches your abdomen. Return to the starting position.

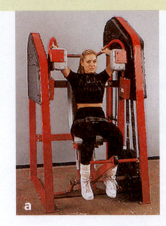
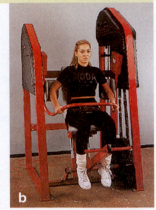

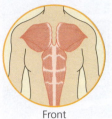
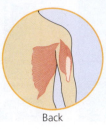

Front   Back

Muscles developed:

Latissimus dorsi, pectoralis major and minor, triceps, rectus abdominis

---

EXERCISE 7

Lateral Raise

Instructions: **(a)** Adjust the seat so the pads rest just above your elbows when your upper arms are at your sides, your elbows are bent, and your forearms are parallel to the floor. Lightly grasp the handles. **(b)** Push outward and up with your arms until the pads are at shoulder height. Lead with your elbows rather than trying to lift the bars with your hands. Return to the starting position.

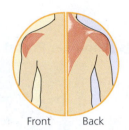

Front   Back

Muscles developed:

Deltoids, trapezius

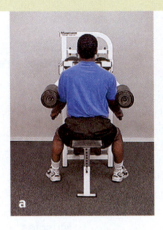
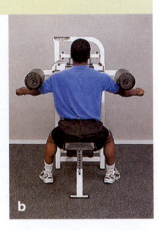

EXERCISE 8

Triceps Extension

Instructions: **(a)** Adjust the seat so your back is straight and your arms rest comfortably against the top and side pads. Place your arms on the support cushions and grasp the hand grips with palms facing inward. **(b)** Keeping your upper body still, extend your elbows as much as possible. Return to the starting position.

Note: *This exercise focuses on some of the same muscles as the Assisted Dip (Exercise 9); choose an appropriate exercise for your program based on your preferences and equipment availability.*

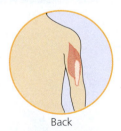

Back

Muscles developed:

Triceps

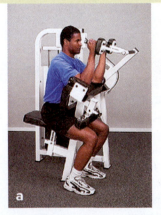
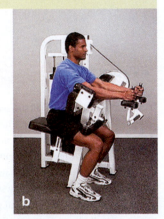

EXERCISE 9　　Assisted Dip

Instructions: Set the weight according to the amount of assistance you need to complete a set of dips—the heavier the weight, the more assistance provided. **(a)** Stand or kneel on the assist platform with your body between the dip bars. With your elbows fully extended and palms facing your body, support your weight on your hands. **(b)** Lower your body until your upper arms are almost parallel with the bars. Then push up until you reach the starting position.

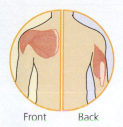

Front　　Back

Muscles developed:
Triceps, deltoids, pectoralis major

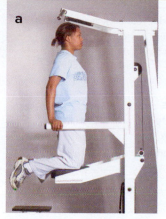

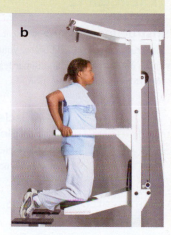

EXERCISE 10　　Leg Press

Instructions: Sit or lie on the seat or bench, depending on the type of machine and the manufacturer's instructions. Your head, back, hips, and buttocks should be pressed against the machine pads. Loosely grasp the handles at the side of the machine. **(a)** Begin with your feet flat on the foot platform about shoulder-width apart. Extend your legs, but do not forcefully lock your knees. **(b)** Slowly lower the weight by bending your knees and flexing your hips until your knees are bent at about a 90-degree angle or your heels start to lift off the foot platform. Keep your lower back flat against the support pad. Then extend your knees and return to the starting position.

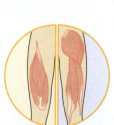

Front　　Back

Muscles developed:
Gluteus maximus, quadriceps, hamstrings

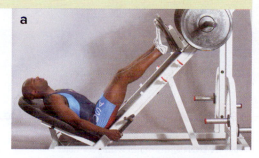

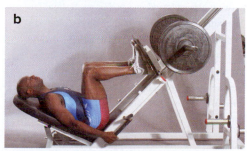

EXERCISE 11　　Leg Extension (Knee Extension)

Instructions: **(a)** Adjust the seat so the pads rest comfortably on top of your lower shins. Loosely grasp the handles. **(b)** Extend your knees until they are almost straight. Return to the starting position.

Knee extensions cause kneecap pain in some people. If you have kneecap pain during this exercise, check with an orthopedic specialist before repeating it.

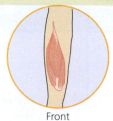

Front

Muscles developed:
Quadriceps

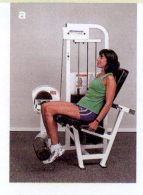

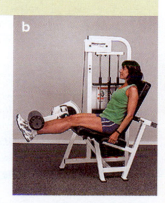

Seated Leg Curl

Instructions: **(a)** Sit on the seat with your back against the back pad and the leg pad below your calf muscles. **(b)** Flex your knees until your lower and upper legs form a 90-degree angle. Return to the starting position.

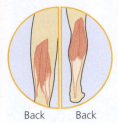

Muscles developed:
Hamstrings, gastrocnemius

Back   Back

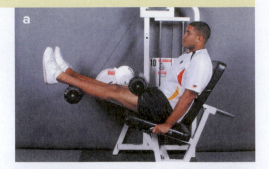
a

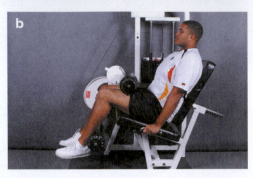
b

EXERCISE 13

Heel Raise

Instructions: **(a)** Stand with your head between the pads and one pad on each shoulder. The balls of your feet should be on the platform. Lightly grasp the handles. **(b)** Press down with your toes while lifting your heels. Return to the starting position. Changing the direction your feet are pointing (straight ahead, inward, and outward) will work different portions of your calf muscles.

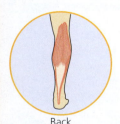

Muscles developed:
Gastrocnemius, soleus

Back

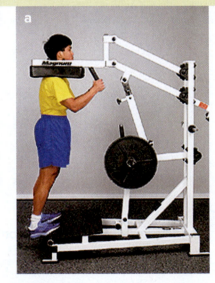
a

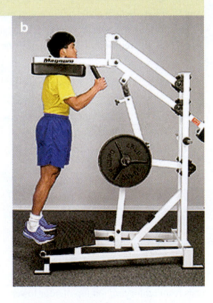
b

Note: *Abdominal machines, low-back machines, and trunk rotation machines are not recommended because of injury risk. Refer to the "Body Weight" and "Free Weights" exercise sections for appropriate exercises to strengthen the abdominal and low-back muscles. For the rectus abdominis, obliques,* *and transverse abdominis, perform curl-ups (Exercise 4 in the "Body Weight" section), and for the erector spinae and quadratus lumborum, perform the spine extension and the isometric side bridge (Exercises 5 and 6 in the "Body Weight" section).*

COMMON QUESTIONS ANSWERED

Q **Will I gain weight if I do resistance exercises?**

A Your weight probably will not change significantly as a result of a general fitness program: one set of 8–12 repetitions of 8–10 exercises, performed on at least two nonconsecutive days per week. You will lose body fat but also increase muscle mass, so your weight will stay about the same. You may notice a change in how your clothes fit, however, because muscle is denser than fat. Increased muscle mass will help you control body fat. Muscle increases your metabolism, which means you burn more calories every day. If you combine resistance exercises with endurance exercises, you will be on your way to developing a healthier body composition. Concentrate on fat loss rather than weight loss.

Q **Do I need more protein in my diet when I train with weights?**

A No. Although there is some evidence that power athletes involved in heavy training have a higher-than-normal protein requirement, there is no reason for most people to consume extra protein. Most Americans take in more protein than they need, so even if there is an increased protein need during heavy training, it is probably supplied by the average diet. Consuming a protein-rich snack before or after training may promote muscle hypertrophy.

Q **What causes muscle soreness the day or two following a weight training workout?**

A The muscle pain you feel a day or two after a heavy weight training workout is caused by injury to the muscle fibers and surrounding connective tissue. Contrary to popular belief, delayed-onset muscle soreness is not caused by lactic acid buildup. Scientists believe that injury to muscle fibers causes inflammation, which in turn causes the release of chemicals that break down part of the muscle tissue and cause pain. After a bout of intense exercise that causes muscle injury and delayed-onset muscle soreness, the muscles produce protective proteins that prevent soreness during future workouts. If you don't work out regularly, you lose these protective proteins and become susceptible to soreness again.

Q **Will strength training improve my sports performance?**

A Strength developed in the weight room does not automatically increase your power in sports such as skiing, tennis, or cycling. Hitting a forehand in tennis and making a turn on skis are precise skills that require coordination between your nervous system and muscles. For skilled people, movements become reflex; you don't think about them when you do them. Increasing strength can disturb this coordination. Only by simultaneously practicing a sport and improving fitness can you expect to become more powerful in the skill. Practice helps you integrate your new strength with your skills, which makes you more powerful. Consequently, you can hit the ball harder in tennis or make more forceful turns on the ski slopes. (Refer to Chapter 2 for more on the concept of specificity in physical training.)

Q **Will I improve faster if I train every day?**

A No. Your muscles need time to recover between training sessions. Doing resistance exercises every day will cause you to become overtrained, which will increase your chance of injury and impede your progress. If your strength training program reaches a plateau, try one of these strategies:

• Vary the number of sets. If you have been performing one set of each exercise, add sets.

• Train less frequently. If you are currently training the same muscle groups three or more times per week, you may not be allowing your muscles to fully recover from intense workouts.

• Change exercises. Using different exercises for the same muscle group may stimulate further strength development.

• Vary the load and number of repetitions. Try increasing or decreasing the loads you are using and changing the number of repetitions accordingly.

• If you are training alone, find a motivated training partner. A partner can encourage you and assist you with difficult lifts, forcing you to work harder.

Q **If I stop training, will my muscles turn to fat?**

A No. Fat and muscle are two different kinds of tissue, and one cannot turn into the other. Muscles that aren't used become smaller (atrophy), and body fat may increase if caloric intake exceeds calories burned. Although the result of inactivity may be smaller muscles and more fat, the change is caused by two separate processes.

Q **Should I wear a weight belt when I lift?**

A Until recently, most experts advised people to wear weight belts. However, several studies have shown that weight belts do not prevent back injuries and may, in fact, increase the risk of injury by encouraging people to lift more weight than they are capable of lifting with good form. Although wearing a belt may allow you to lift more weight in some lifts, you may not get the full benefit of your program because use of a weight belt reduces the effectiveness of the workout on the muscles that help support your spine.

SUMMARY

• Hypertrophy (increased muscle fiber size) occurs when weight training causes the size and number of myofibrils to increase, thereby increasing total muscle size. Strength also increases through muscle learning. Most women do not develop large muscles from weight training.

• Improvements in muscular strength and endurance lead to enhanced physical performance, protection against injury, improved body composition, better self-image, improved muscle and bone health with aging, reduced risk of chronic disease, and decreased risk of premature death.

• Muscular strength can be assessed by determining the amount of weight that can be lifted in one repetition of an exercise. Muscular endurance can be assessed by determining the number of repetitions of a particular exercise that can be performed.

• Static (isometric) exercises involve contraction without movement. They are most useful when a person is recovering from an injury or surgery or needs to overcome weak points in a range of motion.

• Dynamic (isotonic) exercises involve contraction that results in movement. The two most common types are constant resistance (free weights and body weight) and variable resistance (many weight machines).

• Free weights and weight machines have pluses and minuses for developing fitness, although machines tend to be safer.

• Lifting heavy weights for only a few repetitions helps develop strength. Lifting lighter weights for more repetitions helps develop muscular endurance.

• A strength training program for general fitness includes at least one set of 8–12 repetitions (enough to cause fatigue) of 8–10 exercises, along with warm-up and cool-down periods. The program should be carried out at least two nonconsecutive days per week.

• Safety guidelines for strength training include using proper technique, using spotters and collars when necessary, and taking care of injuries.

• Supplements or drugs that are promoted as instant or quick "cures" usually don't work and are either dangerous, expensive, or both.

FOR FURTHER EXPLORATION

American College of Sports Medicine Position Stand: Progression Models in Resistance Training for Healthy Adults. Provides an in-depth look at strategies for setting up a strength training program and making progress based on individual program goals.

http://journals.lww.com/acsm-msse/Fulltext/2009/03000/Progression_Models_in_Resistance_Training_for.26.aspx

Centers for Disease Control and Prevention. Podcast on problems associated with over-consumption of energy drinks.

http://www2c.cdc.gov/podcasts/player.asp?f=8626332

Dan John. An excellent website for people serious about improving strength and fitness, written by a world-class athlete and coach in track and field and Highland games.

http://danjohn.net

Human Anatomy On-line. Provides text, illustrations, and animation about the muscular system, nerve-muscle connections, muscular contraction, and other topics.

http://www.innerbody.com/htm/body.html

Mayo Clinic: Weight Training: Improve Your Muscular Fitness. Provides a basic overview of weight training essentials along with links to many other articles on specific weight training-related topics.

http://www.mayoclinic.com/health/weight-training/HQ01627

National Strength and Conditioning Association. A professional organization that focuses on strength development for fitness and athletic performance.

http://www.nsca-lift.org

Pilates Method Alliance. Provides information about Pilates and about instructor certification; includes a directory of instructors.

http://www.pilatesmethodalliance.org

University of California, San Diego: Muscle Physiology Home Page. Provides an introduction to muscle physiology, including information about types of muscle fibers and energy cycles.

http://muscle.ucsd.edu/index.shtml

University of Michigan: Muscles in Action. Interactive descriptions of muscle movements.

http://www.med.umich.edu/lrc/Hypermuscle/Hyper.html

Yoga Alliance A resource site for yoga instructors and people interested in yoga.

http://www.yogaalliance.org

See also the listings in Chapter 2.

SELECTED BIBLIOGRAPHY

American College of Sports Medicine. 2013. *ACSM's Resource Manual for Guidelines for Exercise Testing and Prescription,* 7th ed. Philadelphia: Lippincott Williams and Wilkins.

American College of Sports Medicine. 2011. American College of Sports Medicine position stand: progression models in resistance training for healthy adults. *Medicine and Science in Sports and Exercise* 43(7): 1334–1359.

American College of Sports Medicine. 2013. *ACSM's Guidelines for Exercise Testing and Prescription,* 9th ed. Philadelphia: Wolters Kluwer/Lippincott Williams & Wilkins Health.

Baechle, T., and R. W. Earl. 2008. *National Strength and Conditioning Association's Essentials of Strength and Conditioning.* Champaign, Ill.: Human Kinetics.

Behm, D. G., et al. 2010. Canadian Society for Exercise Physiology position stand: The use of instability to train the core in athletic and nonathletic conditioning. *Applied Physiology Nutrition and Metabolism* 35(1): 109–112.

Bompa, T., M. Di Pasquale, and L. Cornacchia. 2013. *Serious Strength Training.* Champaign, Ill.: Human Kinetics.

Brooks, G. A., et al. 2005. *Exercise Physiology: Human Bioenergetics and Its Applications,* 4th ed. New York: McGraw-Hill.

Campbell, B. 2013. International Society of Sports Nutrition position stand: energy drinks. *Journal of the International Society of Sports Nutrition* 10:1.

Cermak, N. M., et al. 2013. Perspective: Protein supplementation during prolonged resistance type exercise training augments skeletal muscle mass and strength gains. *Journal American Medical Directors Association* 14(1): 71–72.

Delavier, F. 2010. *Strength Training Anatomy,* 3rd ed. Champaign, Ill.: Human Kinetics.

Deutz, N. E., et al. 2014. Protein intake and exercise for optimal muscle function with aging: recommendations from the ESPEN Expert Group. *Clinical Nutrition* 33(6): 929–936.

Earnest, C. P., et al. 2013. Cardiometabolic risk factors and metabolic syndrome in the Aerobics Center Longitudinal Study. *Mayo Clinics Proceedings.* 88(3): 259–270.

Fahey, T. D. 2011. *Basic Weight Training for Men and Women,* 8th ed. New York: McGraw-Hill.

Farrar, R. E., et al. 2010. Oxygen cost of kettlebell swings. *Journal of Strength and Conditioning Research* 24(4): 1034–1036.

Goldstein, E. R., et al. 2010. International Society of Sports Nutrition position stand: caffeine. *Journal of the International Society of Sports Nutrition* 7: 5.

Goodwill, A. M., et al. 2012. Corticomotor plasticity following unilateral strength training. *Muscle Nerve* 46(3): 384–393.

Gremeaux, V., et al. 2012. Exercise and longevity. *Maturitas* 73(4): 312–317.

Grontved, A., et al. 2012. A prospective study of weight training and risk of type 2 diabetes mellitus in men. *Archives Internal Medicine* 172(17): 1306–1312.

Hackett, D. A., et al. 2012. Training practices and ergogenic aids used by male bodybuilders. *Journal of Strength and Conditioning Research.* Published online.

Heikkinen, A., et al. 2011. Use of dietary supplements in Olympic athletes is decreasing: A follow-up study between 2002 and 2009. *Journal of the International Society of Sports Nutrition* 8(1): 1.

Hoppeler, H. 2013. *Eccentric Exercise: Muscle Physiology in Sport, Rehabilitation and Health.* London: Routledge.

Jay, K., et al. 2011. Kettlebell training for musculoskeletal and cardiovascular health: A randomized controlled trial. *Scandinavian Journal of Work and Environmental Health* 37(3): 196–203.

Jeffreys, I. and J. Moody. 2013. *Strength and Conditioning for Sports Performance.* London: Routledge.

John, D. 2013. *Intervention: Course Correction for the Athlete and Trainer.* Santa Cruz, Calif: On Target Publications.

Kang, J. 2012. *Nutrition and Metabolism in Sports, Exercise, and Health.* London: Routledge.

Karelis, A. D. 2013. Muscle strength during adolescence is associated with longevity. *Evidence Based Medicine.* Published online.

Karelis, A. D. 2013. Muscle strength during adolescence is associated with longevity. *Evidence Based Medicine* 18(5): e48.

Kilgour, A. H., et al. 2014. A systematic review of the evidence that brain structure is related to muscle structure and their relationship to brain and muscle function in humans over the lifecourse. *Biomedical Central (BMC) Geriatrics* 14: 85.

Lee, B. and S. McGill. 2015. The Effect of Long Term Isometric Training on Core/Torso Stiffness. *Journal Strength Conditioning Research,* published online March 23, 2015.

Leopoldino, A. A., et al. 2013. Effect of Pilates on sleep quality and quality of life of sedentary population. *Journal of Bodyworks and Movement Therapy* 17(1): 5–10.

Lundberg, T. R., et al. 2013. Aerobic exercise does not compromise muscle hypertrophy response to short-term resistance training. *Journal of Applied Physiology* 114(1): 81–89.

Maughan, R. J., and S. Shirreffs. 2013. *Food, Nutrition, and Sports Performance III.* London: Routledge.

Oksuzyan, A., et al. 2010. Sex differences in the level and rate of change of physical function and grip strength in the Danish 1905-cohort study. *Journal Aging Health* 22(5): 589–610.

Outram, S. and B. Stewart. 2015. Doping through supplement use: A review of the available empirical data. *International Journal Sports Nutrition Exercise Metabolism* 25(1): 54–59.

Pasiakos, S. M., et al. 2015. The effects of protein supplements on muscle mass, strength, and aerobic and anaerobic power in healthy adults: a systematic review. *Sports Medicine* 45(1): 111–131.

Pattyn, N., et al. 2013. The effect of exercise on the cardiovascular risk factors constituting the metabolic syndrome: a meta-analysis of controlled trials. *Sports Medicine* 43(2): 121–133.

Ruiz, J. R., et al. 2008. Association between muscular strength and mortality in men: Prospective cohort study. *British Medical Journal* 337: a439. Published online.

Saeterbakken, A. H., et al. 2011. A comparison of muscle activity and 1-RM strength of three chest-press exercises with different stability requirements. *Journal of Sports Science:* 1–6.

Saeterbakken, A. H., and M. S. Fimland. 2013. Electromyographic activity and 6RM strength in bench press on stable and unstable surfaces. *Journal of Strength and Conditioning Research* 27(4): 1101–1107.

Sanchis-Gomar, F., et al. 2014. 'Olympic' centenarians: Are they just biologically exceptional? *International Journal Cardiology* 175(1): 216–217.

Sattler, F. R. 2013. Growth hormone in the aging male. *Best Practices & Research Clinical Endocrinology Metabolism* 27(4): 541–555.

Sawyer, B. J., et al. 2015. Predictors of fat mass changes in response to aerobic exercise training in women. *Journal Strength Conditioning Research* 29(2): 297–304.

Senchina, D. S., et al. 2011. BJSM reviews: A–Z of nutritional supplements: dietary supplements, sports nutrition foods and ergogenic aids for health and performance—Part 17. *British Journal Sports Medicine* 45(2): 150–151.

Simao, R., et al. 2012. Exercise order in resistance training. *Sports Medicine* 42(3): 251–265.

Spence, A. L., et al. 2013. A prospective randomized longitudinal study involving 6 months of endurance or resistance exercise. Conduit artery adaptation in humans. *Journal of Physiology* 591(Pt 5): 1265–1275.

Tsatsouline, P. 2010. *Enter the Kettlebell.* Minneapolis, Minn.: Dragon Door Publications.

Tucker, M. A., et al. 2013. The effect of caffeine on maximal oxygen uptake and vertical jump performance in male basketball players. *Journal of Strength and Conditioning Research* 27(2): 382–387.

Vechin, F. C., et al. 2015. Comparisons between low-intensity resistance training with blood flow restriction and high-intensity resistance training on quadriceps muscle mass and strength in elderly. *Journal Strength Conditioning Research* 29(4): 1071–1076.

Villanueva, M. G., et al. 2015. Short rest interval lengths between sets optimally enhance body composition and performance with 8 weeks of strength resistance training in older men. *European Journal Applied Physiology* 115(2): 295–308.

Watanabe, Y., et al. 2013. Increased muscle size and strength from slow-movement, low-intensity resistance exercise and tonic force generation. *Journal of Aging and Physical Activity* 21(1): 71–84.

Wells, C., et al. 2012. Defining Pilates exercise: a systematic review. *Complementary Therapies in Medicine* 20(4): 253–262.

Wilson, J. M., et al. 2013. International Society of Sports Nutrition Position Stand: beta-hydroxy-beta-methylbutyrate (HMB). *Journal International Society Sports Nutrition* 10(1): 6.

Name _____ Section _____ Date _____

LAB 4.1   Assessing Your Current Level of Muscular Strength

For best results, don't do any strenuous weight training within 48 hours of any test. Use great caution when completing 1-RM tests; do not take the maximum bench press test if you have any injuries to your shoulders, elbows, back, hips, or knees. In addition, do not take these tests until you have had at least one month of weight training experience.

The Maximum Bench Press Test

Equipment

The free weights bench press test uses the following equipment

1. Flat bench (with or without racks)
2. Barbell
3. Assorted weight plates with collars to hold them in place
4. One or two spotters
5. Weight scale

If a weight machine is preferred, use the following equipment:

1. Bench press machine
2. Weight scale

Preparation

Try a few bench presses with a small amount of weight so you can practice your technique, warm up your muscles, and, if you use free weights, coordinate your movements with those of your spotters. Weigh yourself and record the results.

Body weight: _____ lb.

Instructions

1. Use a weight that is lower than the amount you believe you can lift. For free weights, men should begin with a weight about two-thirds of their body weight; women should begin with the weight of just the bar (45 lb).

2. Lie on the bench with your feet firmly on the floor. If you are using a weight machine, grasp the handles with palms away from you; the tops of the handles should be aligned with the tops of your armpits.

    If you are using free weights, grasp the bar slightly wider than shoulder width with your palms away from you. If you have one spotter, she or he should stand directly behind the bench; if you have two spotters, they should stand to the side, one at each end of the barbell. Signal to the spotter when you are ready to begin the test by saying, "1, 2, 3." On "3," the spotter should help you lift the weight to a point over your midchest (nipple line).

3. Push the handles or barbell until your arms are fully extended. Exhale as you lift. If you are using free weights, the weight moves from a low point at the chest straight up. Keep your feet firmly on the floor, don't arch your back, and push the weight evenly with your right and left arms. Don't bounce the weight on your chest.

4. Rest for several minutes, then repeat the lift with a heavier weight. It will probably take several attempts to determine the maximum amount of weight you can lift (1 RM).

    1 RM: _____ lb

    Check one: _____ Free weights _____ Universal _____ Other

5. If you used free weights, convert your free weights bench press score to an estimated value for 1 RM on the Universal bench press or other bench press machine using the appropriate formula:

    Males: Estimated Universal 1 RM = (1.016 × free weights 1 RM _____ lb) + 18.41 = _____ lb

    Females: Estimated Universal 1 RM = (0.848 × free weights 1 RM _____ lb) + 21.37 = _____ lb

(Note: this formula might not be accurate on other bench press machines.)

LABORATORY ACTIVITIES

Rating Your Bench Press Result

1. Divide your 1-RM value by your body weight.

   1 RM _____ lb ÷ body weight _____ lb = _____

2. Find this ratio in the table to determine your bench press strength rating. Record the rating here and in the chart at the end of this lab. Bench press strength rating: _____

Strength Ratings for the Maximum Bench Press Test

	Pounds Lifted/Body Weight (lb)					
Men	*Very Poor*	*Poor*	*Fair*	*Good*	*Excellent*	*Superior*
Age: Under 20	Below 0.89	0.89–1.05	1.06–1.18	1.19–1.33	1.34–1.75	Above 1.75
20–29	Below 0.88	0.88–0.98	0.99–1.13	1.14–1.31	1.32–1.62	Above 1.62
30–39	Below 0.78	0.78–0.87	0.88–0.97	0.98–1.11	1.12–1.34	Above 1.34
40–49	Below 0.72	0.72–0.79	0.80–0.87	0.88–0.99	1.00–1.19	Above 1.19
50–59	Below 0.63	0.63–0.70	0.71–0.78	0.79–0.89	0.90–1.04	Above 1.04
60 and over	Below 0.57	0.57–0.65	0.66–0.71	0.72–0.81	0.82–0.93	Above 0.93
Women						
Age: Under 20	Below 0.53	0.53–0.57	0.58–0.64	0.65–0.76	0.77–0.87	Above 0.87
20–29	Below 0.51	0.51–0.58	0.59–0.69	0.70–0.79	0.80–1.00	Above 1.00
30–39	Below 0.47	0.47–0.52	0.53–0.59	0.60–0.69	0.70–0.81	Above 0.81
40–49	Below 0.43	0.43–0.49	0.50–0.53	0.54–0.61	0.62–0.76	Above 0.76
50–59	Below 0.39	0.39–0.43	0.44–0.47	0.48–0.54	0.55–0.67	Above 0.67
60 and over	Below 0.38	0.38–0.42	0.43–0.46	0.47–0.53	0.54–0.71	Above 0.71

SOURCE: Based on norms from The Cooper Institute of Aerobic Research, Dallas, Tex; from *The Physical Fitness Specialist Manual,* revised 2005. Used with permission.

Predicting 1 RM from Multiple-Repetition Lifts Using Free Weights

Instead of doing the 1-RM maximum strength bench press test, you can predict your 1 RM from multiple-repetition lifts.

Instructions

1. Choose a weight you think you can bench press five times.

2. Follow the instructions for lifting the weight given in the maximum bench press test.

3. Do as many repetitions of the bench press as you can. A repetition counts only if done correctly

4. Refer to the chart on p. 131, or calculate predicted 1 RM using the Brzycki equation:

   $1 \text{ RM} = weight ÷ (1.0278 − [0.0278 × number\ of\ repetitions])$

   1 RM = _____ lb ÷ (1.0278 − [0.0278 × _____ repetitions]) = _____

5. Divide your predicted 1-RM value by your body weight.

   1 RM _____ lb ÷ body weight _____ lb = _____

6. Find this ratio in the table above to determine your bench press strength rating. Record the rating here and in the chart at the end of the lab.

   Bench press strength rating: _____

Weight Lifted (lb.)	Repetitions											
	1	2	3	4	5	6	7	8	9	10	11	12
66	66	68	70	72	74	77	79	82	85	88	91	95
77	77	79	82	84	87	89	92	96	99	103	107	111
88	88	91	93	96	99	102	106	109	113	117	122	127
99	99	102	105	108	111	115	119	123	127	132	137	143
110	110	113	116	120	124	128	132	137	141	147	152	158
121	121	124	128	132	136	141	145	150	156	161	168	174
132	132	136	140	144	149	153	158	164	170	176	183	190
143	143	147	151	156	161	166	172	178	184	191	198	206
154	154	158	163	168	173	179	185	191	198	205	213	222
165	165	170	175	180	186	192	198	205	212	220	229	238
176	176	181	186	192	198	204	211	219	226	235	244	254
187	187	192	198	204	210	217	224	232	240	249	259	269
198	198	204	210	216	223	230	238	246	255	264	274	285
209	209	215	221	228	235	243	251	259	269	279	289	301
220	220	226	233	240	248	256	264	273	283	293	305	317
231	231	238	245	252	260	268	277	287	297	308	320	333
242	242	249	256	264	272	281	290	300	311	323	335	349
253	253	260	268	276	285	294	304	314	325	337	350	364
264	264	272	280	288	297	307	317	328	340	352	366	380
275	275	283	291	300	309	319	330	341	354	367	381	396
286	286	294	303	312	322	332	343	355	368	381	396	412
297	297	305	314	324	334	345	356	369	382	396	411	428
308	308	317	326	336	347	358	370	382	396	411	427	444

SOURCE: Brzycki, M. Strength testing—predicting a one-rep max from reps to fatigue. *The Journal of Physical Education, Recreation and Dance* 64 (January 1993): 88–90. A publication of the American Alliance for Health, Physical Education, Recreation and Dance, www.aahperd.org. Reprinted with permission.

Functional Lower Body Movement Tests

The following tests assess functional leg movement skills using squats. Most people do squats improperly, increasing their risk of knee and back pain. Before you add weight-bearing squats to your weight training program, you should determine your functional leg movement skills, check your ability to squat properly, and give yourself a chance to master squatting movements. The following leg strength tests will help you in each of these areas.

These tests are progressively more difficult, so do not move to the next test until you have scored at least a 3 on the current test. On each test, give yourself a rating of 0, 1, 3, or 5, as described in the instructions that follow the last test.

1. Chair Squat

Instructions

1. Sit up straight in a chair with your back resting against the backrest and your arms at your sides. Your feet should be placed more than shoulder-width apart so that you can get them under the body.

2. Begin the motion of rising out of the chair by flexing (bending) at the hips—not the back. Then squat up using a hip hinge movement (no spine movement). Stand without rocking forward, bending your back, or using external support, and keep your head in a neutral position.

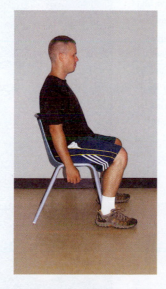
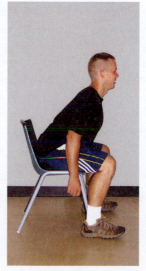
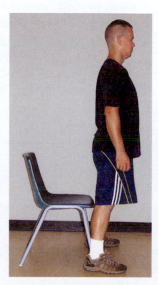

3. Return to the sitting position while maintaining a straight back and keeping your weight centered over your feet. Your thighs should abduct (spread) as you sit back in the chair. Use your rear hip and thigh muscles as much as possible as you sit.

Do five repetitions.

Your rating: _____

(See rating instructions that follow.)

2. Single-Leg Step-Up

Instructions

1. Stand facing a bench, with your right foot placed on the middle of the bench, right knee bent at 90 degrees, and arms at your sides.

2. Step up on the bench until your right leg is straight, maximizing the use of the hip muscles.

3. Return to the starting position. Keep your hips stable, back straight, chest up, shoulders back, and head neutral during the entire movement.

Do five repetitions for each leg.

Your rating: _____

(See rating instructions that follow.)

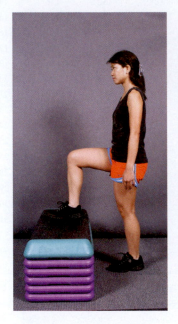
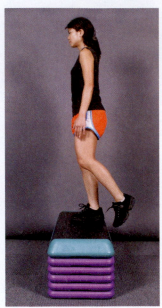

3. Unweighted Squat

Instructions

1. Stand with your feet placed slightly more than shoulder-width apart, toes pointed out slightly, hands on hips or across your chest, head neutral, and back straight. Center your weight over your arches or slightly behind.

2. Squat down, keeping your weight centered over your arches and actively flexing (bending) your hips until your legs break parallel. During the movement, keep your back straight, shoulders back, and chest out, and let your thighs part to the side so that you are "squatting between your legs."

3. Push back up to the starting position, hinging at the hips and not with the spine, maximizing the use of the rear hip and thigh muscles, and maintaining a straight back and neutral head position.

Do five repetitions.

Your rating: _____

(See rating instructions that follow.)

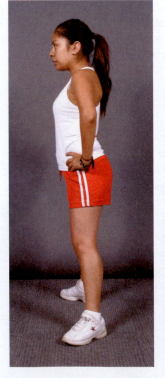
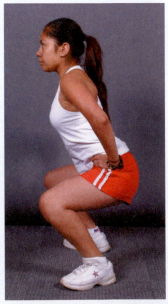

4. Single-Leg Lunge-Squat with Rear-Foot Support

Instructions

1. Stand about three feet in front of a bench (with your back to the bench).

2. Place the top of your left foot on the bench, and put most of your weight on your right leg (your left leg should be bent), with your hands at your sides.

3. Squat on your right leg until your thigh is parallel with the floor. Keep your back straight, chest up, shoulders back, and head neutral.

4. Return to the starting position.

Do three repetitions for each leg.

Your rating: _____

(See rating instructions that follow.)

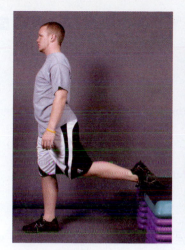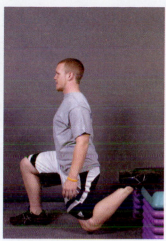

Rating Your Functional Leg Strength Test Results

5 points: Performed the exercise properly with good back and thigh position, weight centered over the middle or rear of the foot, chest out, and shoulders back; good use of hip muscles on the way down and on the way up, with head in a neutral position throughout the movement; maintained good form during all repetitions; abducted (spread) the thighs on the way down during chair squats and double-leg squats; for single-leg exercises, showed good strength on both sides; for single-leg lunge-squat with rear-foot support, maintained straight back, and knees stayed behind toes.

3 points: Weight was forward on the toes, with some rounding of the back; used thigh muscles excessively, with little use of hip muscles; head and chest were too far forward; showed little abduction of the thighs during double-leg squats; when going down for single-leg exercises, one side was stronger than the other; form deteriorated with repetitions; for single-leg lunge-squat with rear-foot support, could not reach parallel (thigh parallel with floor).

1 point: Had difficulty performing the movement, rocking forward and rounding back badly; used thigh muscles excessively, with little use of hip muscles on the way up or on the way down; chest and head were forward; on unweighted squats, had difficulty reaching parallel and showed little abduction of the thighs; on single-leg exercises, one leg was markedly stronger than the other; could not perform multiple repetitions.

0 points: Could not perform the exercise.

Summary of Results

Maximum bench press test from either the 1-RM test or the multiple-repetition test: Weight pressed: _____ lb Rating: _____

Functional leg strength tests (0–5): Chair squat: _____ Single-leg step-up: _____ Unweighted squat: _____

Single-leg lunge-squat with rear-foot support: _____

Remember that muscular strength is specific: Your ratings may vary considerably for different parts of your body.

LABORATORY ACTIVITIES

Using Your Results

How did you score? Are you surprised by your ratings for muscular strength? Are you satisfied with your current ratings?

If you're not satisfied, set realistic goals for improvement:

Are you satisfied with your current level of muscular strength as evidenced in your daily life—for example, your ability to lift objects, climb stairs, and engage in sports and recreational activities?

If you're not satisfied, set realistic goals for improvement:

What should you do next? Enter the results of this lab in the Preprogram Assessment column in Appendix C. If you've set goals for improvement, begin planning your strength training program by completing the plan in Lab 4.3. After several weeks of your program, complete this lab again and enter the results in the Post-program Assessment column of Appendix C. How do the results compare?

Name _____ Section _____ Date _____

LAB 4.2   Assessing Your Current Level of Muscular Endurance

For best results, don't do any strenuous weight training within 48 hours of any test. To assess endurance of the abdominal muscles, perform the curl-up test. To assess endurance of muscles in the upper body, perform the push-up test. To assess endurance of the muscles in the lower body, perform the squat endurance test.

The Curl-Up Test

Equipment

1. Two six-inch strips of self-stick Velcro or heavy tape
2. Ruler
3. Partner
4. Mat (optional)

Preparation

Affix the strips of Velcro or long strips of tape on the mat or testing surface. Place the strips three inches apart.

Instructions

1. Start by lying on your back on the floor or mat, arms straight and by your sides, shoulders relaxed, palms down and on the floor, and fingers straight. Adjust your position so that the longest fingertip of each hand touches the end of the near strip of Velcro or tape. Your knees should be bent about 90 degrees, with your feet about 12–18 inches from your buttocks.

2. To perform a curl-up, flex your spine while sliding your fingers across the floor until the fingertips of each hand reach the second strip of Velcro or tape. Then return to the starting position; the shoulders must be returned to touch the mat between curl-ups, but the head need not touch. Shoulders must remain relaxed throughout the curl-up, and feet and buttocks must stay on the floor. Breathe easily, exhaling during the lift phase of the curl-up; do not hold your breath.

3. Once your partner says "go," perform as many curl-ups as you can at a steady pace with correct form. Your partner counts the curl-ups you perform and calls a stop to the test if she or he notices any incorrect form or drop in your pace.

    Number of curl-ups: _____

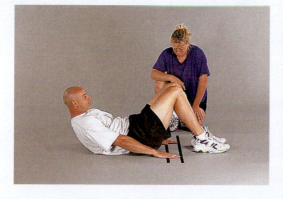 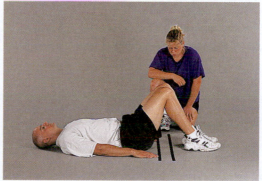

Rating Your Curl-Up Test Result

Your score is the number of completed curl-ups. Refer to the appropriate portion of the table for a rating of your abdominal muscular endurance. Record your rating below and in the summary at the end of this lab.

Rating: _____

LABORATORY ACTIVITIES

Ratings for the Curl-Up Test

			Number of Curl-Ups			
Men	*Very Poor*	*Poor*	*Average*	*Good*	*Excellent*	*Superior*
Age: 16–19	Below 48	48–57	58–64	65–74	75–93	Above 93
20–29	Below 46	46–54	55–63	64–74	75–93	Above 93
30–39	Below 40	40–47	48–55	56–64	65–81	Above 81
40–49	Below 38	38–45	46–53	54–62	63–79	Above 79
50–59	Below 36	36–43	44–51	52–60	61–77	Above 77
60–69	Below 33	33–40	41–48	49–57	58–74	Above 74
Women						
Age: 16–19	Below 42	42–50	51–58	59–67	68–84	Above 84
20–29	Below 41	41–51	52–57	58–66	67–83	Above 83
30–39	Below 38	38–47	48–56	57–66	67–85	Above 85
40–49	Below 36	36–45	46–54	55–64	65–83	Above 83
50–59	Below 34	34–43	44–52	53–62	63–81	Above 81
60–69	Below 31	31–40	41–49	50–59	60–78	Above 78

SOURCE: Ratings based on norms calculated from data collected by Robert Lualhati on 4545 college students, 16–80 years of age, at Skyline College, San Bruno, Calif. Used with permission.

The Push-Up Test

Equipment: Mat or towel (optional)

Preparation

In this test, you will perform either standard push-ups or modified push-ups, in which you support yourself with your knees. The Cooper Institute developed the ratings for this test with men performing push-ups and women performing modified push-ups. Biologically, males tend to be stronger than females; the modified technique reduces the need for upper-body strength in a test of muscular endurance. Therefore, for an accurate assessment of upper-body endurance, men should perform standard push-ups and women should perform modified push-ups. However, in using push-ups as part of a strength training program, individuals should choose the technique most appropriate for increasing their level of strength and endurance—regardless of gender.

Instructions

1. *For push-ups:* Start in the push-up position with your body supported by your hands and feet. *For-modified push-ups:* Start in the modified push-up position with your body supported by your hands and knees. *For both positions,* keep your arms and your back straight and your fingers pointed forward.

2. Lower your chest to the floor with your back straight, and then return to the starting position.

3. Perform as many push-ups or modified push-ups as you can without stopping.

   Number of push-ups: _____ number of modified push-ups: _____

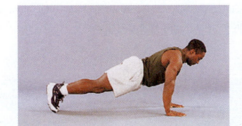 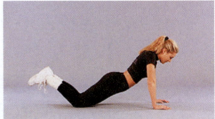

Rating Your Push-Up Test Result

Your score is the number of completed push-ups or modified push-ups. Refer to the appropriate portion of the table for a rating of your upper-body endurance. Record your rating below and in the summary at the end of this lab.

Rating: _____

Men			**Number of Push-Ups**			
	Very Poor	*Poor*	*Fair*	*Good*	*Excellent*	*Superior*
Age: 18–29	Below 22	22–28	29–36	37–46	47–61	Above 61
30–39	Below 17	17–23	24–29	30–38	39–51	Above 51
40–49	Below 11	11–17	18–23	24–29	30–39	Above 39
50–59	Below 9	9–12	13–18	19–24	25–38	Above 38
60 and over	Below 6	6–9	10–17	18–22	23–27	Above 27
Women			**Number of Modified Push-Ups**			
	Very Poor	*Poor*	*Fair*	*Good*	*Excellent*	*Superior*
Age: 18–29	Below 17	17–22	23–29	30–35	36–44	Above 44
30–39	Below 11	11–18	19–23	24–30	31–38	Above 38
40–49	Below 6	6–12	13–17	18–23	24–32	Above 32
50–59	Below 6	6–11	12–16	17–20	21–27	Above 27
60 and over	Below 2	2–4	5–11	12–14	15–19	Above 19

SOURCE: Based on norms from The Cooper Institute of Aerobic Research, Dallas, Tex.; from *The Physical Fitness Specialist Manual*, revised 2002. Used with permission.

The Squat Endurance Test
Instructions

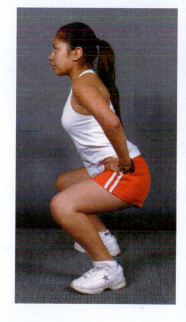

1. Stand with your feet placed slightly more than shoulder width apart, toes pointed out slightly hands on hips or across your chest, head neutral, and back straight. Center your weight over your arches or slightly behind.

2. Squat down, keeping your weight centered over your arches, until your thighs are parallel with the floor. Push back up to the starting position, maintaining a straight back and neutral head position.

3. Perform as many squats as you can without stopping.

Number of squats: _____

Rating Your Squat Endurance Test Result

Your score is the number of completed squats. Refer to the appropriate portion of the table for a rating of your leg muscular endurance. Record your rating below and in the summary at the end of this lab.

Rating: _____

Ratings for the Squat Endurance Test

Men			**Number of Squats Performed**				
	Very Poor	*Poor*	*Below Average*	*Average*	*Above Average*	*Good*	*Excellent*
Age: 18–25	<25	25–30	31–34	35–38	39–43	44–49	>49
26–35	<22	22–28	29–30	31–34	35–39	40–45	>45
36–45	<17	17–22	23–26	27–29	30–34	35–41	>41
46–55	<9	13–17	18–21	22–24	25–38	29–35	>35
56–65	<9	9–12	13–16	17–20	21–24	25–31	>31
65+	<7	7–10	11–14	15–18	19–21	22–28	>28
Women	*Very Poor*	*Poor*	*Below Average*	*Average*	*Above Average*	*Good*	*Excellent*
Age: 18–25	<18	18–24	25–28	29–32	33–36	37–43	>43
26–35	<20	13–20	21–24	25–28	29–32	33–39	>39
36–45	<7	7–14	15–18	19–22	23–26	27–33	>33
46–55	<5	5–9	10–13	14–17	18–21	22–27	>27
56–65	<3	3–6	7–9	10–12	13–17	18–24	>24
65+	<2	2–4	5–10	11–13	14–16	17–23	>23

SOURCE: www.topendsports.com/testing/tests/home-squat.htm

LABORATORY ACTIVITIES

Summary of Results

Curl-up test: Number of curl-ups: _____ Rating: _____

Push-up test: Number of push-ups: _____ Rating: _____

Squat endurance test: Number of squats: _____ Rating: _____

Remember that muscular endurance is specific: Your ratings may vary considerably for different parts of your body.

Using Your Results

How did you score? Are you surprised by your ratings for muscular endurance? Are you satisfied with your current ratings?

If you're not satisfied, set realistic goals for improvement:

Are you satisfied with your current level of muscular endurance as evidenced in your daily life—for example, your ability to carry groceries or your books, hike, and do yard work?

If you're not satisfied, set realistic goals for improvement:

What should you do next? Enter the results of this lab in the Preprogram Assessment column in Appendix C. If you've set goals for improvement, begin planning your strength training program by completing the plan in Lab 4.3. After several weeks of your program, complete this lab again and enter the results in the Post-program Assessment column of Appendix C. How do the results compare?

Name _____ Section _____ Date _____

LAB 4.3 Designing and Monitoring a Strength Training Program

1. *Set goals.* List goals for your strength training program. Your goals can be specific or general, short or long term. In the first section, include specific, measurable goals that you can use to track the progress of your fitness program—for example, raising your upper-body muscular strength rating from fair to good or being able to complete 10 repetitions of a lat pull with 125 pounds of resistance. In the second section, include long-term and more qualitative goals, such as improving self-confidence and reducing your risk for back pain.

Specific Goals: Current Status

_____

_____

_____

Final Goals

_____

_____

_____

Other goals: _____

_____

2. *Choose exercises.* Based on your goals, choose 8–10 exercises to perform during each weight training session. If your goal is general training for wellness, use the sample program in Figure 4.3 on p. 105. List your exercises and the muscles they develop in your program plan.

3. *Frequency: Choose the number of training sessions per week.* Work out at least two nonconsecutive days per week. Indicate the days you will train in your program plan; be sure to include days of rest to allow your body to recover.

4. *Intensity: Choose starting weights.* Experiment with different amounts of weight until you settle on a good starting weight, one that you can lift easily for 10–12 repetitions. As you progress in your program, add more weight. Fill in the starting weight for each exercise in your program plan.

5. *Time: Choose a starting number of sets and repetitions.* Include at least one set of 8–12 repetitions of each exercise. (When you add weight, you may have to decrease the number of repetitions slightly until your muscles adapt to the heavier load.) If your program is focusing on strength alone, your sets can contain fewer repetitions using a heavier load. If you are over approximately age 50–60, your sets should contain more repetitions (10–15) using a lighter load. Fill in the starting number of sets and repetitions of each exercise in your program plan.

6. *Monitor your progress.* Use the workout card on the next page to monitor your progress and keep track of exercises, weights, sets, and repetitions.

Program Plan for Weight Training

Exercise	Muscle(s) Developed	Frequency (✓)							Intensity: Weight (lb.)	Time	
		M	T	W	Th	F	Sa	Su		Repetitions	Sets

WORKOUT CARD FOR _____

Exercise/Date	Wt	Sets	Reps	Wt	Sets	Reps	Wt	Sets	Reps	Wt	Sets	Reps	Wt	Sets	Reps	Wt	Sets	Reps	Wt	Sets	Reps	Wt	Sets	Reps	Wt	Sets	Reps	Wt	Sets	Reps	Wt	Sets	Reps	Wt	Sets	Reps

Flexibility and Low-Back Health

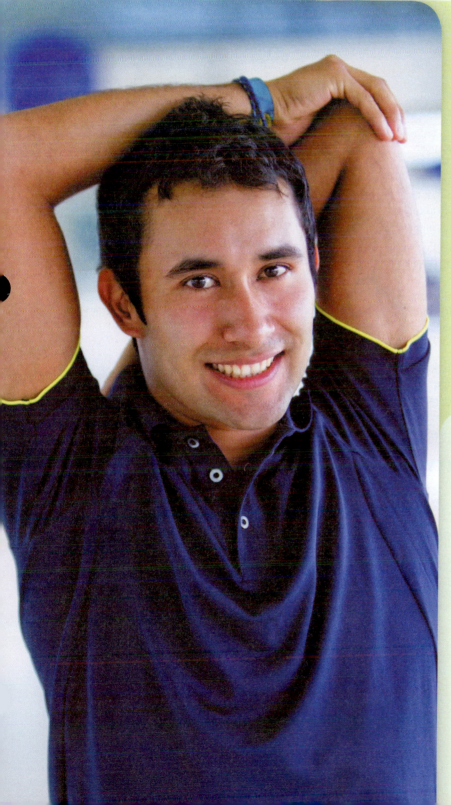

LOOKING AHEAD...

After reading this chapter, you should be able to

- Identify the potential benefits of flexibility and stretching exercises.
- List the factors that affect a joint's flexibility.
- Describe the different types of stretching exercises and how they affect muscles.
- Describe the intensity, duration, and frequency of stretching exercises that will develop the most flexibility with the lowest risk of injury.
- List safe stretching exercises for major joints.
- Explain how low-back pain can be prevented and managed.

TEST YOUR KNOWLEDGE

1. Static stretching exercises should be performed
   a. at the start of a warm-up.
   b. first thing in the morning.
   c. after endurance exercise or strength training.

2. If you injure your back, it's usually best to rest in bed until the pain is completely gone. True or false?

3. It is better to hold a stretch for a short time than to "bounce" while stretching. True or false?

See answers on the next page.

Flexibility—the ability of a joint to move through its normal, full **range of motion**—is important for general fitness and wellness. Flexibility is a highly adaptable physical fitness component: It increases in response to a regular program of stretching exercises and decreases with inactivity. Flexibility is also specific: Good flexibility in one joint doesn't necessarily mean good flexibility in another. You can increase your overall flexibility by doing regular stretching exercises for all your major joints.

This chapter describes the factors that affect flexibility and the benefits of maintaining good flexibility. It provides guidelines for assessing your current level of flexibility and putting together a successful stretching program. It also examines the common problem of low-back pain.

TYPES OF FLEXIBILITY

There are two types of flexibility:

- *Static flexibility* is the ability to hold an extended position at one end or point in a joint's range of motion. For example, static flexibility determines how far you can extend your arm across the front of your body or out to the side. Static flexibility depends on your ability to tolerate stretched muscles, the structure of your joints, and the elasticity of muscles.

- *Dynamic flexibility* is the ability to move a joint through its range of motion with little resistance. It would affect your ability to pitch a ball or swing a golf club. Dynamic flexibility depends on static flexibility, but it also involves strength, coordination, and resistance to movement.

Dynamic flexibility is important for daily activities and sports. But because static flexibility is easier to measure and better researched, most assessment tests and stretching programs target that type of flexibility.

WHAT DETERMINES FLEXIBILITY?

The flexibility of a joint is affected by its structure, by muscle elasticity and length, and by nervous system regulation. Joint structure can't be changed, but other factors, such as the length

of resting muscle fibers, can be changed through exercise; these factors should be the focus of a program to develop flexibility.

Joint Structure

How flexible a joint is depends partly on the nature and structure of the joint (Figure 5.1). Hinge joints such as those in your fingers and knees allow only limited forward and backward movement; they lock when fully extended. Ball-and-socket joints like the hip enable movement in many directions and provide for a greater range of motion. **Joint capsules**, semielastic structures that give joints strength and stability but limit movement, surround the major joints. The bone surfaces within the joint are lined with cartilage and separated by a joint cavity containing *synovial fluid,* which cushions the bones and reduces friction as the joint moves. Ligaments, both inside and outside the joint capsule, strengthen and reinforce the joint. For an illustration of the knee joint and more about its function, see page T4-5 of the color transparency insert "Touring the Musculoskeletal System," in Chapter 4.

Heredity plays a part in joint structure and flexibility. For example, although everyone has a broad range of motion in the

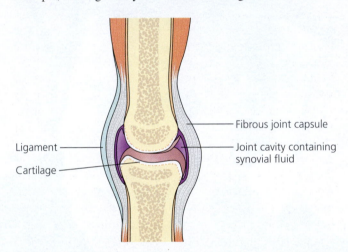

Ligament

Cartilage

Fibrous joint capsule

Joint cavity containing synovial fluid

FIGURE 5.1 **Basic joint structures.**

Answers (Test Your Knowledge)

1. **c.** It's best to do static stretching exercises when your muscles are warm. Intensely stretching muscles before exercise may temporarily reduce their explosive strength and interfere with neuromuscular control.

2. **False.** Prolonged bed rest may actually worsen back pain. Limit bed rest to a day or less, treat pain and inflammation with cold and then heat, and begin moderate physical activity as soon as possible.

3. **True.** "Bouncing" during stretching can damage your muscles. This type of stretching, called ballistic stretching, should be used only by well-conditioned athletes for specific purposes. A person of average fitness should stretch slowly, holding each stretch for 10–30 seconds.

hip joint, not everyone can do a split. Gender may also play a role. Some studies have found that women have greater flexibility in certain joints.

Muscle Elasticity and Length

Soft tissues—including skin, muscles, tendons, and ligaments—also affect the flexibility of a joint. Muscle tissue is the key to developing flexibility because regular stretching can lengthen it. The most important component of muscle tissue related to flexibility is the connective tissue that envelops every part of muscle tissue, from individual muscle fibers to entire muscles. Connective tissue provides structure, elasticity, and bulk and makes up about 30% of muscle mass. Two principal types of connective tissue are **collagen**—white fibers that provide structure and support—and **elastin**—yellow fibers that are elastic and flexible. The collagen and elastin are closely intertwined, so muscle tissue exhibits the properties of both types of fibers. A structural protein in muscles called *titin* also has elastic properties and contributes to flexibility.

When a muscle is stretched, the wavelike elastin fibers straighten; when the stretch is relieved, they rapidly snap back to their resting position. This temporary lengthening is called **elastic elongation**. If stretched gently and regularly, connective tissues may lengthen and flexibility may improve. This long-term lengthening is called **plastic elongation**. Without regular stretching, the process reverses: These tissues shorten, resulting in decreased flexibility. Regular stretching may contribute to flexibility by lengthening muscle fibers through the addition of contractile units called *sarcomeres*.

A muscle can tolerate a limited amount of stretch. As the limits of its flexibility are reached, connective tissue becomes more brittle and may rupture if overstretched. A safe and effective program stretches muscles enough to slightly elongate the tissues but not so much that they are damaged. Research has shown that flexibility is improved best by stretching when muscles are warm (following exercise or the application of heat) and the stretch is applied gradually and conservatively. Sudden, high-stress stretching is less effective and can lead to muscle damage.

Nervous System Regulation

Proprioceptors are nerves that send information about changes in the muscular and skeletal systems to the nervous system, which responds with signals to help control the speed, strength, and coordination of muscle contractions. When a muscle is stretched (lengthened), proprioceptors detect the amount and rate of the change in muscle length. The nerves send a signal to the spinal cord, which then sends a signal back to the muscle, triggering a muscle contraction that resists the change in muscle length. Another signal is sent to the antagonistic, or opposing, muscle, causing it to relax and facilitate contraction of the stretched muscle. These reflexes occur frequently in active muscles and allow for fine control of muscle length and movement. Muscle flexibility is linked to strength. Practicing

lower-body eccentric exercise (lengthening contractions) increases strength and flexibility and might decrease the risk of lower body muscle injury.

Small movements that only slightly stimulate the nerves cause small reflex actions. Rapid, powerful, and sudden changes in muscle length strongly stimulate the nerve receptors and can cause large and powerful reflex muscle contractions. Thus, stretches that involve rapid, bouncy movements can be dangerous and cause injury. Each bounce causes a reflex contraction, which means a muscle might be stretching at the same time it is contracting. Performing a gradual stretch and then holding it allows the proprioceptors to adjust to the new muscle length and to reduce the signals sent to the spine, thereby allowing muscles to lengthen and, over time, improving flexibility.

The stretching technique called *proprioceptive neuromuscular facilitation (PNF)*, described later, takes advantage of nerve activity to improve flexibility. For example, contracting a muscle prior to stretching it can help allow the muscle to stretch farther. The advanced strength training technique called plyometrics (Chapter 4) also takes advantage of the nervous system action in stretching and contracting muscles.

Modifying nervous control through movement and specific exercises is the best way to improve the functional range of motion. Regular stretching trains the proprioceptors to allow the muscles to lengthen. Proprioceptors adapt quickly to stretching (or lack of stretching), so frequent stretching helps develop flexibility. Stretching before exercising, however, can disturb proprioceptors and interfere with motor control during exercise. This is another good reason to stretch *after* exercising.

BENEFITS OF FLEXIBILITY

Good flexibility provides benefits for the entire musculoskeletal system. Flexibility training increases range of motion, and it may prevent muscle strains. As long as you don't overstretch, flexibility training will increase strength and the quality of movement, which might decrease the risk of some sports injuries. Most studies, however, show that stretching does not prevent overuse injuries.

Joint Health

Good flexibility is essential to good joint health. When the muscles and other tissues that support a joint are tight, the joint is subject to abnormal stresses that can cause joint deterioration. For example, tight thigh muscles cause excessive pressure on the kneecap, leading to pain in the knee joint. Poor joint flexibility can also cause abnormalities in joint lubrication, leading to deterioration of the sensitive cartilage cells lining the joint; pain and further joint injury can result.

Improved flexibility can greatly improve your quality of life, particularly as you get older. People tend to exercise less as they age, leading to loss of joint mobility and increased incidence of joint pain. Aging also decreases the natural elasticity of

THE EVIDENCE FOR EXERCISE
Does Physical Activity Increase or Decrease the Risk of Bone and Joint Disease?

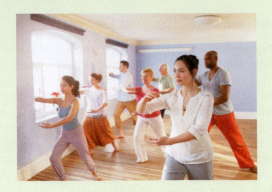

Most college students don't worry much about fall-related fractures or chronic bone-related illnesses, such as osteoporosis (loss of bone mass) or osteoarthritis—(degeneration of the cartilage inside joints). Even so, bone health should be a concern throughout life. This is because girls amass 85% of their adult bone mass by age 18, and boys build the same amount by age 20, but most people begin losing bone mass around age 30. For many, poor diet and lack of exercise accelerate bone loss. According to the National Osteoporosis Foundation, 10 million Americans have osteoporosis. Meantime, 34 million Americans are at risk of the disease because of low bone mass. Overall, osteoporosis is a health threat for about 55% of Americans age 50 and older.

Getting enough nutrients is important for bone health (see Chapter 8), but there is mounting evidence that exercise can also help preserve or improve bone health. For example, several studies have shown an inverse relationship between physical activity and the risk for bone fractures. That is, the more you exercise, the less likely you are to suffer fractures, especially of the upper leg and hip. Research has not determined conclusively how much exercise is required to reduce fracture risk, but people who walk at least four hours per week and devote at least one hour per week to other forms of physical activity appear to reduce that risk. These findings seem to be consistent for women and men, but because some studies disagree on this point, further research is needed.

One way that exercise helps both men and women is by increasing the mineral density of bones, or at least by decreasing the loss of mineral density over time. Several one-year-long studies found that exercise can increase bone mineral density by 1–2% per year, which is significant—especially considering that the same amount of bone mineral density can be lost every one–four years in older persons. Currently, the American College of Sports Medicine recommends that adults perform weight-bearing physical activities (such as walking) three–five days per week and strength training exercises two–three days per week to increase bone mass or avoid loss of mineral density. They also recommend that adults practice neuromotor exercise training exercises, such as yoga or tai chi, to prevent falls and bone fractures. Exercise is particularly important in lactating (breastfeeding) women for preventing bone loss.

The evidence is less conclusive for the effect of exercise on osteoarthritis but still fairly positive. All experts agree that regular, moderate-intensity exercise is necessary for joint health. However, they also warn that vigorous or too-frequent exercise may contribute to joint damage and encourage the onset of osteoarthritis. For this reason, experts try to strike a balance in their exercise recommendations, especially for those with a family history of osteoarthritis. Research seems to support this cautious approach. Some studies have found that regular physical activity (as recommended for general health) at least does not increase osteoarthritis risk. Other studies show that moderate activity may provide some protection against the disease, but this evidence is limited.

A few studies also reveal that the type of exercise you do may increase your risk. For example, competitive or strenuous sports such as ballet, orienteering, football, basketball, soccer, and tennis have been associated with the disease, whereas sports such as cross-country skiing, running, swimming, biking, and walking have not.

The bottom line is that the earlier in life you become physically active, the greater your protection against bone loss and bone-related diseases. However, if you have a family history of osteoporosis or osteoarthritis, or if you have already developed symptoms of one of these ailments, be sure to talk to your physician before beginning an exercise program.

SOURCES: American College of Sports Medicine. 2013. *ACSM's Guidelines for Exercise Testing and Prescription,* 9th ed. Philadelphia: Wolters Kluwer/Lippincott Williams & Wilkins Health; Giangregorio, L. M., et al. 2015. Too Fit To Fracture: Outcomes of a Delphi consensus process on physical activity and exercise recommendations for adults with osteoporosis with or without vertebral fractures. *Osteoporosis International* 26(3): 891–910; American College of Sports Medicine. 2004. ACSM position stand: Physical activity and bone health. *Medicine and Science in Sports and Exercise* 36(11): 1985–1996.

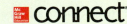

---

muscles, tendons, and joints, resulting in stiffness. The problem is often compounded by arthritis (see the box "Does Physical Activity Increase or Decrease the Risk of Bone and Joint Disease?"). Good joint flexibility may help prevent arthritis, and stretching may lessen pain in people who have the condition. Another benefit of good joint flexibility for older adults is that it increases balance and stability.

Prevention of Low-Back Pain and Injuries

Poor spinal stability puts pressure on the nerves leading out from the spinal column and can lead to low-back pain. Strength and flexibility in the back, pelvis, and thighs may help prevent this type of back pain but may or may not improve back health or reduce the risk of injury. Good hip and knee flexibility protects the spine from excessive motion during the tasks of daily living.

Although scientific evidence is limited, people with either high or low flexibility seem to have an increased risk of injury. Extreme flexibility reduces joint stability, and poor flexibility limits a joint's range of motion. Persons of average fitness should try to attain normal flexibility in joints throughout the body, meaning each joint can move through its normal range of motion with no difficulty. Stretching programs are particularly important for older adults, people engaged in high-power sports that require rapid changes in direction (such as football and tennis), workers involved in brief bouts of intense exertion (such as police officers and firefighters), and people who sit for prolonged periods (such as office workers and students).

However, as we have seen, static stretching *before* a high-intensity activity (such as sprinting or basketball) may increase the risk of injury by interfering with neuromuscular control and reducing muscles' natural ability to stretch and contract. When injuries occur, flexibility exercises can reduce symptoms and help restore normal range of motion in affected joints.

Additional Potential Benefits of Flexibility

• *Relief of aches and pains.* Studying or working in one place for a long time can make your muscles tense. Stretching helps relieve tension and joint stiffness, so you can go back to work refreshed and effective. Stretching reduces the symptoms of exercise-induced muscle damage, and flexible muscles are less susceptible to the damage.

• *Relief of muscle cramps.* Recent research suggests that exercise-related muscle cramps are caused by increased electrical activity within the affected muscle. The best treatment for muscle cramps is gentle stretching, which reduces the electrical activity and allows the muscle to relax.

• *Improved body position and strength for sports (and life).* Good flexibility lets you assume more efficient body positions and exert force through a greater range of motion. For example, swimmers with more flexible shoulders have stronger strokes because they can pull their arms through the water in the optimal position. Some studies also suggest that flexibility training enhances strength development.

• *Maintenance of good posture and balance.* Good flexibility also contributes to body symmetry and good posture. Bad posture can gradually change your body structures. Sitting in a slumped position, for example, can lead to tightness in the muscles in the front of your chest and overstretching and looseness in the upper spine, causing a rounding of the upper back. This condition, called *kyphosis,* is common in older people. Stretching regularly may prevent it.

• *Relaxation.* Flexibility exercises, particularly when practiced in combination with yoga or tai chi, reduce mental tension, slow your breathing rate, and reduce blood pressure.

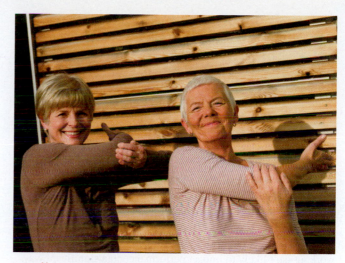

Wellness Tip Flexibility training helps maintain pain-free joints as you age. You don't have to be at the gym to stretch. There are lots of simple, small-movement stretches you can do anywhere—whether at your desk or on the go. For some examples, visit a good health website such as http://www.MayoClinic.com and search for "stretching exercises."

• *Improving impaired mobility.* Stretching often decreases pain and improves functional capacity in people with arthritis, stroke, or muscle and nerve diseases and in people who are recovering from surgery or injury.

ASSESSING FLEXIBILITY

Because flexibility is specific to each joint, there are no tests of general flexibility. The most commonly used flexibility test is the sit-and-reach test, which rates the flexibility of the muscles in the lower back and hamstrings. To assess your flexibility and identify inflexible joints, complete Lab 5.1.

CREATING A SUCCESSFUL PROGRAM TO DEVELOP FLEXIBILITY

A successful program for developing flexibility includes safe exercises executed with the most effective techniques. Your goal should be to attain normal flexibility in the major joints. Balanced flexibility (not too much or too little) provides joint stability and facilitates smooth, economical movement patterns. You can achieve balanced flexibility by performing stretching exercises regularly and by using a variety of stretches and stretching techniques.

Applying the FITT Principle

As with other programs, the acronym FITT can be used to remember key components of a stretching program: Frequency, Intensity, Time, and Type of exercise.

Frequency The American College of Sports Medicine (ACSM) recommends that stretching exercises be performed at least two–three days per week, but more often is even better. To prevent injury and improve flexibility, it's best to stretch when your muscles are warm, either after a warm-up or after cardiorespiratory endurance exercise or weight training.

As described earlier, static stretching can adversely affect muscle performance in the short term. So, if you are planning a workout for which high-performance is important, it is best to perform static stretches after your workout but while your muscles are still warm and your joints are lubricated. Stretching isn't the same thing as a cool-down, so be sure to do the cardiorespiratory cool-down first, so you can transition to a lower level of intensity before stretching. If the plan for your workout includes a moderate activity like walking, then static stretching prior to your workout isn't likely to impact performance in a significant way.

Dynamic stretching, described in the next section, may have less of an impact on muscle performance and so is sometimes included as part of an active warm-up. However, dynamic stretching is more challenging to learn and perform.

Intensity and Time (Duration)
For each exercise, slowly stretch your muscles to the point of slight tension or mild discomfort—but not to the point of pain. Hold the stretch for 10–30 seconds. As you hold the stretch, the feeling of slight tension should slowly subside; at that point, try to stretch a bit farther. Throughout the stretch, try to relax and breathe easily. Rest for about 30–60 seconds between each stretch, and do 2–4 repetitions of each stretch for a total of 60 seconds per exercise. A complete flexibility workout usually takes about 10–30 minutes (Figure 5.2).

Types of Stretching Techniques
Stretching techniques vary from simply stretching the muscles during the course of normal activities to sophisticated methods based on patterns of muscle reflexes. Improper stretching can do more harm than good, so it's important to understand the different types of stretching exercises and how they affect the muscles. Four common techniques are static stretches, ballistic stretches, dynamic stretches, and PNF.

Warm-up 5–10 minutes or following an endurance or strength training workout	Stretching exercises for major joints **Sample program**	
	Exercise	*Areas stretched*
	Head turns and tilts	Neck
	Towel stretch	Triceps, shoulders, chest
	Across-the-body and overhead stretches	Shoulders, upper back, back of arm
	Upper-back stretch	Upper back
	Lateral stretch	Trunk muscles
	Step stretch	Hip, front of thigh
	Side lunge	Inner thigh, hip, calf
	Inner-thigh stretch	Inner thigh, hip
	Hip and trunk stretch	Trunk, outer thigh, hip, buttocks, lower back
	Modified hurdler stretch	Back of thigh, lower back
	Alternate leg stretcher	Back of thigh, hip, knee, ankle, buttocks
	Lower-leg stretch	Calf, soleus, Achilles tendon

Frequency: 2–3 days per week (minimum); 5–7 days per week (ideal)

Intensity: Stretch to the point of mild discomfort, not pain

Time (duration): All stretches should be held for 10–30 seconds and performed 2–4 times, for a total of 60 seconds per exercise.

Type of activity: Stretching exercises that focus on major joints

FIGURE 5.2 **The FITT principle for a flexibility program.**

STATIC STRETCHING In **static stretching**, each muscle is gradually stretched, and the stretch is held for 10–30 seconds. A slow stretch prompts less reaction from proprioceptors, and the muscles can safely stretch farther than usual. Static stretching is the type most often recommended by fitness experts because it is safe and effective.

The key to this technique is to stretch the muscles and joints to the point where a pull is felt, but not to the point of pain. (One note of caution: Excess static stretching can decrease joint stability and increase the risk of injury. This may be a particular concern for women, whose joints are less stable and more flexible than men.) The sample stretching program presented later in this chapter features static stretching exercises.

BALLISTIC STRETCHING In **ballistic stretching**, the muscles are stretched suddenly in a forceful bouncing movement. For example, touching the toes repeatedly in rapid succession is a ballistic stretch for the hamstrings. A problem with this technique is that the heightened activity of proprioceptors caused by the rapid stretches can continue for some time, possibly causing injuries during any physical activities that follow. Another concern is that triggering strong responses from the nerves can cause a reflex muscle contraction that makes it harder to stretch. For these reasons, ballistic stretching is usually not recommended, especially for people of average fitness.

Ballistic stretching trains the muscle dynamically, so it can be an appropriate stretching technique for some well-trained athletes. For example, tennis players stretch their hamstrings and quadriceps ballistically when they lunge for a ball during a

---

> **static stretching** A technique in which a muscle is slowly and gently stretched and then held in the stretched position.
>
> **ballistic stretching** A technique in which muscles are stretched by the force generated as a body part is repeatedly bounced, swung, or jerked.
>
> **dynamic stretching** A technique in which muscles are stretched by moving joints slowly and fluidly through their range of motion in a controlled manner; also called *functional stretching*.
>
> **passive stretching** A technique in which muscles are stretched by force applied by an outside source.
>
> **active stretching** A technique in which muscles are stretched by the contraction of the opposing muscles.

TERMS

tennis match. Because this movement is part of their sport, they might benefit from ballistic training of these muscle groups.

DYNAMIC (FUNCTIONAL) STRETCHING The emphasis in **dynamic stretching** is on functional movements. Dynamic stretching is similar to ballistic stretching in that it includes movement, but it differs in that it does not involve rapid bouncing. Instead, dynamic stretching moves the joints in an exaggerated but controlled manner through the range of motion used in a specific exercise or sport; movements are fluid rather than jerky. An example of a dynamic stretch is the lunge walk, in which a person takes slow steps with an exaggerated stride length and reaches a lunge stretch position with each step.

Slow dynamic stretches can lengthen the muscles in many directions without developing high tension in the tissues. These stretches elongate the tissues and train the neuromuscular system. Because dynamic stretches are based on sports movements or movements used in daily life, they develop functional flexibility that translates well into activities.

Dynamic stretches are more challenging than static stretches because they require balance and coordination and may carry a greater risk of muscle soreness and injury. People just beginning a flexibility program might want to start off with static stretches and try dynamic stretches only after they are comfortable with static stretching and have improved their flexibility. It is also a good idea to seek expert advice on dynamic stretching technique and program development.

Functional flexibility training can be combined with functional strength training. For example, lunge curls, which combine dynamic lunges with free weights biceps curls, stretch the hip, thigh, and calf muscles; stabilize the core muscles in the trunk; and build strength in the arm muscles. Many activities build functional flexibility and strength at the same time, including yoga, Pilates, tai chi, Olympic weight lifting, plyometrics, stability training (including Swiss and Bosu ball exercises), medicine ball exercises, and functional training machines (for example, Life Fitness and Cybex).

PROPRIOCEPTIVE NEUROMUSCULAR FACILITATION (PNF) PNF techniques use reflexes initiated by both muscle and joint nerves to cause greater training effects. The most popular PNF stretching technique is the contract-relax stretching method, in which a muscle is contracted before it is stretched. The contraction activates proprioceptors, causing relaxation in the muscle about to be stretched. For example, in a seated stretch of calf muscles, the first step in PNF is to contract the calf muscles. The individual or a partner can provide resistance for an isometric contraction. Following a brief period of relaxation, the next step is to stretch the calf muscles by pulling the tops of the feet toward the body. A duration of three to six seconds for the contraction at 20 to 75% of maximum effort and 10–30 seconds for the stretch is recommended. PNF appears to be most effective if the individual pushes hard during the isometric contraction.

Another example of a PNF stretch is the contract-relax-contract pattern. In this technique, begin by contracting the muscle to be stretched and then relaxing it. Next, contract the opposing muscle (the antagonist). Finally, stretch the first muscle. For example, using this technique to stretch the

hamstrings (the muscles in the back of the thigh) would require the following steps: Contract the hamstrings, relax the hamstrings, contract the quadriceps (the muscles in the front of the thigh), and then stretch the hamstrings.

PNF appears to allow more effective stretching and greater increases in flexibility than static stretching, but it tends to cause more muscle stiffness and soreness. It also usually requires a partner and takes more time.

PASSIVE VERSUS ACTIVE STRETCHING Stretches can be done either passively or actively. In **passive stretching**, an outside force or resistance provided by yourself, a partner, gravity, or a weight helps your joints move through their range of motion. For example, a seated stretch of the hamstring and back muscles can be done by reaching the hands toward the feet until a pull is felt in those muscles. You can achieve a greater range of motion (a more intense stretch) using passive stretching. However, because the stretch is not controlled by the muscles themselves, there is a greater risk of injury. Communication between partners in passive stretching is important to ensure that joints aren't forced outside their normal functional range of motion.

In **active stretching**, a muscle is stretched by a contraction of the opposing muscle (the muscle on the opposite side of the limb). For example, an active seated stretch of the calf muscles occurs when a person actively contracts the muscles on the top of the shin. The contraction of this opposing muscle produces a reflex that relaxes the muscles to be stretched. The muscle can be stretched farther with a low risk of injury. The only disadvantage of active stretching is that a person may not be able to produce enough stress (enough stretch) to increase flexibility using only the contraction of opposing muscle groups.

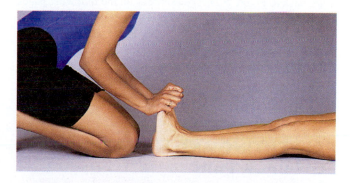

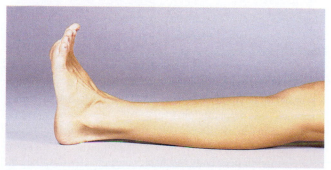

In passive stretching (top), an outside force—such as pressure exerted by another person—helps move the joint and stretch the muscles. In active stretching (bottom), the force to move the joint and stretch the muscles is provided by a contraction of the opposing muscles.

The safest and most convenient technique is *active static stretching,* with an occasional passive assist. For example, you might stretch your calves both by contracting the muscles on the top of your shin and by pulling your feet toward you. This way you combine the advantages of active stretching—safety and the relaxation reflex—with those of passive stretching—greater range of motion. People who are just beginning flexibility training may be better off doing active rather than passive stretches. For PNF techniques, it is particularly important to have a knowledgeable partner.

Making Progress

As with any type of training, you will make progress and improve your flexibility if you stick with your program. Judge your progress by noting your body position while stretching. For example, note how far you can lean forward during a modified hurdler stretch. Repeat the assessment tests that appear in Lab 5.1 periodically and be sure to take the test at the same time of day each time. You will likely notice some improvement after only two to three weeks of stretching, but you may need at least two months to attain significant improvements. By then, you can expect flexibility increases of about 10–20% in many joints.

Exercises to Improve Flexibility: A Sample Program

There are hundreds of exercises that can improve flexibility. Your program should include exercises that work all the major joints of the body by stretching their associated muscle groups (refer back to Figure 5.2). The exercises on the following pages are simple to do and pose a minimum risk of injury. Use these exercises to create a well-rounded program for developing flexibility. Be sure to perform each stretch using the proper technique. Hold each position for 10–30 seconds and perform 2–4 repetitions of each exercise. Complete Lab 5.2 when you're ready to start your program.

PREVENTING AND MANAGING LOW-BACK PAIN

More than 85% of Americans experience back pain by age 50. Low-back pain is the second most common ailment in the United States—headache tops the list—and the second most common reason for absences from work and visits to a physician. Low-back pain is estimated to cost as much as $50 billion a year in lost productivity, medical and legal fees, and disability insurance and compensation.

Back pain can result from sudden traumatic injuries, but it is more often the long-term result of weak and inflexible muscles, poor posture, or poor body mechanics during activities like lifting and carrying. Any abnormal strain on the back can result in pain. Most cases of low-back pain clear up within a few weeks or months, but some people have recurrences or suffer from chronic pain.

Function and Structure of the Spine

The spinal column performs many important functions in the body.

- It provides structural support for the body, especially the thorax (upper-body cavity).
- It surrounds and protects the spinal cord.
- It supports much of the body's weight.
- It serves as an attachment site for a large number of muscles, tendons, and ligaments.
- It allows movement of the neck and back in all directions.

The spinal column is made up of bones called **vertebrae** that provide structural support to the body and protect the spinal cord (Figure 5.3). The spine consists of 7 cervical vertebrae in the neck, 12 thoracic vertebrae in the upper back, and 5 lumbar vertebrae in the lower back. The 9 vertebrae at the base of the spine are fused into two sections and form the sacrum

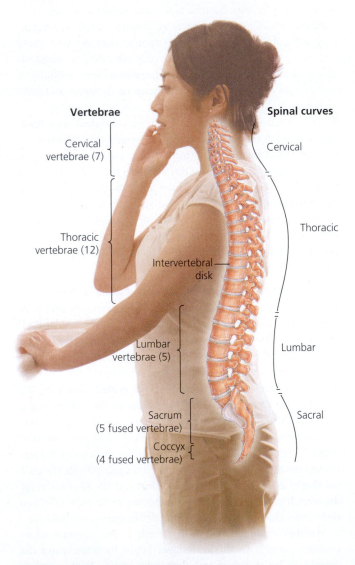

Vertebrae

Cervical vertebrae (7)

Thoracic vertebrae (12)

Intervertebral disk

Lumbar vertebrae (5)

Sacrum (5 fused vertebrae)

Coccyx (4 fused vertebrae)

Spinal curves

Cervical

Thoracic

Lumbar

Sacral

FIGURE 5.3 The spinal column. The spine is made up of five separate regions and has four distinct curves. An intervertebral disk is located between adjoining vertebrae.

FLEXIBILITY EXERCISES

EXERCISE 1 — Head Turns and Tilts

Instructions:

Head turns: Turn your head to the right and hold the stretch. Repeat to the left.

Head tilts: Tilt your head to the right and hold the stretch. Repeat to the left.

Areas stretched: Neck

Variation: Place your right palm on your right cheek; try to turn your head to the right as you resist with your hand. Repeat on the left side.

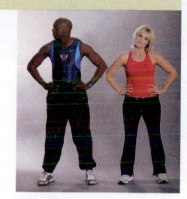

EXERCISE 2 — Towel Stretch

Instructions: Roll up a towel and grasp it with both hands, palms down. With your arms straight, slowly lift the towel back over your head as far as possible. The closer together your hands are, the greater the stretch.

Areas stretched: Triceps, shoulders, chest

Variation: Repeat the stretch with your arms down and the towel behind your back. Grasp the towel with your palms forward and thumbs pointing out. Gently raise your arms behind your back. This exercise can also be done without a towel.

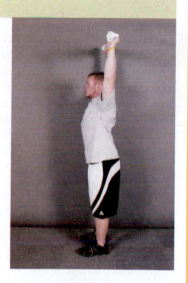

EXERCISE 3 — Across-the-Body and Overhead Stretches

Instructions: **(a)** Keeping your back straight, cross your right arm in front of your body and grasp it with your left hand. Stretch your arm, shoulders, and back by gently pulling your arm as close to your body as possible. Hold. **(b)** Bend your right arm over your head, placing your right elbow as close to your right ear as possible. Grasp your right elbow with your left hand over your head. Stretch the back of your arm by gently pulling your right elbow back and toward your head. Hold. Repeat both stretches on your left side.

Areas stretched: Shoulders, upper back, back of the arm (triceps)

a
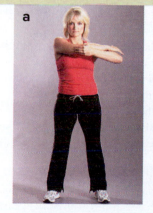
b
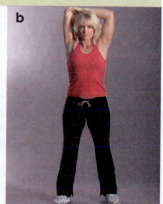

EXERCISE 4 — Upper-Back Stretch

Instructions: Stand with your feet shoulder-width apart, knees slightly bent, and pelvis tucked under. Lace your fingers in front of your body and press your palms forward.

Areas stretched: Upper back

Variation: In the same position, wrap your arms around your body as if you were giving yourself a hug.

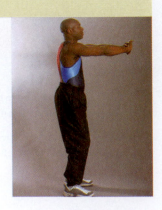

EXERCISE 5 — Lateral Stretch

Instructions: Stand with your feet shoulder-width apart, knees slightly bent, and pelvis tucked under. Raise one arm over your head and bend sideways from the waist. Support your trunk by placing the hand or forearm of your other arm on your thigh or hip for support. Be sure you bend directly sideways and don't move your body below the waist. Repeat on the other side.

Areas stretched: Trunk muscles

Variation: Perform the same exercise in a seated position.

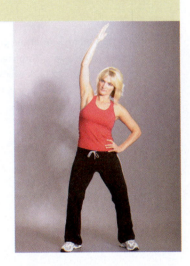

EXERCISE 6 — Step Stretch

Instructions: Step forward and bend your forward knee, keeping it directly above your ankle. Stretch your other leg back so your shin is parallel to the floor. Press your hips forward and down to stretch. Your arms can be at your sides, on top of your knee, or on the ground for balance. Repeat on the other side.

Areas stretched: Hip, front of thigh (quadriceps)

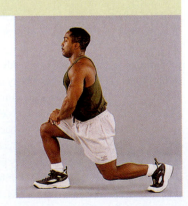

EXERCISE 7 — Side Lunge

Instructions: Stand in a wide straddle with your legs turned out from your hip joints and your hands on your thighs. Lunge to one side by bending one knee and keeping the other leg straight. Keep your bent knee directly over your ankle; do not bend it more than 90 degrees. Repeat on the other side.

Areas stretched: Inner thigh, hip, calf

Variation: In the same position, lift the heel of the bent knee to provide additional stretch. The exercise may also be performed with your hands on the floor for balance.

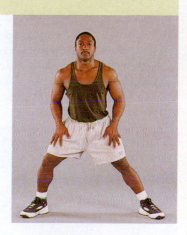

EXERCISE 8 — Inner-Thigh Stretch

Instructions: Sit on the floor with the soles of your feet together. Push your knees toward the floor using your hands or forearms.

Areas stretched: Inner thigh, hip

Variation: When you first begin to push your knees toward the floor, use your legs to resist the movement. Then relax and press your knees down as far as they will go.

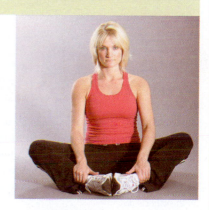

EXERCISE 9 — Hip and Trunk Stretch

Instructions: Sit on the floor with your left leg straight, right leg bent and crossed over the left knee, and right hand on the floor next to your right hip. Turn your trunk as far as possible to the right by pushing against your right leg with your left forearm or elbow. Keep your right foot on the floor. Repeat on the other side.

Areas stretched: Trunk, outer thigh and hip, buttocks, lower back

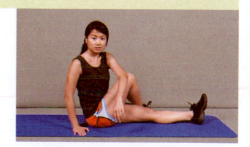

EXERCISE 10 — Modified Hurdler Stretch (Seated Single-Leg Hamstring)

Instructions: Sit on the floor with your left leg straight and your right leg tucked close to your body. Reach toward your left ankle as far as possible. Repeat for the other leg.

Areas stretched: Back of the thigh (hamstring), lower back

Variation: As you stretch forward, alternately flex and point the foot of your extended leg.

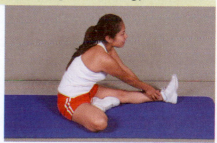

EXERCISE 11 — Leg Stretcher

Instructions: Lie flat on your back with both legs straight. **(a)** Grasp your left leg behind the thigh, and pull it in to your chest. **(b)** Hold this position, and then extend your left leg toward the ceiling. **(c)** Hold this position, and then bring your left knee back to your chest and pull your toes toward your shin with your left hand. Stretch the back of the leg by attempting to straighten your knee. Repeat for the other leg.

Areas stretched: Back of the thigh (hamstring), hip, knee, ankle, and buttocks

Variation: Perform the stretch on both legs at the same time.

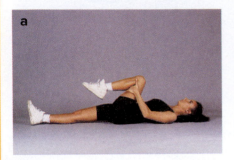

a

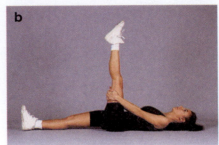

b

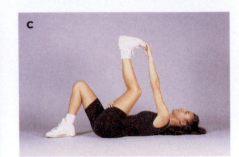

c

EXERCISE 12 — Lower-Leg Stretch

Instructions: Stand with one foot about one–two feet in front of the other, with both feet pointing forward. **(a)** Keeping your back leg straight, lunge forward by bending your front knee and pushing your rear heel backward. Hold. **(b)** Then pull your back foot in slightly and bend your back knee. Shift your weight to your back leg. Hold. Repeat on the other side.

Areas stretched: Back of the lower leg (calf, soleus, Achilles tendon)

Variation: Place your hands on a wall and extend one foot back, pressing your heel down to stretch, or stand with the balls of your feet on a step or bench and allow your heels to drop below the level of your toes.

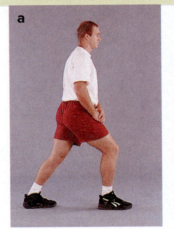

a

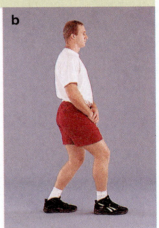

b

EXERCISE 13 — Single-Leg Deadlift

Instructions: Start with a dumbbell or kettlebell placed slightly outside the foot of one leg. Bend down to the weight by hinging at the hips and bending at the knee. Your other leg should be bent and relaxed. Pick up the weight and tighten your body and extend the hip and knee as you stand straight, locking out your hip and contracting your glute. Repeat with the other leg.

Areas stretched: This exercise stretches and loads the hamstrings and glute muscles both eccentrically and concentrically (lengthening and shortening contractions).

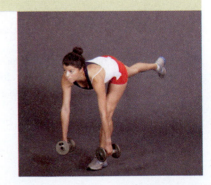

and the coccyx (tailbone). The spine has four curves: the cervical, thoracic, lumbar, and sacral curves (see Figure 5.3). These curves help bring the body weight supported by the spine in line with the axis of the body.

Although the structure of vertebrae depends on their location on the spine, the different types of vertebrae share common characteristics. Each consists of a body, an arch, and several bony processes (Figure 5.4). The vertebral body is cylindrical, with flattened surfaces where **intervertebral disks** are attached. The vertebral body is designed to carry the stress of body weight and physical activity. The vertebral arch surrounds and protects the spinal cord. Irregularly shaped bony outgrowths serve as joints for adjacent vertebrae and attachment sites for muscles and ligaments. **Nerve roots** from the spinal cord pass through notches in the vertebral arch.

Intervertebral disks, which absorb and disperse the stresses placed on the spine, separate vertebrae from one another. Disks are made up of a gel- and water-filled nucleus surrounded by a series of fibrous rings. The liquid nucleus can change shape when it is compressed, allowing the disk to absorb shock. The intervertebral disks also help maintain the spaces between vertebrae where the spinal nerve roots are located.

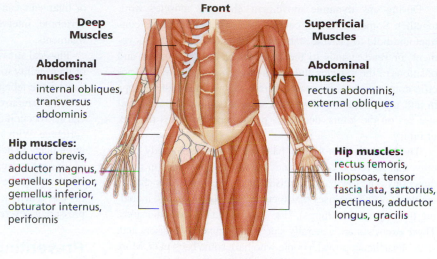

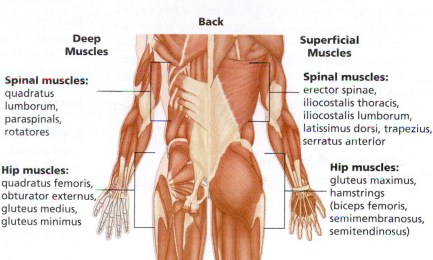

Front

Deep Muscles

Abdominal muscles: internal obliques, transversus abdominis

Hip muscles: adductor brevis, adductor magnus, gemellus superior, gemellus inferior, obturator internus, periformis

Superficial Muscles

Abdominal muscles: rectus abdominis, external obliques

Hip muscles: rectus femoris, Iliopsoas, tensor fascia lata, sartorius, pectineus, adductor longus, gracilis

Back

Deep Muscles

Spinal muscles: quadratus lumborum, paraspinals, rotatores

Hip muscles: quadratus femoris, obturator externus, gluteus medius, gluteus minimus

Superficial Muscles

Spinal muscles: erector spinae, iliocostalis thoracis, iliocostalis lumborum, latissimus dorsi, trapezius, serratus anterior

Hip muscles: gluteus maximus, hamstrings (biceps femoris, semimembranosus, semitendinosus)

FIGURE 5.5 Major core muscles.

Core Muscle Fitness

The **core muscles** are the trunk muscles extending from the hips to the upper back, including those in the abdomen, pelvic floor, sides of the trunk, back, buttocks, hip, and pelvis (Figure 5.5). These muscles are attached to the ribs, hips, spinal column, and other bones in the trunk of the body. The core muscles stabilize the spine and help transfer force between the upper body and lower body. They stabilize the midsection when you sit, stand, reach, walk, jump, twist, squat, throw, or bend. The muscles on the front, back, and sides of your trunk support your spine when you sit in a chair and fix your midsection as you use your legs to stand up. When hitting a forehand in tennis or batting a softball, most of the force is transferred from the legs and hips, across the core muscles, to the arms. Strong core muscles make movements more forceful and help prevent back pain.

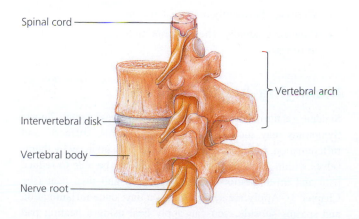

Spinal cord

Vertebral arch

Intervertebral disk

Vertebral body

Nerve root

FIGURE 5.4 Vertebrae and an intervertebral disk.

vertebrae Bony segments composing the spinal column that provide structural support for the body and protect the spinal cord. **TERMS**

intervertebral disk An elastic disk located between adjoining vertebrae, consisting of a gel- and water-filled nucleus surrounded by fibrous rings; serves as a shock absorber for the spinal column.

nerve roots The bases of the 31 pairs of spinal nerves that branch off the spinal cord through spaces between vertebrae.

core muscles The trunk muscles extending from the hips to the upper back.

During any dynamic movement, the core muscles work together. Some shorten to cause movement, while others contract and hold to provide stability, lengthen to brake the movement, or send signals to the brain about the movements and positions of the muscles and bones (proprioception). When specific core muscles are weak or tired, the nervous system steps in and uses other muscles. This substitution causes abnormal stresses on the joints, decreases power, and increases the risk of injury.

The best exercises for low-back health are whole-body exercises that force the core muscles to stabilize the spine in many directions. The low-back exercises presented later in this chapter include several exercises that focus on the core muscles, including the step stretch (lunge), side bridges, and spine extensions. These exercises are generally safe for beginning exercisers and, with physician approval, people who have some back pain. More challenging core exercises utilize stability balls or free weights. Stability ball exercises require the core muscles to stabilize the ball (and the body) while performing nearly any type of exercise. Many traditional exercises with free weights can strengthen the core muscles if you do them in a standing position. Weight machines train muscles in isolation, while exercises with free weights done while standing help train the body for real-world movements—an essential principle of core training.

Causes of Back Pain

Back pain can occur at any point along your spine. The lumbar area, because it bears the majority of your weight, is the most common site. Any movement that puts excessive stress on the spinal column can cause injury and pain. The spine is well equipped to bear body weight and the force or stress of body movements along its long axis. However, it is less capable of bearing loads at an angle to its long axis or when the trunk is flexed (bent). You do not have to carry a heavy load or participate in a vigorous contact sport to injure your back. Picking a pencil up from the floor while using poor body mechanics—reaching too far out in front of you or bending over with your knees straight, for example—can also result in back pain.

Risk factors associated with low-back pain include age greater than 34 years, degenerative diseases such as arthritis or osteoporosis, a family or personal history of back pain or trauma, a sedentary lifestyle, low job satisfaction, low socioeconomic status, excess body weight, smoking (which appears to hasten degenerative changes in the spine), and psychological stress or depression (which can cause muscle tension and back pain). Occupations and activities associated with low-back pain are those requiring physically hard work, such as frequent lifting, twisting, bending, standing up, or straining in forced positions; those requiring high concentration demands while seated (such as computer programming); and those involving vibrations affecting the entire body (such as truck driving).

Underlying causes of back pain include poor muscle endurance and strength in the core muscles; excess body weight; poor posture or body position when standing, sitting, or sleeping; and poor body mechanics when performing actions like lifting and carrying or sports movements. Strained muscles, tendons,

or ligaments can cause pain and, over time, lead to injuries to vertebrae, intervertebral disks, and surrounding muscles and ligaments.

Physical stress can cause disks to break down and lose some of their ability to absorb shock. A damaged disk may bulge out between vertebrae and put pressure on a nerve root, a condition commonly referred to as a *slipped disk*. Painful pressure on nerves can also occur if damage to a disk narrows the space between two vertebrae. With age, you lose fluid from the disks, making them more likely to bulge and put pressure on nerve roots. Depending on the amount of pressure on a nerve, symptoms may include numbness in the back, hip, leg, or foot; radiating pain; loss of muscle function; depressed reflexes; and muscle spasm. If the pressure is severe enough, loss of function can be permanent.

Preventing Low-Back Pain

Incorrect posture is responsible for many back injuries. Strategies for maintaining good posture are presented in the box "Good Posture and Low-Back Health." Follow the same guidelines when you engage in sports or recreational activities. Control your movements, and warm up thoroughly before you exercise. Take special care when lifting weights.

The role of exercise in preventing and treating back pain is still being investigated. However, many experts recommend exercise, especially for people who have already experienced an episode of low-back pain. The exercise can take the form of a workout aimed at increasing muscle endurance and strength in the back and abdomen or just regular lifestyle physical activity such as walking. Movement helps lubricate your spinal joints and increases muscle fitness in your trunk and legs. Other lifestyle recommendations for preventing back pain include the following:

- Maintain a healthy weight. Excess fat contributes to poor posture, which can place harmful stresses on the spine.
- Stop smoking, and reduce stress.
- Avoid sitting, standing, or working in the same position for too long. Stand up every hour or half-hour and move around.
- Use a supportive seat and a medium-firm mattress.
- Use lumbar support when driving, particularly for long distances, to prevent muscle fatigue and pain.
- Warm up thoroughly before exercising.
- Progress gradually when attempting to improve strength or fitness.

Managing Acute Back Pain

Sudden (acute) back pain usually involves tissue injury. Symptoms may include pain, muscle spasms, stiffness, and inflammation. Many cases of acute back pain go away by themselves within a few days or weeks. You may be able to reduce pain and inflammation by applying cold and then heat (see Chapter 3). Apply ice several times a day; once inflammation and spasms subside, you can apply heat using a heating pad or a warm bath. If the pain is bothersome, an over-the-counter

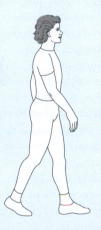

Changes in everyday posture and behavior can help prevent and alleviate low-back pain.

- **Lying down.** When resting or sleeping, lie on your side with your knees and hips bent. If you lie on your back, place a pillow under your knees. However, do not elevate your knees so much that the curve in your lower spine is flattened. Don't lie on your stomach. Use a medium-firm mattress.

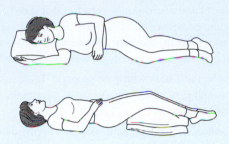

- **Sitting at a computer.** Sit in a slightly reclined position of 100–110 degrees, not an upright 90-degree position. Adjust your chair so your knees are slightly lower than your hips. If your back flattens as you sit, try using a lumbar roll to maintain your back's natural curvature. Place your feet flat on the floor or on a footrest. Place the monitor directly in front of you and adjust it so your eyes are level with the top of the screen; you should be looking slightly downward at the middle of the screen. Adjust the keyboard and mouse so your forearms and wrists are in a neutral position, parallel with the floor.

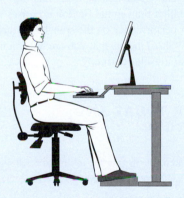

- **Lifting.** If you need to lower yourself to grasp an object, bend at the knees and hips rather than at the waist. Your feet should be about shoulder-width apart. Lift gradually, keeping your arms straight, by standing up or by pushing with your hip muscles. Keep the object close to your body. Don't twist; if you have to turn with the object, change the position of your feet so that you pivot your body as a whole rather than twisting at your waist or shoulders.

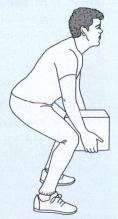

- **Standing.** When you are standing, a straight line should run from the top of your ear through the center of your shoulder, the center of your hip, the back of your kneecap, and the front of your ankle bone. Support your weight mainly on your heels, with one or both knees slightly bent. Don't let your pelvis tip forward or your back arch. Shift your weight back and forth from foot to foot. Avoid prolonged standing.

To check your posture, stand normally with your back to a wall. Your upper back and buttocks should touch the wall; your heels may be a few inches away. Slide one hand into the space between your lower back and the wall. It should slide in easily but should almost touch both your back and the wall. Adjust your posture as needed, and try to hold this position as you walk away from the wall.

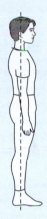

- **Walking.** Walk with your toes pointed straight ahead. Keep your back flat, head up and centered over your body, and chin in. Swing your arms freely. Don't wear tight or high-heeled shoes. Walking briskly is better for back health than walking slowly.

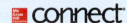

nonsteroidal anti-inflammatory medication such as ibuprofen or naproxen may be helpful. Stronger pain medications and muscle relaxants are available by prescription.

Bed rest immediately following the onset of back pain may make you feel better, but it should be of very short duration. Prolonged bed rest—five days or more—was once thought to be an effective treatment for back pain, but most physicians now advise against it because it may weaken muscles and actually worsen pain. Limit bed rest to one day and begin moderate physical activity as soon as possible. Exercise can increase muscular endurance and flexibility and protect disks from loss of fluid. Three of the back exercises discussed later in the chapter may be particularly helpful following an episode of acute back pain: curl-ups, side bridges, and spine extensions ("bird dogs").

See your physician if acute back pain doesn't resolve within a short time. Other warning signals of a more severe problem that requires a professional evaluation include severe pain, numbness, pain that radiates down one or both legs, problems with bladder or bowel control, fever, and rapid weight loss.

Managing Chronic Back Pain

Low-back pain is considered chronic if it persists for more than three months. Symptoms vary—some people experience stabbing or shooting pain, and others a steady ache accompanied by stiffness. Sometimes pain is localized; in other cases, it radiates to another part of the body. Underlying causes of chronic back pain include injuries, infection, muscle or ligament strains, and disk herniations.

Because symptoms and causes are so varied, different people benefit from different treatment strategies, and researchers have found that many treatments have only limited benefits. Potential treatments include over-the-counter or prescription medications; exercise; physical therapy, massage, yoga, or chiropractic care; acupuncture; percutaneous electrical nerve stimulation (PENS), in which acupuncture-like needles deliver an electrical current; education and advice about posture, exercise, and body mechanics; and surgery (see the box "Yoga for Relaxation and Pain Relief").

Psychological therapy may also be beneficial in some cases. Reducing emotional stress that causes muscle tension can provide direct benefits, and other therapies can help people deal better with chronic pain and its effects on their daily lives. Support groups and expressive writing are beneficial for people with chronic pain and other conditions.

Exercises for the Prevention and Management of Low-Back Pain

The tests in Lab 5.3 can help you assess low-back muscular endurance. The exercises that follow are designed to help you maintain a healthy back by stretching and strengthening the major muscle groups that affect the back—the abdominal muscles, the muscles along your spine and sides, and the muscles of your hips and thighs. If you have back problems, check with your physician before beginning any exercise program. Perform the exercises slowly and progress very gradually. Stop and consult your physician if any exercise causes back pain. General guidelines for back exercise programs include the following:

- Do low-back exercises at least three days per week. Most experts recommend daily back exercises.

- Emphasize muscular endurance rather than muscular strength—endurance is more protective.

- Don't do spine exercises involving a full range of motion early in the morning. Because your disks have a high fluid content early in the day, injuries may result.

- Engage in regular endurance exercise such as cycling or walking in addition to performing exercises that specifically build muscular endurance and flexibility. Brisk walking with a natural arm swing may help relieve back pain. Start with fast walking if your core muscles are weak or you have back pain.

- Be patient and stick with your program. Increased back fitness and pain relief may require as long as three months of regular exercise.

- The adage "no pain, no gain" does not apply to back exercises. Always use good form and stop if you feel pain.

- Build core stiffness through stabilization exercises because they strengthen muscles, improve muscular endurance, reduce low back pain, and boost sports performance. Greater core stiffness transfers strength and speed to the limbs, increases the load bearing capacity of the spine, and protects the internal organs during sports movements. When working on abdominal muscles, emphasize stabilization exercises, such as side-bridges, carry exercises, planks, bird-dogs, and the "stir-the-pot" exercise rather than spinal flexion exercises such as sit-ups. Poor performance on the spinal endurance labs (see pages 171–174) means that you are not training your abdominal muscles correctly.

TIPS FOR TODAY AND THE FUTURE

To improve and maintain your flexibility, perform stretches that work the major joints at least twice a week.

RIGHT NOW YOU CAN

- Stand up and stretch—do either the upper-back stretch or the across-the-body stretch shown in the chapter.
- Practice the recommended sitting and standing postures described in the chapter. If needed, adjust your chair or find something to use as a footrest.

IN THE FUTURE YOU CAN

- Build up your flexibility by incorporating more sophisticated stretching exercises into your routine.
- Increase the frequency of your flexibility workouts to five or more days per week.
- Increase the efficiency of your workouts by adding stretching exercises to the cool-down period of your endurance or strength workouts.

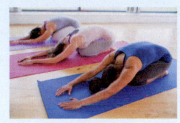

Exercise, such as yoga and tai chi, can provide relief from back pain, depending on the pain's underlying cause. Effective exercises stretch the muscles and connective tissue in the hips, stabilize the spine, and strengthen and build endurance in the core muscles of the back and abdomen.

Yoga may be an option for many back pain sufferers because it offers a variety of exercises that target the spine and the core muscles. Yoga is an ancient practice involving slow, gentle movements performed with controlled breathing and focused attention. Yoga practitioners slowly move into a specific posture (called an *asana*) and hold the posture for up to 60 seconds. There are hundreds of asanas, many of which are easy to do and provide good stretches.

Yoga also involves simple breathing exercises that gently stretch the muscles of the upper back while helping the practitioner focus. Yoga experts say that breathing exercises not only encourage relaxation but also clear the mind and can help relieve mild to moderate pain. Yoga enthusiasts end their workouts energized and refreshed but calm and relaxed.

Many medical professionals now recommend yoga for patients with back pain, particularly asanas that arch and gently stretch the back, such as the cat pose (similar to the cat stretch shown on p. 156) and the child pose (shown here). These are basic asanas that most people can perform repeatedly and hold for a relatively long time.

Because asanas must be performed correctly to be beneficial, qualified instruction is recommended. For those with back pain, physicians advise choosing an instructor who is not only accomplished in yoga but also knowledgeable about back pain and its causes. Such instructors can steer students away from exercises that do more harm than good. It is especially important to choose postures that will benefit the back without worsening the underlying problem. Some asanas can aggravate an injured or painful back if they are performed incorrectly or too aggressively. In fact, people with back pain should avoid a few yoga postures, such as a standing forward bend.

If you have back pain, see your physician to determine its cause before beginning any type of exercise program.

Even gentle exercise or stretching can be bad for an already injured back, especially if the spinal disks or nerves are involved. For some back conditions, rest or therapy may be a better option than exercise, at least in the short term.

Wellness Tip When practicing yoga, it is important to choose postures, such as this child pose, that will benefit the back without worsening the underlying problem. Some asanas can aggravate an injured or painful back if they are performed incorrectly or too aggressively. In fact, people with back pain should avoid a few yoga postures, such as a standing forward bend.

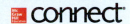

SUMMARY

- Flexibility, the ability of a joint to move through its full range of motion, is highly adaptable and specific to each joint.

- Range of motion can be limited by joint structure, muscle inelasticity, and proprioceptor activity.

- Developing flexibility depends on stretching the elastic tissues within muscles regularly and gently until they lengthen. Overstretching can make connective tissue brittle and lead to rupture.

- Signals sent between muscle and tendon nerves and the spinal cord can enhance flexibility.

- The benefits of flexibility include preventing abnormal stresses that lead to joint deterioration and possibly reducing the risk of injuries.

- Stretches should be held for 10–30 seconds and performed with 2–4 repetitions. Flexibility training should be done a minimum of two–three days per week, preferably following activity, when muscles are warm.

- Static stretching is slow and held to the point of mild tension; ballistic stretching, consisting of bouncing stretches, can lead to injury.

Dynamic stretching moves joints slowly and fluidly through their range of motions. Proprioceptive neuromuscular facilitation uses muscle receptors in contracting and relaxing a muscle.

- Passive stretching, using an outside force to move muscles and joints, achieves a greater range of motion (and has a higher injury risk) than active stretching, which uses opposing muscles to initiate a stretch.

- The spinal column consists of vertebrae separated by intervertebral disks. It provides structure and support for the body and protects the spinal cord. The core muscles stabilize the spine and transfer force between the upper and lower body.

- Acute back pain can be treated as a soft tissue injury, with cold treatment followed by application of heat (once swelling subsides); prolonged bed rest is not recommended. A variety of treatments have been suggested for chronic back pain, including regular exercise, physical therapy, acupuncture, education, and psychological therapy.

- In addition to good posture, proper body mechanics, and regular physical activity, a program for preventing low-back pain includes exercises that develop flexibility, strength, and endurance in the muscle groups that affect the lower back.

LOW-BACK EXERCISES

EXERCISE 1 — Cat Stretch

Instructions: Begin on all fours with your knees below your hips and your hands below your shoulders. Slowly and deliberately move through a cycle of extension and flexion of your spine. **(a)** Begin by slowly pushing your back up and dropping your head slightly until your spine is extended (rounded). **(b)** Then slowly lower your back and lift your chin slightly until your spine is flexed (relaxed and slightly arched). *Do not press at the ends of the range of motion.* Stop if you feel pain. Do 10 slow, continuous cycles of the movement.

Target: Improved flexibility, relaxation, and reduced stiffness in the spine

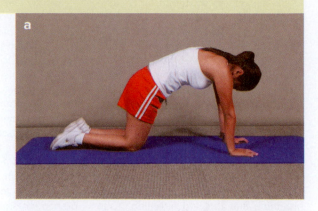

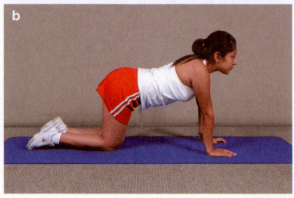

EXERCISE 2 — Step Stretch (See Exercise 6 in the flexibility program, p. 148)

Instructions: Hold each stretch for 10–30 seconds and do 2–4 repetitions on each side.

Target: Improved flexibility, strength, and endurance in the muscles of the hip and the front of the thigh

EXERCISE 3 — Leg Stretcher (See Exercise 11 in the flexibility program, p. 150)

Instructions: Hold each stretch for 10–30 seconds and do 2–4 repetitions on each side.

Target: Improved flexibility in the back of the thigh, hip, knee, and buttocks

EXERCISE 4 — Trunk Twist

Instructions: Lie on your side with top knee bent, lower leg straight, lower arm extended in front of you on the floor, and upper arm at your side. Push down with your upper knee while you twist your trunk to the opposite side. Try to get your shoulders and upper body flat on the floor, turning your head as well. Return to the starting position, and then repeat on the other side. Hold the stretch for 10–30 seconds and do 2–4 repetitions on each side.

Target: Improved flexibility in the lower back and sides

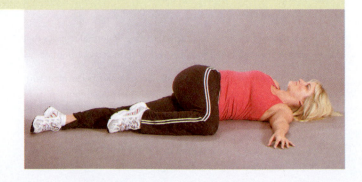

EXERCISE 5 — Curl-Up (See Exercise 4 in the body weight program in Chapter 4, p. 111)

Instructions: Lie on your back with one or both knees bent and arms crossed on your chest or hands under your lower back. Maintain a neutral spine. Tuck your chin in and slowly curl up, one vertebra at a time, as you use your abdominal muscles to lift your head first and then your shoulders. Stop when you can see your knees and hold for 5–10 seconds before returning to the starting position. Do 10 or more repetitions.

Target: Improved strength and endurance in the abdomen

Variation: Add a twist to develop other abdominal muscles. When you have curled up so that your shoulder blades are off the floor, twist your upper body so that one shoulder is higher than the other; reach past your knee with your upper arm. Hold and then return to the starting position. Repeat on the opposite side. Curl-ups can also be done using an exercise ball.

EXERCISE 6 — Isometric Side Bridge (See Exercise 6 in the body weight program in Chapter 4, p. 112)

Instructions: Hold the bridge position for 10 seconds, breathing normally. Work up to a 60-second hold. Perform one or more repetitions on each side.

Target: Increased strength and endurance in the muscles along the sides of the abdomen

Variation: You can make the exercise more difficult by keeping your legs straight and supporting yourself with your feet and forearm (see Lab 5.3) or with your feet and hand (with elbow straight).

EXERCISE 7 — Spine Extensions ("Bird dogs"; see Exercise 5 in the body weight program in Chapter 4, p. 112)

Instructions: Hold each position for 10–30 seconds. Begin with one repetition on each side, and work up to several repetitions.

Target: Increased strength and endurance in the back, buttocks, and back of the thighs

Variation: If you have experienced back pain in the past or if this exercise is difficult for you, do the exercise with both hands on the ground rather than with one arm lifted. You can make this exercise more difficult by doing it balancing on an exercise ball. Find a balance point on your chest while lying face down on the ball with one arm and the opposite leg on the ground. Tense your abdominal muscles while reaching and extending with one arm and reaching and extending with the opposite leg. Repeat this exercise using the other arm and leg.

EXERCISE 8 — Wall Squat (Phantom Chair)

Instructions: Lean against a wall and bend your knees as though you are sitting in a chair. Support your weight with your legs. Begin by holding the position for 5–10 seconds. Squeeze your gluteal muscles together as you do the exercise. Build up to one minute or more. Perform one or more repetitions.

Target: Increased strength and endurance in the lower back, thighs, and abdomen

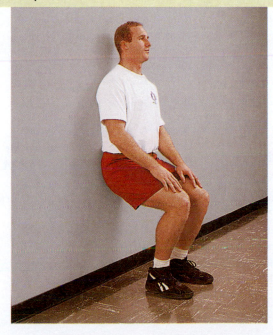

| EXERCISE 9 | Pelvic Tilt |

Instructions: Lie on your back with knees bent and arms extended to the side. Tilt your pelvis under and try to flatten your lower back against the floor. Tighten your buttock and abdominal muscles while you hold this position for 5–10 seconds. Don't hold your breath. Work up to 10 repetitions of the exercise. Pelvic tilts can also be done standing or leaning against a wall. *Note:* Although this is a popular exercise with many therapists, some experts question the safety of pelvic tilts. Stop if you feel pain in your back at any time during the exercise.

Target: Increased strength and endurance in the abdomen and buttocks

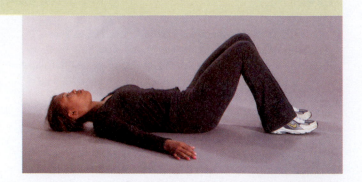

| EXERCISE 10 | Back Bridge |

Instructions: Lie on your back with knees bent and arms extended to the side. Tuck your pelvis under; contract your gluteal muscles; then lift your tailbone, buttocks, and lower back from the floor. Hold this position for 5–10 seconds with your weight resting on your feet, arms, and shoulders, and then return to the starting position. Work up to 10 repetitions of the exercise.

Target: Increased strength and endurance in the hips and buttocks

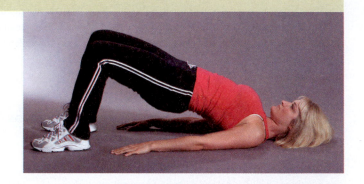

| EXERCISE 11 | Stir the Pot |

Instructions: Assume a plank position on an exercise ball, with forearms on the ball and legs extended to the rear. Maintaining a stiff torso and neutral spine, rotate on the ball in a clockwise direction for 10 repetitions and then repeat in a counterclockwise direction for 10 repetitions.

Target: Increased strength and endurance in the core muscles and shoulders.

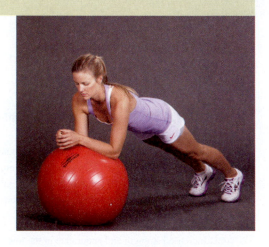

| EXERCISE 12 | Kettlebell or Dumbbell Carry (Suitcase Carry; see Exercise 11 in the body weight program in Ch. 4, p. 118) |

Instructions: This is an excellent exercise for building the core muscles. Pick up a dumbbell or kettlebell in one or both hands. Maintaining good posture, walk 20 to 100 yards carrying the weights. Carry 10 to several hundred pounds, depending on your fitness.

Target: Core muscles, trapezius, leg and hip muscles

COMMON QUESTIONS ANSWERED

Q **Is stretching the same as warming up?**

A No. They are two distinct activities. A warm-up is light exercise that involves moving the joints through the same motions used during a more intense activity; it increases body temperature so your metabolism works better when you're exercising at high intensity. Stretching increases the movement capability of your joints, so you can move more easily with less risk of injury. It is best to stretch when your muscles are warm. Warmed muscles stretch better than cold ones and are less prone to injury.

Q **How much flexibility do I need?**

A This question is not always easy to answer. If you're involved in a sport such as gymnastics, figure skating, or ballet, you are often required to reach extreme joint motions to achieve success. However, nonathletes do not need to reach these extreme joint positions. In fact, too much flexibility may, in some cases, create joint instability and increase your risk of injury. As with other types of fitness, moderation is the key. You should regularly stretch your major joints and muscle groups but not aspire to reach extreme flexibility.

Q **Can I stretch too far?**

A Yes. As muscle tissue is progressively stretched, it reaches a point where it becomes damaged and may rupture. The greatest danger occurs during passive stretching when a partner is doing the stretching for you. It is critical that your stretching partner not force your joint outside its normal functional range of motion.

Q **Can physical training limit flexibility?**

A When done properly, weight training increases flexibility. However, because of the limited range of motion used during the running stride, jogging tends to compromise flexibility. It is important for runners to do flexibility exercises for the hamstrings and quadriceps regularly.

Q **Does static stretching affect muscular strength?**

A Flexibility training increases muscle strength over time, but several recent studies have found that stretching causes short-term decreases in strength, power, and motor control. This is one reason some experts suggest that people not stretch as part of their exercise warm-up, particularly if they plan to engage in a high-performance activity. It is important to warm up before any workout by engaging in 5–10 minutes of light exercise such as walking or slow jogging.

FOR FURTHER EXPLORATION

American Academy of Orthopaedic Surgeons. Provides information about a variety of joint problems.
http://orthoinfo.aaos.org

Back Fit Pro. A website maintained by Dr. Stuart McGill, a professor of spine biomechanics at the University of Waterloo, which provides evidence-based information on preventing and treating back pain.
http://www.backfitpro.com

CUErgo: Cornell University Ergonomics Website. Provides information about how to arrange a computer workstation to prevent back pain and repetitive strain injuries, as well as other topics related to ergonomics.
http://ergo.human.cornell.edu

FIFA 11+. Provides information about a specialized warm-up and conditioning programming that includes dynamic stretches; designed to reduce injuries among soccer players.
http://f-marc.com/11plus/home

Georgia State University: Flexibility. Provides information about the benefits of stretching and ways to develop a safe and effective program; includes illustrations of stretches.
http://www2.gsu.edu/~wwwfit/flexibility.html

International Yoga Federation. A good resource for yoga organizations around the world.
http://www.internationalyogafederation.net

Mayo Clinic: Focus on Flexibility. Presents an easy-to-use program of basic stretching exercises for beginners, with a focus on the benefits of greater flexibility.
http://www.mayoclinic.com/health/stretching/HQ01447

NIH Back Pain Fact Sheet. Provides basic information on the prevention and treatment of back pain.
http://www.ninds.nih.gov/disorders/backpain/backpain.htm

Southern California Orthopedic Institute. Provides information on a variety of orthopedic problems, including back injuries; also has illustrations of spinal anatomy.
http://www.scoi.com

Stretching and Flexibility. Provides information on the physiology of stretching and different types of stretching exercises.
http://www.ifafitness.com/stretch/stretch5.htm

See also the listings for Chapters 2 and 4.

SELECTED BIBLIOGRAPHY

Aguilar, A. J., et al. 2012. A dynamic warm-up model increases quadriceps strength and hamstring flexibility. *Journal of Strength and Conditioning Research* 26(4): 1130–1141.

American College of Sports Medicine. 2012. *ACSM's Health/Fitness Facility Standards and Guidelines,* 4th ed. Champaign, Ill.: Human Kinetics.

American College of Sports Medicine. 2013. *ACSM's Guidelines for Exercise Testing and Prescription,* 9th ed. Philadelphia: Wolters Kluwer/Lippincott Williams & Wilkins Health.

Anderson, B., and J. Anderson. 2010. *Stretching,* 30th anniversary ed. Bolinas, Calif.: Shelter Publications.

Armiger, P., and M. A. Martyn. 2010. *Stretching for Functional Flexibility.* Philadelphia: Lippincott Williams & Wilkins.

Avloniti, A., et al. 2015. The effects of static stretching on speed and agility: One or multiple repetition protocols? *European Journal Sport Science,* published online April 4, 2015, doi:10.1080/17461391.2015.1028467.

Barengo, N. C., et al. 2014. The impact of the FIFA 11+ training program on injury prevention in football players: A systematic review. *International Journal of Environmental Research and Public Health* 11(11): 1198–2000.

Barroso, R., et al. 2012. Maximal strength, number of repetitions, and total volume are differently affected by static-, ballistic-, and proprioceptive neuromuscular facilitation stretching. *Journal of Strength and Conditioning Research* 26(9): 2432–2437.

Bedard, R. J., et al. 2013. Increased active hamstring stiffness after exercise in women with a history of low back pain. *Journal of Sports Rehabilitation* 22(1): 47–52.

Bidwell, A. J., et al. 2012. Yoga training improves quality of life in women with asthma. *Journal of Alternative Complementary Medicine* 18(8): 749–755.

Blahnik, J. 2011. *Full-Body Flexibility,* 2nd ed. Champaign, Ill.: Human Kinetics.

Brito, L. B., et al. 2013. Does flexibility influence the ability to sit and rise from the floor? *American Journal of Physical Medicine and Rehabilitation* 92(3): 241–247.

Cabido, C. E., et al. 2014. Acute effect of constant torque and angle stretching on range of motion, muscle passive properties, and stretch discomfort perception. *Journal Strength Conditioning Research* 28(4): 1050–1057.

Castanharo, R., et al. 2014. Corrective sitting strategies: An examination of muscle activity and spine loading. *Journal Electromyographic Kinesiology* 24(1): 114–119.

Chatzopoulos, D., et al. 2014. Acute effects of static and dynamic stretching on balance, agility, reaction time and movement time. *Journal of Sports Science and Medicine* 13(2): 403–409.

Chen, C. H., et al. 2013. Two stretching treatments for the hamstrings: proprioceptive neuromuscular facilitation versus kinesio taping. *Journal of Sports Rehabilitation* 22(1): 59–66.

Costa, P. B., et al. 2014. Effects of dynamic stretching on strength, muscle imbalance, and muscle activation. *Medicine Science Sports Exercise* 46(3): 586–593.

Cramer, H., et al. 2013. Randomized-controlled trial comparing yoga and home-based exercise for chronic neck pain. *Clinical Journal of Pain* 29(3): 216–223.

Cramer, H., et al. 2014. A systematic review and meta-analysis of yoga for hypertension. *American Journal Hypertension* 27(9): 1146–1151.

Cramer, H., et al. 2015. A systematic review of yoga for heart disease. *European Journal Preventive Cardiology* 22(3): 284–295.

Delavier, F., and M. Gundill. *Delavier's Core Training Anatomy.* 2012. Champaign, Ill.: Human Kinetics.

Delavier, F., J. P. Clemenceau, and M. Gundill. 2012. *Delavier's Stretching Anatomy.* Champaign, Ill.: Human Kinetics.

Dhananjai, S., et al. 2013. Reducing psychological distress and obesity through Yoga practice. *International Journal of Yoga* 6(1): 66–70.

Franca, F. R., et al. 2012. Effects of muscular stretching and segmental stabilization on functional disability and pain in patients with chronic low back pain: a randomized, controlled trial. *Journal of Manipulative and Physiological Therapy* 35(4): 279–285.

Frost, D. M., et al. 2012. Is there a low-back cost to hip-centric exercise? Quantifying the lumbar spine joint compression and shear forces during movements used to overload the hips. *Journal of Sports Science* 30(9): 859–870.

Garber, C. E., et al. 2011. Quantity and quality of exercise for developing and maintaining cardiorespiratory, musculoskeletal, and neuromotor fitness in apparently healthy adults: guidance for prescribing exercise. *Medicine and Science in Sports and Exercise* 43(7): 1334–1359.

Giangregorio, L. M., et al. 2015. Too fit to fracture: Outcomes of a Delphi consensus process on physical activity and exercise recommendations for adults with osteoporosis with or without vertebral fractures. *Osteoporosis International* 26(3): 891–910.

Gonzalez-Rave, J. M., et al. 2012. Efficacy of two different stretch training programs (passive vs. proprioceptive neuromuscular facilitation) on shoulder and hip range of motion in older people. *Journal of Strength and Conditioning Research* 26(4): 1045–1051.

Guo, Y. H., et al. 2014. Effect of high temperature yoga exercise on improving physical and mental well-being of overweight middle-aged and young women. *International Journal Clinical Experimental Medicine* 7(12): 5842–5846.

Haddad, M., et al. 2014. Static stretching can impair explosive performance for at least 24 hours. *Journal Strength Conditioning Research* 28(1): 140–146.

Haladay, D. E., et al. 2013. Quality of systematic reviews on specific spinal stabilization exercise for chronic low back pain. *Journal of Orthopedic Sports Physical Therapy.* In press.

Halpern, J., et al. 2014. Yoga for improving sleep quality and quality of life for older adults. *Alternative Therapies Health Medicine* 20(3): 37–46.

Hayes, B. T., et al. 2012. Lack of neuromuscular origins of adaptation after a long-term stretching program. *Journal of Sports Rehabilitation* 21(2): 99–106.

Heinrich, K. M., et al. 2012. Mission essential fitness: comparison of functional circuit training to traditional Army physical training for active duty military. *Military Medicine* 177(10): 1125–1130.

Herman, K., et al. 2012. The effectiveness of neuromuscular warm-up strategies, that require no additional equipment, for preventing lower limb injuries during sports participation: A systematic review. *BMC Medicine* 10: 75.

Howley, E., and D. Thompson. 2012. *Fitness Professional's Handbook.* 6th ed. Champaign, Ill.: Human Kinetics.

Husu, P., and J. Suni. 2012. Predictive validity of health-related fitness tests on back pain and related disability: a 6-year follow-up study among high-functioning older adults. *Journal of Physical Activity and Health* 9(2): 249–258.

Inami, T., et al. 2015. Acute changes in peripheral vascular tonus and systemic circulation during static stretching. *Research in Sports Medicine* 23(2): 167–178.

Judge, L. W., et al. 2012. An examination of pre-activity and post-activity stretching practices of cross country and track and field distance coaches. *Journal of Strength and Conditioning Research.* In press.

Junqueira, D.R.G., et al. 2014. Heritability and lifestyle factors in chronic low back pain: Results of the Australian Twin Low Back Pain Study (The AUTBACK study). *European Journal of Pain* 18: 1410–1418.

Kanaya, A. M., et al. 2014. Restorative yoga and metabolic risk factors: The Practicing Restorative Yoga vs. Stretching for the Metabolic Syndrome (PRYSMS) randomized trial. *Journal Diabetes Complications* 28(3): 406–412.

Kirmizigil, B., et al. 2014. Effects of three different stretching techniques on vertical jumping performance. *Journal Strength Conditioning Research* 28(5): 1263–1271.

Konrad, A. and M. Tilp. 2014. Increased range of motion after static stretching is not due to changes in muscle and tendon structures. *Clinical Biomechanics* 29(6): 636–642.

Lam, L. C., et al. 2012. A 1-year randomized controlled trial comparing mind body exercise (tai chi) with stretching and toning exercise on cognitive function in older Chinese adults at risk of cognitive decline. *Journal of the American Medical Directors Association* 13(6): 568 e515–520.

LEE, B. C. Y. and S. M. McGill. 2015. Effect of long-term isometric training on core/torso stiffness. *Journal Strength Conditioning Research* 29(6): 1515–1526.

Lowery, R. P., et al. 2014. Effects of static stretching on 1-mile uphill run performance. *Journal Strength Conditioning Research* 28(1): 161–167.

Maddigan, M. E., et al. 2012. A comparison of assisted and unassisted proprioceptive neuromuscular facilitation techniques and static stretching. *Journal of Strength and Conditioning Research* 26(5): 1238–1244.

Malliaropoulos, N., et al. 2012. Hamstring exercises for track and field athletes: injury and exercise biomechanics, and possible implications for exercise selection and primary prevention. *British Journal of Sports Medicine* 46(12): 846–851.

Mandroukas, A., et al. 2014. Acute partial passive stretching increases range of motion and muscle strength. *Journal Sports Medicine Physical Fitness* 54(3): 289–297.

Mannion, A. F., et al. 2012. Spine stabilisation exercises in the treatment of chronic low back pain: a good clinical outcome is not associated with improved abdominal muscle function. *European Spine Journal* 21(7): 1301–1310.

Markil, N., et al. 2012. Yoga Nidra relaxation increases heart rate variability and is unaffected by a prior bout of Hatha yoga. *Journal of Alternative Complementary Medicine* 18(10): 953–958.

Matsuo, S., et al. 2015. Changes in force and stiffness after static stretching of eccentrically damaged hamstrings. *European Journal Applied Physiology* 115(5): 981–991.

McBain, K., et al. 2012. Prevention of sports injury I: a systematic review of applied biomechanics and physiology outcomes research. *British Journal of Sports Medicine* 46(3): 169–173.

McBain, K., et al. 2012. Prevention of sport injury II: a systematic review of clinical science research. *British Journal of Sports Medicine* 46(3): 174–179.

McGill, S. 2007. *Low Back Disorders: Evidence-Based Prevention and Rehabilitation,* 2nd ed. Champaign, Ill.: Human Kinetics.

McGill, S. 2012. *Ultimate Back: Enhancing Performance* (DVD). Waterloo, Canada: Backfit Pro.

McGill, S. 2014. *Ultimate Back Fitness and Performance,* 5th ed. Waterloo, Canada: Backfit Pro.

McGill, S., et al. 2013. Movement quality and links to measures of fitness in firefighters. *Work.* 45(3): 357–366.

McGill, S., et al. 2014. *Assessing Movement: A Contrast in Approaches and Future Directions* (DVD). Waterloo, Canada: Backfit Pro.

McGill, S. M., and L. W. Marshall. 2012. Kettlebell swing, snatch, and bottoms-up carry: back and hip muscle activation, motion, and low back loads. *Journal of Strength and Conditioning Research* 26(1): 16–27.

McGill, S. M., et al. 2009. Comparison of different strongman events: trunk muscle activation and lumbar spine motion, load, and stiffness. *Journal of Strength and Conditioning Research* 23(4): 1148–1161.

McGill, S. M., et al. 2013. Low back loads while walking and carrying: comparing the load carried in one hand or in both hands. *Ergonomics* 56(2): 293–302.

McGill, S. M., et al. 2014. Analysis of pushing exercises: Muscle activity and spine load while contrasting techniques on stable surfaces with a labile suspension strap training system. *Journal Strength Conditioning Research* 28(1): 105–116.

McGill, S., M. Belore, I. Crosby, and C. Russell. 2010. Clinical tools to quantify torso flexion endurance: Normative data from student and firefighter populations. *Occupational Ergonomics* 9 (1): 55–61.

Miles, S. C., et al. 2013. Arterial blood pressure and cardiovascular responses to yoga practice. *Journal of Alternative Complementary Medicine* 19(1): 38–45.

Miller, K. C. and J. A. Burne. 2014. Golgi tendon organ reflex inhibition following manually applied acute static stretching. *Journal Sports Science* 32(15): 1491–1497.

Mizuno, T., et al. 2014. Stretching-induced deficit of maximal isometric torque is restored within 10 minutes. *Journal Strength Conditioning Research* 28(1): 147–153.

Molacek, Z. D., et al. 2010. Effects of low- and high-volume stretching on bench press performance in collegiate football players. *Journal of Strength and Conditioning Research* 24(3): 711–716.

Muyor, J. M., et al. 2012. Effect of stretching program in an industrial workplace on hamstring flexibility and sagittal spinal posture of adult women workers: a randomized controlled trial. *Journal of Back and Musculoskeletal Rehabilitation* 25(3): 161–169.

Myer, G. D., et al. 2014. The back squat: A proposed assessment of functional deficits and technical factors that limit performance *Strength Conditioning Journal* 36(6): 4–27.

Nelson, A. G., and J. Kokkonen. 2014. *Stretching Anatomy,* 2nd ed. Champaign, Ill.: Human Kinetics.

Newton, K. M., et al. 2014. Efficacy of yoga for vasomotor symptoms: A randomized controlled trial. *Menopause* 21(4): 339–346.

Nieman, D. C. 2011. *Exercise Testing and Prescription: A Health-Related Approach,* 7th ed. New York: McGraw-Hill.

Norasteh, A. A., ed. 2012. *Low Back Pain.* InTech, www.intechopen.com/books/low-back-pain/.

O'Sullivan, K., et al. 2012. The effects of eccentric training on lower limb flexibility: a systematic review. *British Journal of Sports Medicine* 46(12): 838–845.

Peck, E., et al. 2014. The effects of stretching on performance. *Current Sports Medicine Reports* 13(3): 179–185.

Pinto, M. D., et al. 2014. Differential effects of 30- vs. 60-second static muscle stretching on vertical jump performance. *Journal Strength Conditioning Research* 28(12): 3440–3446.

Plouvier, S. et al. 2015. Occupational biomechanical exposure predicts low back pain in older age among men in the Gazel Cohort. *International Archives Occupational Environmental Health* 88: 501–510.

Prado, E. T., et al. 2014. Hatha yoga on body balance. *International Journal Yoga* 7(2): 133–137.

Qui, P., and W. Zhu. 2013. *Tai Chi Illustrated.* Champaign, Ill.: Human Kinetics.

Ribeiro, A. S., et al. 2014. Static stretching and performance in multiple sets in the bench press exercise. *Journal Strength Conditioning Research* 28(4): 1158–1163.

Ryan, E. D., et al. 2014. Acute effects of different volumes of dynamic stretching on vertical jump performance, flexibility and muscular endurance. *Clinical Physiology and Functional Imaging.* 34(6): 485–492.

Samuel, M. N., et al. 2008. Acute effects of static and ballistic stretching on measures of strength and power. *Journal of Strength and Conditioning Research* 22(5): 1422–1428.

Sartor, C. D., et al. 2012. Effects of a combined strengthening, stretching and functional training program versus usual-care on gait biomechanics and foot function for diabetic neuropathy: a randomized controlled trial. *BMC Musculoskeletal Disorders* 13: 36.

Scannell, J. P., et al. 2009. Disc prolapse: Evidence of reversal with repeated extension. *Spine* 34(4): 344–350.

Shnayderman, I., and M. Katz-Leurer. 2013. An aerobic walking programme versus muscle strengthening programme for chronic low back pain: a randomized controlled trial. *Clinical Rehabilitation* 27(3): 207–214.

Shrier, I., and M. McHugh. 2012. Does static stretching reduce maximal muscle performance? A review. *Clinical Journal of Sports Medicine* 22(5): 450–451.

Siddarth, D., et al. 2014. An observational study of the health benefits of yoga or tai chi compared with aerobic exercise in community-dwelling middle-aged and older adults. *American Journal Geriatric Psychiatry.* 22(3): 272–273.

Sidorkewicz N and S.M. McGill. 2015. Documenting female spine motion during coitus with a commentary on the implications for the low back pain patient. *European Spine Journal.* 24(3): 513–520.

Signorelli, G. R., et al. 2012. A pre-season comparison of aerobic fitness and flexibility of younger and older professional soccer players. *International Journal of Sports Medicine* 33(11): 867–872.

Stathokostas, L., et al. 2012. Flexibility training and functional ability in older adults: a systematic review. *Journal of Aging Research* 2012: 306818.

Suni, J. H., et al. 2013. Neuromuscular exercise and counseling decrease absenteeism due to low back pain in young conscripts: a randomized, population-based primary prevention study. *Spine* 38(5): 375–384.

Swain, D. P. 2013. *ACSM's Resource Manual for Guidelines for Exercise Testing and Prescription,* 7th ed. Philadelphia: Wolters Kluwer/Lippincott Williams & Wilkins Health.

Taniguchi, K., et al. 2015. Acute decrease in the stiffness of resting muscle belly due to static stretching. *Scandinavian Journal Medicine Science Sports.* 25(1): 32–40.

Tracy, B. L., and C. E. Hart. 2013. Bikram yoga training and physical fitness in healthy young adults. *Journal of Strength and Conditioning Research* 27(3): 822–830.

Trajano, G., et al. 2015. Static stretching increases muscle fatigue during submaximal sustained isometric contractions. *Journal Sports Medicine Physical Fitness.* 55(1–2): 43–50.

Wajswelner, H., et al. 2012. Clinical Pilates versus general exercise for chronic low back pain: randomized trial. *Medicine and Science in Sports and Exercise* 44(7): 1197–1205.

Wang, X. Q., et al. 2012. A meta-analysis of core stability exercise versus general exercise for chronic low back pain. *PLoS One* 7(12): e52082.

Wells, C., et al. 2012. Defining Pilates exercise: a systematic review. *Journal of Alternative Complementary Medicine* 20(4): 253–262.

Wells, C., et al. 2013. Effectiveness of Pilates exercise in treating people with chronic low back pain: a systematic review of systematic reviews. *BMC Medical Research Methodology* 13: 7.

Wicke, J., et al. 2014. A comparison of self-administered proprioceptive neuromuscular facilitation to static stretching on range of motion and flexibility. *Journal Strength Conditioning Research.* 28(1): 168–172.

Wong, A. and A. Figueroa. 2014. Eight weeks of stretching training reduces aortic wave reflection magnitude and blood pressure in obese postmenopausal women. *Journal Human Hypertension.* 28(4): 246–250.

Yamaguchi, T., K. Takizawa, and K. Shibata. 2015. Acute effect of dynamic stretching on endurance running performance in well-trained male runners. *Journal of Strength and Conditioning Research* 29 April [epub ahead of print]

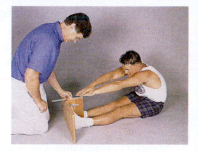
Name _____ Section _____ Date _____

LAB 5.1 Assessing Your Current Level of Flexibility

Part I Sit-and-Reach Test

Equipment

Use a modified Wells and Dillon flexometer or construct your own measuring device using a firm box or two pieces of wood about 30 centimeters (12 inches) high attached at right angles to each other. Attach a metric ruler to measure the extent of reach. With the low numbers of the ruler toward the person being tested, set the 26-centimeter mark of the ruler at the footline of the box. Individuals who cannot reach as far as the footline will have scores below 26 centimeters; those who can reach past their feet will have scores above 26 centimeters. Most studies show no relationship between performance on the sit-and-reach test and the incidence of back pain.

Preparation

Warm up your muscles with a low-intensity activity such as walking or easy jogging. Then perform slow stretching movements.

Instructions

1. Remove your shoes and sit facing the flexibility measuring device with your knees fully extended and your feet flat against the device about 10 centimeters (4 inches) apart.

2. Reach as far forward as you can, with palms down, arms evenly stretched, and knees fully extended; hold the position of maximum reach for about two seconds.

3. Perform the stretch 2 times, recording the distance of maximum reach to the nearest 0.5 centimeters:
   _____ cm

Rating Your Flexibility

Find the score in the table below to determine your flexibility rating. Record it here and on the final page of this lab.

Rating: _____

Ratings for Sit-and-Reach Test

	Rating/Score (cm)*				
Men	*Needs Improvement*	*Fair*	*Good*	*Very Good*	*Excellent*
Age: 15–19	Below 24	24–28	29–33	34–38	Above 38
20–29	Below 25	25–29	30–33	34–39	Above 39
30–39	Below 23	23–27	28–32	33–37	Above 37
40–49	Below 18	18–23	24–28	29–34	Above 34
50–59	Below 16	16–23	24–27	28–34	Above 34
60–69	Below 15	15–19	20–24	25–32	Above 32
Women					
Age: 15–19	Below 29	29–33	34–37	38–42	Above 42
20–29	Below 28	28–32	33–36	37–40	Above 40
30–39	Below 27	27–31	32–35	36–40	Above 40
40–49	Below 25	25–29	30–33	34–37	Above 37
50–59	Below 25	25–29	30–32	33–38	Above 38
60–69	Below 23	23–26	27–30	31–34	Above 34

*Footline is set at 26 cm.

SOURCE: Canadian Society for Exercise Physiology. 2003. *The Canadian Physical Activity, Fitness & Lifestyle Approach: CSEP-Health & Fitness Program's Health-Related Appraisal and Counseling Strategy,* 3rd ed. Adapted with permission from the Canadian Society for Exercise Physiology.

LABORATORY ACTIVITIES

Part II Range-of-Motion Assessment

This portion of the lab can be completed by doing visual comparisons or by measuring joint range of motion with a goniometer or other instrument.

Equipment

1. A partner to do visual comparisons or to measure the range of motion of your joints. (You can also use a mirror to perform your own visual comparisons.)
2. For the measurement method, you need a goniometer, flexometer, or other instrument to measure range of motion.

Preparation

Warm up your muscles with some low-intensity activity such as walking or easy jogging.

Instructions

On the following pages, the average range of motion is illustrated and listed quantitatively for some of the major joints. Visually assess the range of motion in your joints, and compare it to that shown in the illustrations. For each joint, note (with a check mark) whether your range of motion is above average, average, or below average and in need of improvement. Average values for range of motion are given in degrees for each joint in the assessment. You can also complete the assessment by measuring your range of motion with a goniometer, flexometer, or other instrument. If you are using this measurement method, identify your rating (above average, average, or below average) and record your range of motion in degrees next to the appropriate category. Although the measurement method is more time-consuming, it allows you to track the progress of your stretching program more precisely and to note changes within the broader ratings categories (below average, above average).

Record your ratings on the following pages and on the chart on the final page of this lab. (Ratings were derived from several published sources.)

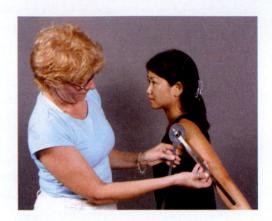

Assessment of range of motion using a goniometer

1. Shoulder Abduction and Adduction

For each position and arm, check one of the following; fill in degrees if using the measurement method.

Shoulder abduction—raise arm up to the side.

Right   Left

_____   _____   Below average/needs improvement

_____   _____   Average (92–95°)

_____   _____   Above average

Shoulder adduction—move arm down and in front of body.

Right   Left

_____   _____   Below average/needs improvement

_____   _____   Average (124–127°)

_____   _____   Above average

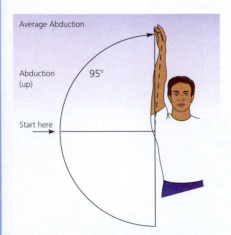

Average Abduction

Abduction (up)   95°

Start here

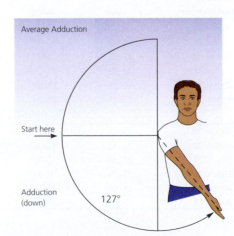

Average Adduction

Start here

Adduction (down)   127°

2. Shoulder Flexion and Extension

For each position and arm, check one of the following; fill in degrees if using the measurement method.

Shoulder flexion—raise arm up in front of the body.

Right	Left	
_____	_____	Below average/needs improvement
_____	_____	Average (92–95°)
_____	_____	Above average

Shoulder extension—move arm down and behind the body.

Right	Left	
_____	_____	Below average/needs improvement
_____	_____	Average (145–150°)
_____	_____	Above average

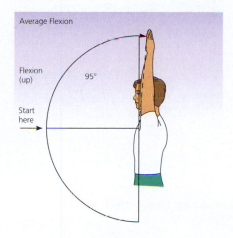

Average Flexion

Flexion (up) 95°

Start here

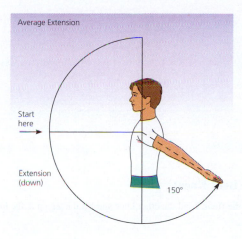

Average Extension

Start here

Extension (down) 150°

3. Trunk/Low-Back Lateral Flexion

Bend directly sideways at your waist. To prevent injury, keep your knees slightly bent, and support your trunk by placing your hand or forearm on your thigh. Check one of the following for each side; fill in degrees if using the measurement method.

Right	Left	
_____	_____	Below average/needs improvement
_____	_____	Average (36–40°)
_____	_____	Above average

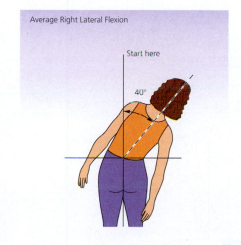

Average Right Lateral Flexion

Start here

40°

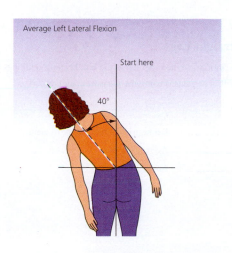

Average Left Lateral Flexion

Start here

40°

4. Hip Abduction

Raise your leg to the side at the hip. Check one of the following for each leg; fill in degrees if using the measurement method.

Right   Left

_____   _____   Below average/needs improvement

_____   _____   Average (40–45°)

_____   _____   Above average

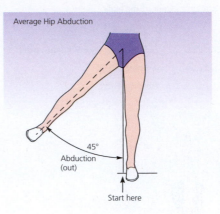

5. Hip Flexion (Bent Knee)

With one leg flat on the floor, bend the other knee and lift the leg up at the hip. Check one of the following for each leg; fill in degrees if using the measurement method.

Right   Left

_____   _____   Below average/needs improvement

_____   _____   Average (121–125°)

_____   _____   Above average

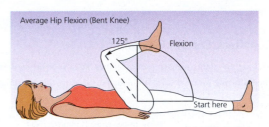

6. Hip Flexion (Straight Leg)

With one leg flat on the floor, raise the other leg at the hip, keeping both legs straight. Take care not to put excess strain on your back. Check one of the following for each leg; fill in degrees if using the measurement method.

Right   Left

_____   _____   Below average/needs improvement

_____   _____   Average (79–81°)

_____   _____   Above average

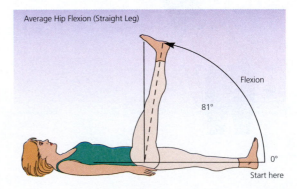

7. Ankle Dorsiflexion and Plantar Flexion

For each position and foot, check one of the following; fill in degrees if using the measurement method.

Ankle dorsiflexion—pull your toes toward your shin.

Right   Left

_____   _____   Below average/needs improvement

_____   _____   Average (9–13)

_____   _____   Above average

Plantar flexion—point your toes.

Right   Left

_____   _____   Below average/needs improvement

_____   _____   Average (50–55)

_____   _____   Above average

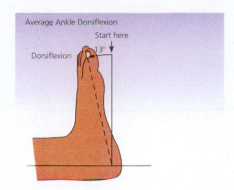

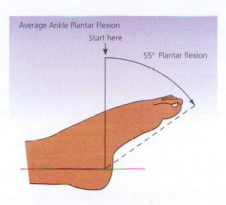

Rating Your Flexibility

Sit-and-reach test: Score: _____ cm Rating: _____

Range-of-Motion Assessment

Identify your rating for each joint on each side of the body. If you used the comparison method, put check marks in the appropriate categories; if you measured range of motion, enter the degrees for each joint in the appropriate category.

Joint/Assessment		Right Below Average	Right Average	Right Above Average	Left Below Average	Left Average	Left Above Average
1. Shoulder abduction and adduction	Abduction						
	Adduction						
2. Shoulder flexion and extension	Flexion						
	Extension						
3. Trunk/low-back lateral flexion	Flexion						
4. Hip abduction	Abduction						
5. Hip flexion (bent knee)	Flexion						
6. Hip flexion (straight leg)	Flexion						
7. Ankle dorsiflexion and plantar flexion	Dorsiflexion						
	Plantar flexion						

LABORATORY ACTIVITIES

Using Your Results

How did you score? Do your scores for the flexibility tests surprise you? Are you satisfied with your current ratings?

If you're not satisfied, set a realistic goal for improvement:

Are you satisfied with your current level of flexibility as expressed in your daily life—for example, your ability to maintain good posture and move easily and without pain?

If you're not satisfied, set some realistic goals for improvement:

What should you do next? Enter the results of this lab in the Preprogram Assessment column in Appendix C. If you've set goals for improvement, begin planning your flexibility program by completing the plan in Lab 5.2. After several weeks of your program, complete this lab again and enter the results in the Post-program Assessment column of Appendix C. How do the results compare?

Name _____ Section _____ Date _____

LAB 5.2 Creating a Personalized Program for Developing Flexibility

1. *Goals.* List goals for your flexibility program. On the left, include specific, measurable goals that you can use to track the progress of your fitness program. These goals might be things like raising your sit-and-reach score from fair to good or your bent-leg hip flexion rating from below average to average. On the right, include long-term and more qualitative goals, such as reducing your risk for back pain.

Specific Goals: Current Status   Final Goals

_____   _____

_____   _____

_____   _____

Other Goals: _____

_____

2. *Exercises.* The exercises in the program plan below are from the general stretching program presented in Chapter 5. You can add or delete exercises depending on your needs, goals, and preferences. For any exercises you add, fill in the areas of the body affected.

3. *Frequency.* A minimum frequency of two–three days per week is recommended; five–seven days per week is ideal. You may want to do your stretching exercises the same days you plan to do cardiorespiratory endurance exercise or weight training because muscles stretch better following exercise, when they are warm.

4. *Intensity.* All stretches should be done to the point of mild discomfort, not pain.

5. *Time/duration.* All stretches should be held for 10–30 seconds. (PNF techniques should include a 6-second contraction followed by a 10–30-second assisted stretch.) All stretches should be performed 2–4 times, for a total of 60 seconds per exercise.

Program Plan for Flexibility

Exercise	Areas Stretched	Frequency (check ✓)						
		M	T	W	Th	F	Sa	Su
Head turns and tilts	Neck							
Towel stretch	Triceps, shoulders, chest							
Across-the-body and overhead stretches	Shoulders, upper back, back of the arm							
Upper-back stretch	Upper back							
Lateral stretch	Trunk muscles							
Step stretch	Hip, front of thigh							
Side lunge	Inner thigh, hip, calf							
Inner-thigh stretch	Inner thigh, hip							
Hip and trunk stretch	Trunk, outer thigh and hip, lower back							
Modified hurdler stretch	Back of the thigh, lower back							
Leg stretcher	Back of the thigh, hip, knee, ankle, buttocks							
Lower-leg stretch	Back of the lower leg							
Single-leg deadlift	Hamstrings and gluteal muscles							

You can monitor your program using a chart like the one on the next page.

LABORATORY ACTIVITIES

Flexibility Program Chart

Fill in the dates you perform each stretch, the number of seconds you hold each stretch (should be 10–30), and the number of repetitions of each (should be 2–4). For an easy check on the duration of your stretches, count "one thousand one, one thousand two," and so on. You will probably find that over time you'll be able to hold each stretch longer (in addition to being able to stretch farther).

Exercise/Date																		
	Duration																	
	Reps																	
	Duration																	
	Reps																	
	Duration																	
	Reps																	
	Duration																	
	Reps																	
	Duration																	
	Reps																	
	Duration																	
	Reps																	
	Duration																	
	Reps																	
	Duration																	
	Reps																	
	Duration																	
	Reps																	
	Duration																	
	Reps																	
	Duration																	
	Reps																	
	Duration																	
	Reps																	
	Duration																	
	Reps																	
	Duration																	
	Reps																	
	Duration																	
	Reps																	
	Duration																	
	Reps																	
	Duration																	
	Reps																	

Name _____ **Section** _____ **Date** _____

LAB 5.3 Assessing Muscular Endurance for Low-Back Health

The four tests in this lab evaluate the muscular endurance of major spine-stabilizing muscles. These tests are the trunk flexor endurance test, back extensor endurance test, side bridge endurance test, and the front plank endurance test.

Trunk Flexor Endurance Test (also called the V-sit–Flexor Endurance Test)

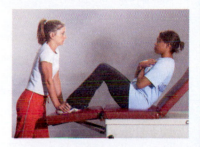

Equipment

1. Stopwatch or clock with a second hand
2. Exercise mat or padded exercise table
3. Two helpers
4. A wedge angled at 55 degrees from the floor or padded bench (optional)

Preparation

Warm up with some low-intensity activity such as walking or easy jogging.

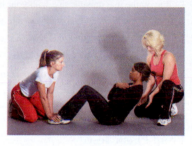

Instructions

1. To start, assume a sit-up posture with your back supported at an angle of 55 degrees from the floor; support can be provided by a wedge, a padded bench, or a spotter (see photos). Your knees and hips should both be flexed at 90 degrees, and your arms should be folded across your chest with your hands placed on the opposite shoulders. Your toes should be secured under a toe strap or held by a partner.

2. Your goal is to hold the starting position (isometric contraction) as long as possible after the support is pulled away. To begin the test, a helper should pull the wedge or other support back about 10 centimeters (4 inches). The helper should keep track of the time; if a spotter is acting as your support, she or he should be ready to support your weight as soon as your torso begins to move back. Your final score is the total time you are able to hold the contraction—from the time the support is removed until any part of your back touches the support or you request to discontinue the test. Remember to breathe normally throughout the test.

3. Record your time here and on the chart at the end of the lab. Trunk flexors endurance time: _____ sec

Back Extensor Endurance Test (also called the Biering-Sorensen extension test)

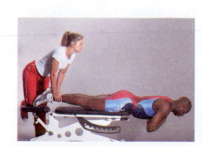

Equipment

1. Stopwatch or clock with a second hand
2. Extension bench with padded ankle and hip support or any padded bench
3. Partner

Preparation

Warm up with some low-intensity activity such as walking or easy jogging.

Instructions

1. Lie face down on the test bench with your upper body extending out over the end of the bench and your pelvis, hips, and knees flat on the bench. Your arms should be folded across your chest with your hands placed on the opposite shoulders. Your legs and hips should be secured under padded straps or held by a partner.

2. Your goal is to hold your upper body in a straight horizontal line with your lower body as long as possible. Keep your neck straight and neutral; don't raise your head and don't arch your back. Breathe normally. Your partner should keep track of the time and watch your form. Your final score is the total time you are able to hold the horizontal position—from the time you assume the position until your upper body drops from the horizontal position.

3. Record your time here and on the chart below. Back extensors endurance time: _____ sec

Side Bridge Endurance Test

Equipment

1. Stopwatch or clock with a second hand
2. Exercise mat
3. Partner

Preparation

Warm up your muscles with some low-intensity activity such as walking or easy jogging. Practice assuming the side bridge position described below.

Instructions

1. Lie on the mat on your side with your legs extended. Place your top foot in front of your lower foot for support. Lift your hips off the mat so you are supporting yourself on one elbow and your feet (see photo). Your body should maintain a straight line. Breathe normally; don't hold your breath.

2. Hold the position as long as possible. Your partner should keep track of the time and make sure that you maintain the correct position. Your final score is the total time you are able to hold the side bridge with correct form—from the time you lift your hips until your hips return to the mat.

3. Rest for five minutes and then repeat the test on the other side. Record your times here and on the chart at the end of the lab.
Right side bridge time: _____ sec
Left side bridge time: _____ sec

Front Plank Test

Equipment

1. Stopwatch or clock with a second hand
2. Exercise mat
3. Partner

Preparation

Warm up your muscles with some low-intensity activity such as walking or easy jogging. Practice assuming the front plank position described below.

Instructions

1. Assume a front plank position by lying on your front and then lifting your hips, supporting your weight on your forearms and toes and keeping the torso rigid (see photo). Your body should maintain a straight line; keep your hands together and elbows directly under your shoulders. Breathe normally and don't hold your breath.

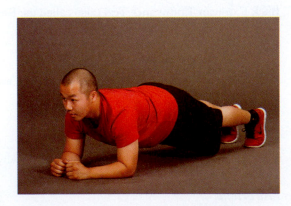

2. Hold the position as long as possible. Your partner should keep track of the time and make sure that you maintain the correct position. Your final score is the total time you are able to hold the front plank with correct form—from the time you lift your hips until your hips return to the mat.

3. Record your time here and on the chart at the end of the lab. Front plank time: _____ sec

Rating Your Test Results for Muscular Endurance for Low-Back Health

The table below shows percentiles for torso endurance tests for healthy young college students, ages 17 to 25, based on a study of 181 university students. Compare your scores with the times shown in the table. Your percentile on each test tells you the percent of the students in the study scored at or below your score.

Percentiles Ranks for Torso Muscle Endurance Tests for College-Age Men and Women (age 17–25)

Percentiles	Trunk flexor test (sec)		Back extensor test (sec)		Side bridge test, right (sec)		Side bridge test, left (sec)		Front plank test (sec)	
	Men	Women	Men	Women	Men	Women	Men	Women	Men	Women
99%	276	246	246	265	193	130	187	133	400	213
95%	234	208	215	232	164	112	160	114	336	181
90%	211	188	199	215	149	102	146	104	302	165
85%	196	174	188	204	140	96	137	97	280	154
80%	184	163	179	194	131	91	129	92	261	145
75%	174	154	171	186	124	86	122	87	245	137
70%	164	145	164	179	118	83	116	83	231	130
65%	156	138	159	173	113	79	111	79	219	124
60%	148	130	152	167	107	76	106	75	206	118
55%	140	123	147	161	102	72	101	72	195	112
50%	132	116	141	155	97	69	96	68	183	106
45%	124	109	135	149	92	66	91	64	171	100
40%	117	102	130	143	87	63	86	61	160	95
35%	108	94	123	137	81	59	81	57	147	88
30%	100	87	118	131	76	55	76	53	135	82
25%	90	78	111	124	70	52	70	49	121	75
20%	80	69	103	116	63	47	63	44	105	67
15%	68	58	94	106	54	42	55	39	86	58
10%	53	44	83	95	45	36	46	32	64	47
5%	30	24	67	78	30	26	32	22	30	31
1%	0	0	36	45	1	8	5	3	0	0

NOTE: The percentiles were based on data collected on 181 university kinesiology students ages 17–25. The results might not be representative of other populations.

SOURCE: Percentile charts calculated from the data of McGill, S., M. Belore, I. Crosby, and C. Russell. 2010. Clinical tools to quantify torso flexion endurance: Normative data from student and firefighter populations. *Occupational Ergonomics* 9(1): 55–61.

Record Your Scores

Test	Time	Percentile
Trunk Flexor Test		
Back Extensor Test		
Side Bridge Test, right side		
Side Bridge Test, left side		
Front Plank Test		

LABORATORY ACTIVITIES

Using Your Results

How did you score? Are you surprised by your scores for the low-back tests? Are you satisfied with your current ratings?

If you're not satisfied, set a realistic goal for improvement. The norms in this lab are based on healthy young adults, so a score above the mean may or may not be realistic for you. Instead, you may want to set a specific goal based on time rather than rating; for example, set a goal of improving your time by 10%. Imbalances in muscular endurance have been linked with back problems, so if your rating is significantly lower for one of the three tests, you should focus particular attention on that area of your body.

Goal:

What should you do next? Enter the results of this lab in the Preprogram Assessment column in Appendix C. If you've set a goal for improvement, begin a program of low-back exercises such as that suggested in this chapter. After several weeks of your program, complete this lab again and enter the results in the Post-Program Assessment column of Appendix C. How do the results compare?

Body Composition

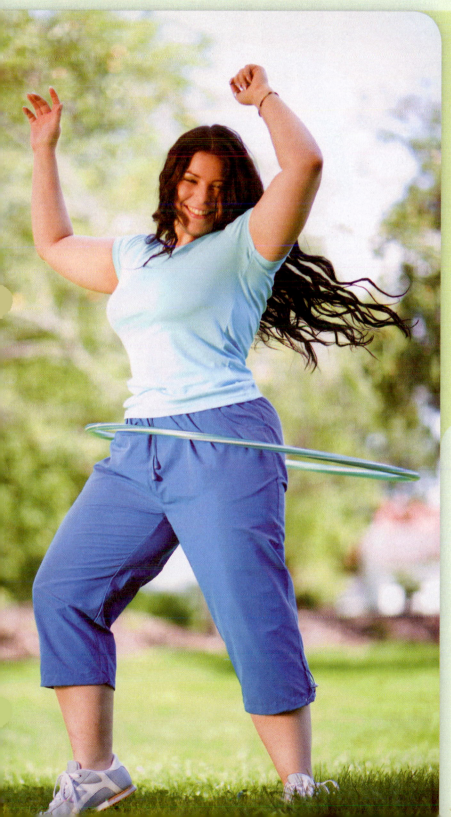

LOOKING AHEAD...

After reading this chapter, you should be able to

- Define fat-free mass and body fat, and describe their functions in the body.
- Explain how body composition affects overall health and wellness.
- Describe how body mass index, body composition, and body fat distribution are measured and assessed.
- Explain how to determine recommended body weight and body fat distribution.

TEST YOUR KNOWLEDGE

1. Exercise helps reduce the risks associated with overweight and obesity even if it doesn't result In improvements in body composition. True or false?

2. Which of the following is the most significant risk factor for the most common type of diabetes (type 2 diabetes)?
   a. smoking
   b. low-fiber diet
   c. overweight or obesity
   d. inactivity

3. In women, excessive exercise and low energy (calorie) intake can cause which of the following?
   a. unhealthy reduction in body fat levels
   b. amenorrhea (absent menstruation)
   c. bone density loss and osteoporosis
   d. muscle wasting and fatigue

See answers on the next page.

ody composition, the body's relative amounts of fat and fat-free mass, is an important component of fitness for health and wellness. People with an optimal body composition tend to be healthier, to move more efficiently, and to feel better about themselves. They also have a lower risk of many chronic diseases.

Many people, however, don't succeed in their efforts to obtain a fit and healthy body because they set unrealistic goals and emphasize short-term weight loss rather than permanent lifestyle changes that lead to fat loss and a healthy body composition. Successful management of body composition requires the long-term, consistent coordination of many aspects of a wellness program. Even in the absence of changes in body composition, an active lifestyle improves wellness and decreases the risk of disease and premature death (see the box "Why Is Physical Activity Important Even If Body Composition Doesn't Change?").

This chapter focuses on defining and measuring body composition. The aspects of lifestyle that affect body composition are discussed in detail in other chapters: physical activity and exercise in Chapters 2–5 and 7, nutrition in Chapter 8, weight management in Chapter 9, and stress management in Chapter 10.

WHAT IS BODY COMPOSITION, AND WHY IS IT IMPORTANT?

The human body can be divided into fat-free mass and body fat. As defined in Chapter 2, fat-free mass comprises all the body's nonfat tissues: bone, water, muscle, connective tissue, organ tissues, and teeth.

Body fat is incorporated into the nerves, brain, heart, lungs, liver, mammary glands, and other body organs and tissues. A certain amount of body fat is necessary for the body to function. It is the main source of stored energy in the body; it also cushions body organs and helps regulate body temperature. This **essential fat** makes up about 3–5% of total body weight in men and about 8–12% in women (Figure 6.1). The percentage is higher in women due to fat deposits in the breasts, uterus, and other gender-specific sites.

Most of the fat in the body is stored in fat cells, or **adipose tissue**, located under the skin (**subcutaneous fat**) and around major organs (**visceral fat** or *intra-abdominal fat*). People have a genetically determined number of fat cells, but these cells can become larger or smaller depending on how much fat is being stored. The amount of stored fat depends on several factors, including age, gender, metabolism, diet, and activity

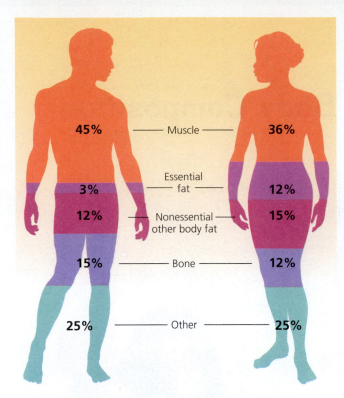

FIGURE 6.1   Body composition of a typical man and woman, 20–24 years old.

SOURCE: Adapted from Brooks, G. A., et al. 2005. *Exercise Physiology: Human Bioenergetics and Its Applications*, 4th ed. New York: McGraw-Hill; Santos, D.A., et al. 2014. *Reference Values for body composition and anthropometric measurements in athletes*. PLoS ONE 9(5): e97846.

level. The primary source of excess body fat is excess calories consumed in the diet—that is, calories consumed beyond what are expended in metabolism, physical activity, and exercise. A pound of body fat is equal to 3500 calories, so an intake of just 100 calories a day in excess of calories expended will result in a 10-pound weight gain over the course of a year. Excess stored body fat is associated with increased risk of chronic diseases like diabetes and cardiovascular disease, as described later in this chapter.

Answers (Test Your Knowledge)

1. **True.** Regular physical activity provides protection against the health risks of overweight and obesity. It lowers the risk of death for people who are overweight or obese as well as for those at a normal weight.
2. **c.** All four are risk factors for diabetes, but overweight/obesity is the most significant. It's estimated that 90% of cases of type 2 diabetes could be prevented if people adopted healthy lifestyle behaviors.
3. **All four.** Very low levels of body fat, and the behaviors used to achieve them, have serious health consequences for both men and women.

Why Is Physical Activity Important Even If Body Composition Doesn't Change?

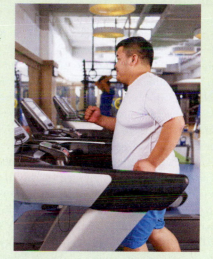

Physical activity is important for health even if it produces no changes in body composition—that is, even if a person remains overweight or obese. Physical activity confers benefits no matter how much you weigh; conversely, physical inactivity operates as a risk factor for health problems independently of body composition.

Regular physical activity and exercise block many of the destructive effects of obesity. For example, physical activity improves blood pressure, blood glucose levels, cholesterol levels, and body fat distribution. It also lowers the risk of cardiovascular disease, diabetes, and premature death. Although physical activity and exercise produce these improvements quickly in some people and slowly in others, due to genetic differences, the improvements do occur. Physical activity is particularly important for the many people who have metabolic syndrome or prediabetes, both of which are characterized by insulin resistance. Exercise encourages the body's cells to take up and use insulin efficiently for converting nutrients into usable energy. Being physically inactive for just one day decreases the capacity of the cells to take up and use blood sugar. Exercise makes fat cells fit by improving the function of their mitochondria (powerhouses of the cell) and decreasing inflammation.

Although being physically active and not being sedentary may sound identical, experts describe them as different dimensions of the same health issue. Data suggest that it is important not only to be physically active but also to avoid prolonged sitting. In one study, people who watched TV or used a computer four or more hours a day had twice the risk of having metabolic syndrome as those who spent less than one hour a day in these activities; other studies reported similar results. Thus, in addition to increasing physical activity, avoiding or reducing sedentary behavior is an important—and challenging—health goal.

Physical activity, then, is important even if it doesn't change body composition. But at a certain level, physical activity and exercise do improve body composition (meaning less fat and more lean muscle mass). Evidence supports a *dose-response* relation between exercise and fat loss: The more you exercise, the more fat you will lose. This includes both total body fat and abdominal fat. In addition, the more body fat a person has, the greater the loss of abdominal fat with exercise. Studies show that, even without calorie reduction, walking 150 minutes per week at a pace of four miles per hour, or jogging 75 minutes a week at six miles per hour, decreases total fat and abdominal fat and improves metabolic health.

Studies also show, however, that combining exercise with an appropriate reduction in calories is an even better way to reduce levels of body fat and increase lean muscle mass. The results of combining exercise and calorie reduction may not show up as expected on the scale because the weight of body fat lost is partially offset by the weight of muscle mass gained. Still, your body composition, physical fitness, and overall health have improved.

The question is sometimes asked: Which is more important in combating the adverse health effects of obesity—physical activity or physical fitness? Many studies suggest that both are important; the more active and fit you are, the lower your risk of having health problems and dying prematurely. Of the two, however, physical activity appears to be more important for health than physical fitness.

SOURCES: Earnest, C. P., et al. 2013. Cardiometabolic risk factors and metabolic syndrome in the Aerobics Center Longitudinal Study. *Mayo Clinics Proceedings* 88(3): 259–270; Loprinzi, P., et al. 2014. The "fit but fat" paradigm addressed using accelerometer-determined physical activity data. *North American Journal of Medical Sciences* 6(7): 295–301; Vieira-Potter, V. J., et al. 2015. Exercise (and estrogen) make fat cells "fit." *Exercise Sport Sciences Reviews*, 43(3):172–178.

Overweight and Obesity Defined

When looking at body composition, the most important consideration is the proportion of the body's total weight that is fat—the **percent body fat**. For example, two women may both be 5 feet, 5 inches tall and weigh 130 pounds. But one woman may have only 15% of her body weight as fat, whereas the other woman could have 34% body fat. Although neither woman is overweight by most standards, the second woman is considered overfat. Too much body fat (not just total weight) has a negative effect on health and well-being. Just as the amount of body fat is important, so is its location on your body. Visceral fat is more harmful to health than subcutaneous fat.

Overweight is usually defined as total body weight above the recommended range for good health as determined by large-scale population surveys. **Obesity** is defined as a more serious degree of overweight that carries multiple major health risks. The cutoff point for obesity may be set in terms of percent body fat or in terms of some measure of total body weight.

Prevalence of Overweight and Obesity among Americans

Americans are getting fatter. Since 1960, the average American man's weight has increased from 166 to 196 pounds, and the average American woman's weight has increased from 140 to 166 pounds. The prevalence of obesity has increased from about 13% in 1960 to 27.7–34.9% today—depending on whether measures are self-reported or measured by health-care professionals. By any measure, 62–69% of Americans are overweight (Figures 6.2 and 6.3). In 2012, according to the National Health and Nutrition Examination Survey (NHANES), about 33.5% of adult men and 36.1% of adult women were obese. The general trend recorded by NHANES since 1960 has been for a significant overall increase in the proportion of Americans who are above the normal weight classification defined by body mass index (see Figure 6.2). Looking at how self-reported obesity rates have changed in recent years, certain demographic patterns are clear, including higher rates of obesity in certain geographic regions (Midwest) and among people with lower income. Between 2008 and 2014, increases in self-reported obesity rates were lowest among Hispanics, young adults, and blacks (see Figure 6.3). However, the self-reported obesity rate among blacks is higher than in most groups, at 35.5%. Obesity rates increased most among middle-aged and older adults.

Possible explanations for this increase include more time spent in sedentary work and leisure activities, fewer short trips on foot and more by automobile, fewer daily gym classes for students, more meals eaten outside the home, greater consumption of fast food, increased portion sizes, and increased consumption of soft drinks and convenience foods. According to NHANES, energy intake increased from 1955 calories per day in 1971 to 2269 calories per day in 2003 and then declined to 2195 calories per day in 2010. In spite of this decline, overweight and obesity rates have continued to increase. People are not losing weight because they are doing less daily physical activity.

Excess Body Fat and Wellness

As rates of overweight and obesity increase, so do the problems associated with them. Obesity doubles mortality rates and can reduce life expectancy by 10–20 years. In fact, if the current trends in overweight and obesity (and their related health problems) continue, scientists believe the average American's life expectancy will soon decline by five years.

Metabolic Syndrome and Premature Death Many overweight and obese people—especially those who are sedentary and eat a poor diet—suffer from a group of symptoms called **metabolic syndrome** (or *insulin resistance syndrome*). Metabolic syndrome is diagnosed if a person has at least 3 out of 5 of these key factors: large waistline (fat deposits in the abdominal region), high blood pressure, high fasting blood sugar, high triglycerides, and low HDL ("good" cholesterol). Associated conditions include **chronic inflammation**, erectile dysfunction, and **fatty liver** disease. Metabolic syndrome increases the risk of heart disease, more so in men than in women. According to the American Heart Association, about 34% of adult Americans have metabolic syndrome.

Obesity is also associated with increased risk of death from many types of cancer. Other health problems associated with

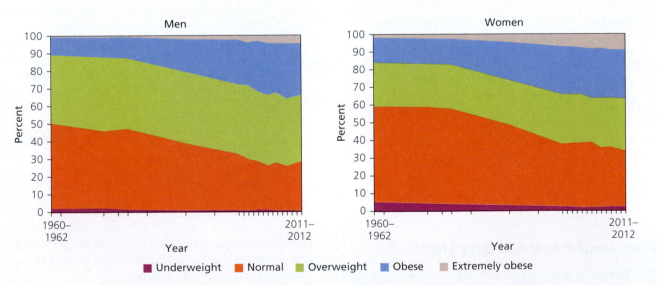

FIGURE 6.2 **Trends in overweight and obesity in adults age 20–74, by sex, in the United States, 1960–2012.** Since 1960, the proportion of American adults who are overweight but not obese (BMI 25.0–29.9) has remained fairly stable. However, during this same period, the proportion of adults who are obese (BMI ≥ 30), especially extremely obese (BMI ≥ 40) has increased significantly. Since 1960, the proportion of adults classified as at a normal weight (BMI 18.5–24.9) has dropped over 40%.

SOURCES: Centers for Disease Control and Prevention, National Center for Health Statistics. 2014. Health E-Stat: Prevalence of Overweight, Obesity, and Extreme Obesity Among Adults: United States, 1960–1962 Through 2011–2012, http://www.cdc.gov/nchs/data/hestat/obesity_adult_11_12/obesity_adult_11_12.htm; Centers for Disease Control and Prevention, National Center for Health Statistics. 2014. Health E-Stat: Prevalence of Underweight Among Adults Aged 20 and Over: United States, 1960–1962 Through 2011–2012, http://www.cdc.gov/nchs/data/hestat/underweight_adult_11_12/underweight_adult_11_12.htm.

Percentage Obese

	2008	2014	Difference (% points)
All adults	25.5	27.7	2.2
Ages 18–29	17.4	17.7	0.3
Ages 30–44	27.0	29.3	2.3
Ages 45–64	29.5	33.0	3.5
Ages 65+	23.4	27.4	4.0
Women	23.9	26.7	2.8
Men	27.0	28.7	1.7
Whites	24.3	26.7	2.4
Hispanics	28.8	28.3	−0.5
Blacks	35.0	35.5	0.5
Annual income less than $36,000	30.0	32.3	2.3
Annual income $36,000–$89,999	25.8	27.7	1.9
Annual income $90,000+	21.1	23.1	2.0
Midwest	26.8	29.7	2.9
South	26.9	29.2	2.3
East	24.7	26.6	1.9
West	22.8	24.6	1.8

FIGURE 6.3   Percentage of self-reported obesity (BMI ≥ 30) among various demographic groups, adults 18 and older, in the United States, 2008 and 2014. The self-reported values differ from those collected by the CDC, but the trend toward increasing obesity in nearly all groups is clear. The association between obesity and lower income is particularly strong. Since 2008, the largest increases in obesity rates were among older adults, adults aged 45–64, those living in the Midwest, and women.

SOURCE: Data from Jenna Levy. January 26, 2015. U.S. obesity rate inches up to 27.7% in 2014. *Gallup-Healthways Well-Being Index.* http://www.gallup.com /poll/181271/obesity-rate-inches-2014.aspx.

obesity include hypertension, impaired immune function, gallbladder and kidney diseases, skin problems, sleep and breathing disorders, erectile dysfunction, pregnancy complications, back pain, arthritis, and other bone and joint disorders.

Body Fat Distribution and Health   The distribution of body fat (the locations of fat on the body) is also an important indicator of health. Men and postmenopausal women tend to store fat in the upper regions of their bodies, particularly in the abdominal area (the "apple shape"). Premenopausal women

usually store fat in the hips, buttocks, and thighs (the "pear shape"). Excess fat in the abdominal area increases risk of high blood pressure, diabetes, early-onset heart disease, stroke, certain cancers, and mortality. The reason for this increase in risk is not entirely clear, but it appears that abdominal fat is more easily mobilized and sent into the bloodstream, increasing disease-related blood fat levels.

A measure of waist circumference helps assess the risks of unhealthy body fat distribution. A total waist measurement of more than 40 inches (102 cm) for men and more than 35 inches (88 cm) for women is associated with a significantly increased risk of disease. In the United States, waist circumference increased by about 1 inch in men and women between 1999 and 2010.

Waist circumference tends to be higher in taller people, so waist-to-height ratio is a more accurate measure than waist circumference alone. Your waist measurement should be less than half your height. Using this index, a person who is 5 feet 8 inches (68 inches) tall should have a waist circumference of less than 34 inches. A person who is 6 feet 4 inches (76 inches) tall should have a waist circumference of less than 38 inches.

Performance of Physical Activities   Too much body fat makes physical activity difficult because moving the body through everyday activities entails working harder and using more energy. In general, overfat people are less fit than others and don't have the muscular strength, endurance, and flexibility that make normal activity easy. Because exercise is more difficult, they do less of it, depriving themselves of an effective way to improve body composition.

Emotional Wellness and Self-Image   Obesity can affect psychological as well as physical wellness. Being perceived as fat can be a source of judgment, ostracism, and sometimes discrimination by others; it can contribute to psychological problems such as depression, anxiety, and low self-esteem.

The popular image of the "ideal" body has changed greatly in the past 50 years, evolving from slightly plump to unhealthily thin. The ideal body—as presented by the media—is an unrealistic goal for most Americans. This is because one's ability to change body composition depends on heredity as well

metabolic syndrome   A cluster of symptoms present in many overweight and obese people that greatly increases their risk of heart disease, diabetes, and other chronic illnesses; symptoms include insulin resistance, abnormal blood fats, abdominal fat deposition, type 2 diabetes, high blood pressure, and high blood glucose.

chronic inflammation   A response of blood vessels to harmful substances, such as germs, damaged cells, or irritants; can lead to heart disease, cancer, allergies, and muscle degeneration.

fatty liver   Increased fat storage in the liver that can lead to liver inflammation and failure.

TERMS

as diet and exercise. Body image, problems with body image, and unhealthy ways of dealing with a negative body image are all discussed in Chapter 9. We need to change popular perceptions so that active obese people are regarded as more fit, and normal-weight sedentary people as less fit.

Diabetes and Excess Body Fat

Even mild to moderate overweight is associated with a substantial increase in the risk of type 2 diabetes. Obese people are more than three times as likely as nonobese people to develop type 2 diabetes, and the incidence of this disease among Americans has increased dramatically as the rate of obesity has climbed (see the depiction of diabetes on page T3-5 of the color transparency insert "Touring the Cardiorespiratory System" in Chapter 3).

Diabetes mellitus is a disease that disrupts normal metabolism. The pancreas normally secretes the hormone insulin, which stimulates cells to take up glucose (blood sugar) to produce energy. Diabetes interferes with this process, causing a buildup of glucose in the bloodstream. Diabetes is associated with kidney failure; nerve damage; circulation problems; retinal damage and blindness; and increased rates of heart attack, stroke, and hypertension. Diabetes is currently the seventh leading cause of death in the United States.

Types of Diabetes About 29.1 million Americans (9.3% of the population) have one of two major forms of diabetes—more than double the number of people affected in 1995. About 5–10% of people with diabetes have the more serious form, known as *type 1 diabetes*. In this type of diabetes, the pancreas produces little or no insulin, which means a person can lapse into a coma. Daily doses of insulin are required, and other medications to control blood sugar levels and other complications of the disease may also be necessary. Type 1 diabetes usually strikes before age 30.

The remaining 90–95% of Americans with diabetes have *type 2 diabetes*. This condition can develop slowly, and about 25% of affected individuals are unaware of their condition. In type 2 diabetes, the pancreas doesn't produce enough insulin, cells are resistant to insulin, or both. This condition is usually diagnosed in people over age 40, although there has been a tenfold increase in type 2 diabetes in children in the past two decades. About one-third of people with type 2 diabetes must take insulin; others may take medications that increase insulin production or stimulate cells to take up glucose.

A third type of diabetes occurs in 2–10% of women during pregnancy. *Gestational diabetes* usually disappears after pregnancy, but 5–10% of women with gestational diabetes go on to have type 2 diabetes immediately after pregnancy. Women who had gestational diabetes during pregnancy have up to a 60% chance of developing diabetes within 10–20 years.

The term *prediabetes* describes blood glucose levels that are higher than normal but not high enough for a diagnosis of full-blown diabetes. According to a 2014 estimate from the American Diabetes Association, about 86 million Americans have prediabetes. Experts warn that most people with the

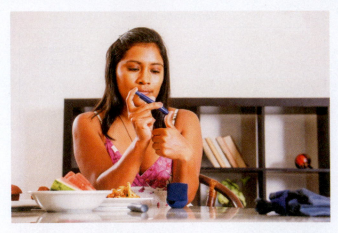

Wellness Tip Most cases of type 2 diabetes can be prevented through lifestyle measures such as regular physical activity and modest weight loss. For those who have type 2 diabetes, careful management to keep blood sugar levels within a healthy range through diet, exercise, and, if needed, medication can reduce the rate of complications from the disorder.

condition will develop type 2 diabetes unless they adopt preventive lifestyle measures.

The major factors involved in the development of diabetes are age, obesity, physical inactivity, a family history of diabetes, and lifestyle. Excess body fat reduces cell sensitivity to insulin, and insulin resistance is usually a precursor of type 2 diabetes. Ethnicity also plays a role. According to the Centers for Disease Control and Prevention (CDC), the rate of diagnosed diabetes cases is highest among Native Americans and Alaska Natives, followed by blacks, Hispanics, Asian Americans, and white Americans. Across all races, about 26% of Americans age 65 and older have diabetes, either diagnosed or undiagnosed.

Treatment There is no cure for diabetes, but it can be managed successfully by keeping blood sugar levels within safe limits through diet, exercise, and, if necessary, medication. Blood sugar levels can be monitored with a home test; close control of glucose levels can significantly reduce the rate of serious complications.

Nearly 90% of people with type 2 diabetes are overweight when diagnosed, including 55% who are obese. An important step in treatment is to lose weight. Even a small amount of exercise and weight loss can be beneficial. Regular exercise and a healthy diet are often sufficient to control type 2 diabetes.

Prevention It is estimated that 90% of cases of type 2 diabetes could be prevented if people adopted healthy lifestyle behaviors, including regular physical activity, a moderate diet, and modest weight loss. For people with prediabetes, lifestyle measures are more effective than medication for delaying or preventing the development of diabetes. Studies of people with prediabetes show that a 5–7% weight loss can lower diabetes onset by nearly 60%. Exercise

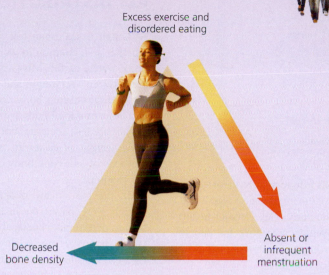

Excess exercise and disordered eating

Decreased bone density

Absent or infrequent menstruation

Even while obesity is at epidemic levels in the United States, many girls and women strive for unrealistic thinness in response to pressure from peers and a society obsessed with appearance. This quest for thinness has led to an increasingly common, underreported condition called the **female athlete triad**.

The triad consists of three interrelated disorders: abnormal eating patterns (and excessive exercising), followed by lack of menstrual periods (amenorrhea), followed by decreased bone density (premature osteoporosis). Left untreated, the triad can lead to decreased physical performance, reproductive problems, increased incidence of bone fractures, disturbances of heart rhythm and metabolism, and even death.

Abnormal eating leads to the other two components of the triad. Abnormal eating ranges from moderately restricting food intake, to binge eating and purging (bulimia), to severely restricting food intake (anorexia nervosa). Whether serious or relatively mild, eating disorders prevent women from getting enough calories to meet their bodies' needs.

Disordered eating, combined with intense exercise and emotional stress, can suppress the hormones that control the menstrual cycle. If the menstrual cycle stops for three consecutive months, the condition is called amenorrhea. Prolonged amenorrhea can lead to osteoporosis. Bone density may erode to the point that a woman in her twenties has the bone density of a woman in her sixties. Women with osteoporosis have fragile, easily fractured bones. Some researchers have found that even a few missed menstrual periods can decrease bone density.

All physically active women and girls have the potential to develop one or more components of the female athlete triad. For example, it is estimated that 5–20% of women who exercise regularly and vigorously may develop amenorrhea. But the triad is most prevalent among athletes who participate in certain sports: those in which appearance is highly important, those that emphasize a prepubertal body shape, those that require contour-revealing clothing for competition, those that require endurance, and those that use weight categories for participation. Such sports include gymnastics, figure skating, swimming, distance running, cycling, cross-country skiing, track, volleyball, rowing, horse racing, and cheerleading.

The female athlete triad can be life-threatening. Typical signs of the eating disorders that trigger the condition are extreme weight loss, dry skin, loss of hair, brittle fingernails, cold hands and feet, low blood pressure and heart rate, swelling around the ankles and hands, and weakening of the bones. Female athletes who have repeated stress fractures may be suffering from the condition.

Early intervention is the key to stopping this series of interrelated conditions. Unfortunately, once the condition has progressed, long-term consequences, especially bone loss, are unavoidable. Teenagers may need only to learn about good eating habits; college-age women with a long-standing problem may require psychological counseling.

SOURCES: Joy, E., et al. 2014. 2014 Female Athlete Triad coalition consensus statement on treatment and return to play of the Female Athlete Triad. *Current Sports Medicine Reports* 13(4): 219–232; Mallinson, R. J., and M. J. De Souza. 2014. Current perspectives on the etiology and manifestation of the "silent" component of the Female Athlete Triad. *International Journal Women's Health* 6: 451–467; Mountjoy, M., et al. 2014. The IOC consensus statement: Beyond the Female Athlete Triad–Relative Energy Deficiency in Sport (RED-S). *British Journal Sports Medicine* 48(7): 491–497.

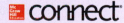

(endurance and/or strength training) makes cells more sensitive to insulin and helps stabilize blood glucose levels; it also helps keep body fat at healthy levels.

A moderate diet to control body fat is perhaps the most important dietary recommendation for the prevention of diabetes. However, the composition of the diet may also be important. Studies have linked diets low in fiber and high in sugar, refined carbohydrates, saturated fat, red meat, and high-fat dairy products to increased risk of diabetes. Specific foods linked to higher diabetes risk include soft drinks, white bread, white rice, French fries, processed meats, and sugary desserts. Diets rich in whole grains, fruits, vegetables, legumes, fish, and poultry may be protective.

female athlete triad   A condition consisting of three interrelated disorders: abnormal eating patterns (and excessive exercising) followed by lack of menstrual periods (amenorrhea) and decreased bone density (premature osteoporosis).

TERMS

Warning Signs and Testing Be alert for the warning signs of diabetes:

- Frequent urination
- Extreme hunger or thirst
- Unexplained weight loss
- Extreme fatigue
- Blurred vision
- Frequent infections
- Cuts and bruises that are slow to heal
- Tingling or numbness in the hands or feet
- Generalized itching with no rash

The best way to avoid complications is to recognize these symptoms and get early diagnosis and treatment. Because type 2 diabetes is often asymptomatic in the early stages, major health organizations now recommend routine screening for people over age 45 and anyone younger who is at high risk, including those who are obese.

Screening involves a blood test to check glucose levels after either a period of fasting or the administration of a set dose of glucose. A fasting glucose level of 126 mg/dl or higher indicates diabetes; a level of 100–125 mg/dl indicates prediabetes. If you are concerned about your risk for diabetes, talk with your physician about being tested.

Problems Associated with Very Low Levels of Body Fat

Though not as prevalent a problem as overweight or obesity, having too little body fat is also dangerous. Essential fat is necessary for the functioning of the body, and health experts generally view too little body fat—less than 8–12% for women and 3–5% for men—as a threat to health. Extreme leanness is linked with reproductive, respiratory, circulatory, and immune system disorders and with premature death. Extremely lean people may experience muscle wasting and fatigue. They are also more likely to have eating disorders (described in more detail in Chapter 9). For women, an extremely low percentage of body fat is associated with loss of bone mass and **amenorrhea**—absent or infrequent menstruation (see the box "The Female Athlete Triad"). In older adults, having a low level of lean body mass is a better predictor of premature death than BMI.

---

amenorrhea Absent or infrequent menstruation, sometimes related to unhealthily low levels of body fat and excessive quantity or intensity of exercise.

TERMS

body mass index (BMI) A measure of relative body weight correlating highly with more direct measures of body fat, calculated by dividing total body weight (in kilograms) by the square of body height (in meters).

ASSESSING BODY MASS INDEX, BODY COMPOSITION, AND BODY FAT DISTRIBUTION

Although a scale can tell your total weight, it can't reveal whether a fluctuation in weight is due to a change in muscle, body water, or fat. Most important, a scale can't differentiate between overweight and overfat. Some methods of assessing and classifying body composition are based on body fat and others on total body weight. Methods based on total body weight are less accurate, but they are commonly used because body weight is easier to measure than body fat. (Various methods of assessing body composition are described later in the chapter.)

In the past, many people relied on height/weight tables (which were based on insurance company mortality statistics) to determine whether they were at a healthy weight. Such tables, however, can be highly inaccurate for some people. Because muscle tissue is denser and heavier than fat, a fit person can easily weigh more than the recommended weight on a height/weight table. For the same reason, an unfit person may weigh less than the table's recommended weight.

There are a number of simple, inexpensive ways to estimate healthy body weight and healthy body composition. These assessments can provide you with information about the health risks associated with your current body weight and body composition. They can also help you establish reasonable goals and set a starting point for current and future decisions about weight loss and weight gain.

Calculating Body Mass Index

Body mass index (BMI) is useful for classifying the health risks of body weight if you don't have access to more sophisticated methods. Though more accurate than height-weight tables, body mass index is also based on the concept that weight should be proportional to height. BMI is easy to calculate and rate. Researchers frequently use BMI in conjunction with waist circumference in studies that examine the health risks associated with body weight.

BMI is calculated by dividing your body weight (expressed in kilograms) by the square of your height (expressed in meters). The following example is for a person who is 5 feet, 3 inches tall (63 inches) and weighs 130 pounds:

1. Divide body weight in pounds by 2.2 to convert weight to kilograms:
   $130 \div 2.2 = 59.1$

2. Multiply height in inches by 0.0254 to convert height to meters:
   $63 \times 0.0254 = 1.6$

3. Multiply the result of step 2 by itself to get the square of the height measurement:
   $1.6 \times 1.6 = 2.56$

4. Divide the result of step 1 by the result of step 3 to determine BMI:

59.1 ÷ 2.56 = 23

An alternative equation, based on pounds and inches, is

$$BMI = [weight/(height \times height)] \times 703$$

Space for your own calculations can be found in Lab 6.1, and a complete BMI chart appears in Lab 6.2.

A BMI between 18.5 and 24.9 is considered normal and desirable under separate standards from the National Institutes of Health (NIH) and the World Health Organization (WHO). A person with a BMI of 25 or above is classified as overweight, and someone with a BMI of 30 or above is classified as obese (Table 6.1). A person with a BMI below 18.5 is classified as underweight, although low BMI values may be healthy in some cases if they are not the result of smoking, an eating disorder, or an underlying disease. A BMI of 17.5 or less is sometimes used as a diagnostic criterion for the eating disorder anorexia nervosa (Chapter 9).

A meta-analysis from the National Center for Health Statistics, pooling data from studies of nearly 3 million people, found that those with severe obesity (BMI greater than 34.9) had a higher death rate from all causes than did people with normal weight (BMI = 18.5–24.9). However, overweight people (BMI = 25–29.9) had a *lower* all-cause death rate than normal weight people, and moderately obese people (BMI = 30–34.9)

had similar death rates to normal weight people. These controversial results showed that there are problems associated with using BMI to predict health and longevity. Other factors, such as amount of physical activity, lean mass, level of stress, dietary composition, and social factors, might account for the results.

Fat percentage varies for people with a given BMI. In the NHANES, for example, people with BMIs less than 25 had fat percentages ranging from 10% to nearly 32%. Factors influencing fat percentage at a given BMI included age, race, gender, and physical activity.

In classifying the health risks associated with overweight and obesity, the NIH and WHO guidelines consider body fat distribution and other disease risk factors in addition to BMI. As described earlier, excess fat in the abdomen is of greater concern than excess fat in other areas. Measurement of waist circumference (see Table 6.1) is one method of assessing body fat distribution. At a given level of overweight, people with a large waist circumference and/or additional disease risk factors are at risk for health problems. For example, a man with a BMI of 27, a waist circumference of more than 40 inches, and high blood pressure is at greater risk for health problems than another man who has a BMI of 27 but a smaller waist circumference and no other risk factors.

Thus, optimal BMI for good health depends on many factors; if your BMI is 25 or above, consult a physician for help in determining a healthy BMI for you. While BMI and waist circumference are important measures of health, they must be considered with other factors such as high blood pressure, diabetes, blood fats, and insulin resistance.

Because BMI doesn't distinguish between fat weight and fat-free weight, it is inaccurate for some groups. For example, athletes who weight train have more muscle mass—and thus weigh more—than average people and may be classified as overweight by the BMI scale. Because their "excess" weight is in the form of muscle, however, it is healthy. Further, BMI is not particularly useful for tracking changes in body composition—gains in muscle mass and losses of fat. BMI also does not take into account differences in gender; women are likely to have more body fat for a given BMI than men. BMI measurements have also over- and underestimated the prevalence of obesity in several ethnic groups, such as Hispanics and blacks, because of racial and ethnic differences in muscle mass and muscle density. Finally, BMI is a poor predictor of health in people short in stature, whose gene function may have been altered by environmental factors early in life. If you are an athlete, a serious weight trainer, or a person of short stature, do not use BMI as your primary means of assessing whether your current weight is healthy. Instead, try one of the methods described in the next section for estimating percent body fat.

Estimating Percent Body Fat

Assessing body composition involves estimating percent body fat. Unfortunately, an autopsy—the dissection and chemical analysis of the body—is the only method for directly measuring the percentage of body weight that is fat. However, there

---

Table 6.1	Classifications from the World Health Organization

Body Mass Index (Bmi) Classifications

WEIGHT STATUS CLASSIFICATION	BODY MASS INDEX
Underweight	<18.5
Severe thinness	<16.0
Moderate thinness	16.0–16.9
Mild thinness	17.0–18.4
Normal	18.5–24.9
Overweight	25.0–29.9
Obese, Class I	30.0–34.9
Obese, Class II	35.0–39.9
Obese, Class III	≥40.0

Waist Circumference Classifications

	WAIST CIRCUMFERENCE IN INCHES (CENTIMETERS)	
RISK CLASSIFICATION	WOMEN	MEN
Normal	<32 in. (80 cm)	<37 in. (94 cm)
Increased	≥32 in. (80 cm)	≥37 in. (94 cm)
Substantially increased	≥35 in. (88 cm)	≥40 in. (102 cm)

SOURCE: Adapted from World Health Organization. 2008. *Waist Circumference and Waist-to-Hip Ratio. Report of a WHO Expert Consultation.* Geneva: WHO.

are indirect techniques that can provide an *estimate* of percent body fat. One of the most accurate is underwater weighing. Other techniques include skinfold measurements, the Bod Pod, bioelectrical impedance analysis, and dual-energy X-ray absorptiometry.

All of these methods have a margin of error, so it is important not to focus too much on precise values. For example, underwater weighing has a margin of error of about ±3%, meaning that if a person's percent body fat is actually 17%, the test result could range from 14–20%. The results of different methods may also vary. If you plan to track changes in body composition over time, be sure to perform the assessment using the same method each time. See Table 6.2 for body composition ratings based on percent body fat as a criterion for obesity. It should be noted, however, that the National Institutes of Health has not developed an official standard linking body fat percentage with obesity.

Underwater Weighing In hydrostatic (underwater) weighing, an individual is submerged and weighed under water. The percentages of fat and fat-free weight are calculated from body density. Muscle has a higher density and fat a lower density than water. Therefore, people with more body fat tend to float and weigh less under water, and lean people tend to sink and weigh more under water. Many university exercise physiology departments or sports medicine laboratories have an underwater weighing facility. For an accurate assessment of your body composition, find a place that does underwater weighing or has a BodPod (described in the next section).

The Bod Pod The Bod Pod, a small chamber containing computerized sensors, measures body composition by air displacement. The technique's technical name is *plethysmography*. It determines the percentage of fat by calculating body density from how much air is displaced by the person sitting inside the chamber. The Bod Pod has an error rate of about ±2–4% in determining percent body fat.

Skinfold Measurements Skinfold measurement is a simple, inexpensive, and practical way to assess body composition. Equations can link the thickness of skinfolds at various sites to percent body fat calculations from more precise laboratory techniques.

Skinfold assessment typically involves measuring the thickness of skinfolds at several different places on the body. You can sum the skinfold values as an indirect measure of body fatness. For example, if you plan to create a fitness (and dietary change) program to improve body composition, you can compare the sum of skinfold values over time as an indicator of your program's progress and of improvements in body composition. You can also plug your skinfold values into equations like those in Lab 6.1 that predict percent body fat. When using these equations, however, remember that they have a fairly substantial margin of error (±4% if performed by a skilled technician), so don't focus too much on specific values. The sum represents only a relative measure of body fatness.

Skinfolds are measured with a device called a **caliper**, which is a pair of spring-loaded, calibrated jaws. High-quality calipers are made of metal and have parallel jaw surfaces and constant spring tension. Inexpensive plastic calipers are also available, but you need to make sure they are spring-loaded and have metal jaws to ensure accuracy. Refer to Lab 6.1 for instructions on how to take skinfold measurements.

Taking accurate measurements with calipers requires patience, experience, and considerable practice. It's best to take several measurements at each site (or have several different people take each measurement). Be sure to take the measurements in the exact location called for in the procedure. Because the

Table 6.2	Percent Body Fat Classification						
	PERCENT BODY FAT (%)				**PERCENT BODY FAT (%)**		
	20–39 YEARS	*40–59 YEARS*	*60–79 YEARS*		*20–39 YEARS*	*40–59 YEARS*	*60–79 YEARS*
Women				**Men**			
Essential*	8–12	8–12	8–12	Essential*	3–5	3–5	3–5
Low/athletic**	13–20	13–22	13–23	Low/athletic**	6–7	6–10	6–12
Recommended	21–32	23–33	24–35	Recommended	8–19	11–21	13–24
Overfat[†]	33–38	34–39	36–41	Overfat[†]	20–24	22–27	25–29
Obese[†]	≥39	≥40	≥42	Obese[†]	≥25	≥28	≥30

NOTE: The cutoffs for recommended, overfat, and obese ranges in this table are based on a study that linked body mass index classifications from the National Institutes of Health with predicted percent body fat (measured using dual-energy X-ray absorptiometry).

*Essential body fat is necessary for the basic functioning of the body.

**Percent body fat in the low/athletic range may be appropriate for some people as long as it is not the result of illness or disordered eating habits.

[†]Health risks increase as percent body fat exceeds the recommended range.

SOURCES: Gallagher, D., et al. 2009. Healthy percentage body fat ranges: An approach for developing guidelines based on body mass index. *American Journal of Clinical Nutrition* 72: 694–701; Swain, D. P. 2013. *ACSM's Resource Manual for Guidelines for Exercise Testing and Prescription*, 7th ed. Philadelphia: Wolters Kluwer/Lippincott Williams & Wilkins Health.

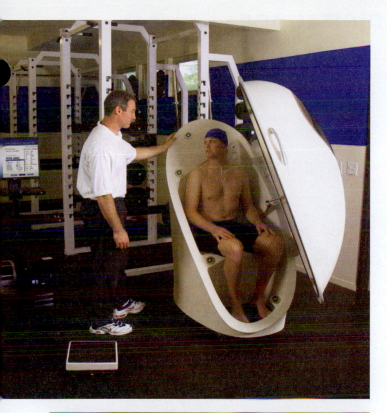

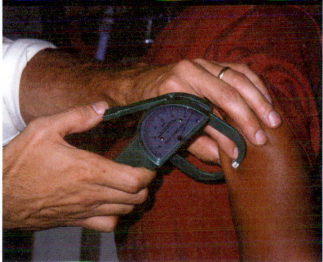

Fitness Tip If you plan to track body composition, be sure to use the same assessment method each time. In addition, don't become overly focused on precise values, because even the most accurate methods have a margin of error. The Bod Pod estimates body composition by air displacement and has a margin of error of about ±2–4%. Skinfold assessment is based on measurement of the thickness of several skinfolds, including the back of the arm, as shown here; equations translate these measurements into a percent body fat estimate, with about a ±4% margin of error.

amount of water in your body changes during the day, skinfold measurements taken in the morning and evening often differ. If you repeat the measurements in the future to track changes in your body composition, measure skinfolds at approximately the same time of day.

Bioelectrical Impedance Analysis (BIA) The BIA technique works by sending a small electrical current through the body and measuring the body's resistance to it. Fat-free tissues, where most body water is located, are good conductors of electrical current, whereas fat is not (see the box "Using BIA at Home"). Thus, the amount of resistance to electrical current is related to the amount of fat-free tissue in the body (the lower the resistance, the greater the fat-free mass) and can be used to estimate percent body fat.

Bioelectrical impedance analysis has an error rate of about ±4–5%. To reduce error, follow the manufacturer's instructions carefully and avoid overhydration or underhydration (more or less body water than normal). Because measurement varies with the type of BIA analyzer, use the same instrument to compare measurements over time.

Advanced Techniques: DEXA and TOBEC Dual-energy X-ray absorptiometry (DEXA) works by measuring the tissue absorption of high- and low-energy X-ray beams. The procedure has an error rate of about ±2%. Total body electrical conductivity (TOBEC) estimates lean body mass by passing a body through a magnetic field. These methods are often used in sophisticated research projects but are seldom available to the average person. We mention them because they are often used for comparison with some of the field tests described in this chapter.

Assessing Body Fat Distribution

Researchers have studied many different methods for measuring body fat distribution. Two of the simplest to perform are waist circumference measurement and waist-to-hip ratio calculation. In the first method, you measure your waist circumference; in the second, you divide your waist circumference by your hip circumference. Waist circumference has been found to be a better indicator of abdominal fat than waist-to-hip ratio. More research is needed to determine the precise degree of risk associated with specific values for these two assessments of body fat distribution. However, as noted earlier, a total waist measurement of more than 40 inches (102 cm) for men and 35 inches (88 cm) for women and a waist-to-hip ratio above 0.94 for young men and 0.82 for young women are associated with a significantly increased risk of heart disease and diabetes. Lab 6.1 shows you how to measure your body fat distribution.

Somatotype

As discussed in Chapter 2, somatotype describes your basic body build. The three somatotypes are endomorph, mesomorph, and ectomorph. Endomorphs are round and pear shaped, with wide hips and shoulders. They gain weight easily and will typically regain weight rapidly if they resume their normal lifestyle

> **caliper** A pressure-sensitive measuring instrument with two jaws that can be adjusted to determine thickness of the skinfold. **TERMS**

WELLNESS IN THE DIGITAL AGE
Using BIA at Home

Scientists can use several techniques to accurately measure body composition. As described in the chapter, these techniques include underwater weighing, air displacement, and Dual-energy X-ray absorptiometry (DEXA). These methods, however, are costly and require technical expertise.

You can estimate your body fat and fat-free weight simply and accurately, at home, without the help of a technician. All you need is a digital home scale with a built-in bioelectrical impedance analyzer (BIA) or a hand-held BIA unit. BIA works by measuring the resistance in the body to a small electric current. Electricity flows more slowly through fat tissue than through muscle, so the more fat you have, the more slowly such a current will flow through your body. Conversely, a current will pass through your body more quickly if you have more fat-free (muscle) weight.

To use a BIA scale or hand-held unit, just stand on the scale with bare feet or grasp the handles with each hand. As it checks your weight, the BIA unit sends a low-voltage electrical current through your body and analyzes the speed at which the current travels. Checking your weight and body composition takes no longer than checking your weight alone. Most BIA units can remember your last weight and body composition measurement, making it easy to compare the measurements from day to day or week to week. Some scales can remember measurements for multiple people, as well.

A study of 22 weight-trained men showed that BIA compared favorably to underwater weighing for measuring body composition. Measurements of fat and lean mass are most valuable for measuring changes in body composition during diet and exercise programs.

Popular BIA scales and hand-held BIA devices are manufactured by Taylor, Whynter, Omron, RemedyT, and Tanita. These scales and devices are available in most department stores and online, and cost between $30 and $200, depending on features.

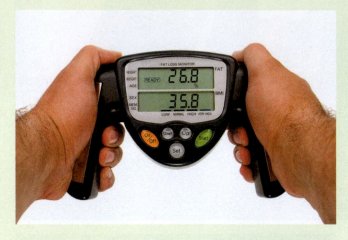

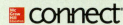

after losing weight. Endomorphs often excel at weight lifting and might enjoy weight-supported aerobic exercises such as swimming or cycling. Conversely, they might find distance running difficult and painful.

Mesomorphs are lean and muscular and respond well to exercise. They have wedged-shaped bodies, broad shoulders, narrow hips, and little body fat. They gain fitness easily and usually excel at almost any kind of physical activity or sport.

Ectomorphs are thin and linear, with narrow hips and shoulders. They typically have little muscle or fat. Their light frame helps make them successful in activities such as distance running and gymnastics.

Few people have extreme body types—most of us are a mixture of all three. People with every body type can benefit from some form of physical activity.

SETTING BODY COMPOSITION GOALS

If assessment tests indicate that fat loss would be beneficial for your health, your first step is to establish a goal. You can use the ratings in Table 6.1 or Table 6.2 to choose a target value for BMI or percent body fat (depending on which assessment you completed).

Set a realistic goal that will ensure good health. Heredity limits your capacity to change your body composition, and few people can expect to develop the body of a fashion model or competitive bodybuilder. However, you can improve your body composition through a program of regular exercise and a healthy diet. If your body composition is in or close to the recommended range, you may want to set a lifestyle goal rather than a specific percent body fat or BMI goal. For example, you might set a goal of increasing your daily

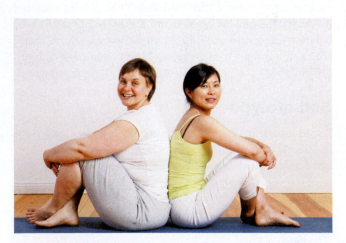

Wellness Tip Many body shapes and sizes are associated with good health. Focus on positive lifestyle behaviors rather than on unrealistic goals related to body weight or shape.

physical activity from 20 to 60 minutes or beginning a program of weight training, and then let any improvements in body composition occur as a secondary result of your primary target (physical activity). Remember, a lifestyle that includes regular exercise may be more important for health than trying to reach any ideal weight.

If you are significantly overfat or if you have known risk factors for disease (such as high blood pressure or high cholesterol), consult your physician to determine a body composition goal for your individual risk profile. For people who are obese, even small losses of body weight (5–15%) over a 6- to 12-month period can result in significant health improvements.

After you've established a body composition goal, you can then set a target range for body weight. Although body weight is not an accurate method of assessing body composition, it's a useful method for tracking progress in a program to change body composition. If you're losing a small or moderate amount of weight and exercising, you're probably losing fat while building muscle mass. Lab 6.2 will help you determine a range for recommended body weight.

Using percent body fat or BMI will generate a fairly accurate target body weight for most people. However, it's best not to stick rigidly to a recommended body weight calculated from any formula; individual genetic, cultural, and lifestyle factors are also important. Decide whether the body weight that the formulas generate for you is realistic, meets all your goals, is healthy, *and* is reasonable for you to maintain.

MAKING CHANGES IN BODY COMPOSITION

Chapter 9 includes specific strategies for losing or gaining weight and improving body composition. In general, lifestyle should be your focus—regular physical activity, endurance exercise, strength training, and a moderate energy intake. Making significant cuts in food intake in order to lose weight and body fat is a difficult strategy to maintain; focusing on increased physical activity is a better approach for many people. In studies of people who have lost weight and maintained the loss, physical activity was the key to long-term success.

You can track your progress toward your target body composition by checking your body weight regularly. Also, focus on how much energy you have and how your clothes fit.

To get a more accurate idea of your progress, you should directly reassess your body composition occasionally during your program: Body composition changes as weight changes. Losing a lot of weight usually includes losing some muscle mass no matter how hard a person exercises, partly because carrying less weight requires the muscular system to bear a smaller burden. Conversely, a large gain in weight without exercise still causes some gain in muscle mass because muscles are working harder to carry the extra weight.

TIPS FOR TODAY AND THE FUTURE

A wellness lifestyle can lead naturally to a body composition that is healthy and appropriate for you.

RIGHT NOW YOU CAN
- Find out what types of body composition assessment techniques are available at facilities on your campus or in your community.
- Do 30 minutes of physical activity five days per week—walk, jog, bike, swim, or climb stairs.
- Drink a glass of water instead of a soda, and include a high-fiber food such as whole-grain bread or cereal, popcorn, apples, berries, or beans in your next snack or meal.

IN THE FUTURE YOU CAN
- Think about your image of the ideal body type for your sex. Consider where your idea comes from, whether you use this image to judge your own body, and whether it is a realistic goal for you.
- Be aware of media messages (especially visual images) that make you feel embarrassed or insecure about your body. Remind yourself that these messages are usually designed to sell a product; they should not form the basis of your body image.

SUMMARY

- The human body is composed of fat-free mass (which includes bone, muscle, organ tissues, and connective tissues) and body fat.

- Having too much body fat has negative health consequences, especially in terms of cardiovascular disease and diabetes. Distribution of fat is also a significant factor in health.

- A fit and healthy looking body, with the right body composition for a particular person, develops from habits of proper nutrition and exercise.

- Measuring body weight alone is not an accurate way to assess body composition because this measure does not differentiate between muscle weight and fat weight.

- Body mass index (calculated from weight and height measurements) and waist circumference can help classify the health risks associated with being overweight. BMI is sometimes inaccurate, however, particularly in muscular people.

- Techniques for estimating percent body fat include underwater weighing, the Bod Pod, skinfold measurements, bioelectrical impedance analysis (BIA), dual-energy X-ray absorptiometry (DEXA), and total body electrical conductivity (TOBEC).

- Body fat distribution can be assessed through waist measurement or the waist-to-hip ratio.

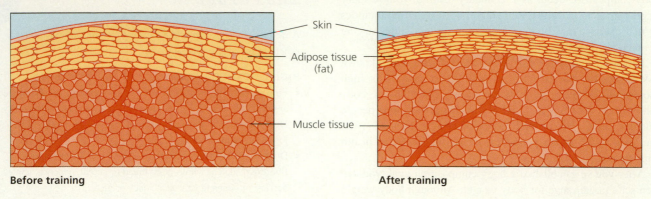

Before training

After training

EFFECTS OF EXERCISE ON BODY COMPOSITION. Endurance exercise and strength training both reduce body fat and increase muscle mass.

Labels: Skin; Adipose tissue (fat); Muscle tissue

Q Is spot reducing effective?

A *Spot reducing* refers to attempts to lose body fat in specific parts of the body by doing exercises for those parts. Danish researchers have shown that fat use increases in adipose tissue surrounding active muscle, but it is not known if short-term fat use helps reduce fat in specific sites. Most studies show that spot-reducing exercises contribute to fat loss only to the extent that they burn calories. The best way to reduce fat in any specific area is to create an overall negative energy balance: Take in less energy (food) than you use through exercise and metabolism.

Q How does exercise affect body composition?

A Cardiorespiratory endurance exercise burns calories, thereby helping create a negative energy balance. Weight training does not use many calories and therefore is of little use in creating a negative energy balance. However, weight training increases muscle mass, which maintains a higher metabolic rate (the body's rate of energy use) and helps improve body composition. To minimize body fat and increase muscle mass, thereby improving body composition, combine cardiorespiratory endurance exercise and weight training (see figure above).

Q Are people who have a desirable body composition physically fit?

A Having a healthy body composition is not necessarily associated with overall fitness. For example, many bodybuilders have very little body fat but have poor cardiorespiratory capacity and flexibility. Some athletes, such as NFL linemen, weigh 300 pounds or more; they have to lose the weight when they retire if they don't want to jeopardize their health. To be fit, you must rate high on all the components of fitness.

Q What is liposuction, and will it help me lose body fat?

A Suction lipectomy, popularly known as *liposuction,* has become the most popular type of elective surgery in the world. The procedure involves removing limited amounts of fat from specific areas. Typically, no more than 2.5 kilograms (5.5 pounds) of adipose tissue are removed at a time. The procedure is usually successful if the amount of excess fat is limited and skin elasticity is good. The procedure is most effective if integrated into a program of dietary restriction and exercise. Side effects include infection, dimpling, and wavy skin contours. Liposuction has a death rate of 1 in 5000 patients, primarily from pulmonary thromboembolism (a blood clot in the lungs) or fat embolism (circulatory blockage caused by a dislodged piece of fat). Other serious complications include shock, bleeding, and impaired blood flow to vital organs.

Q What is cellulite, and how do I get rid of it?

A *Cellulite* is the name commonly given to rippling, wavy fat deposits that collect just under the skin. The "cottage cheese" appearance stems from the breakdown of tissues supporting the fat. These rippling fat deposits are really the same as fat deposited anywhere else in the body. The only way to control them is to create a negative energy balance—that is, burn more calories than you take in. There are no creams or lotions that will rub away surface (subcutaneous) fat deposits, and spot reducing is also ineffective. The solution is sensible eating habits and exercise.

- Somatotype—endomorph (round), mesomorph (muscular), ectomorph (linear)—is a useful tool for describing basic body characteristics.

- You can determine a recommended body composition and weight by choosing a target BMI or target body fat percentage. Keep heredity in mind when setting a goal, and focus on positive changes in lifestyle.

FOR FURTHER EXPLORATION

American Diabetes Association. Provides information, a free newsletter, and referrals to local support groups; the website includes an online diabetes risk assessment.

http://www.diabetes.org

American Heart Association: Body Composition Tests. Offers detailed information about body composition, testing and analysis, and the impact of body composition on heart health.

http://www.heart.org/HEARTORG/GettingHealthy/NutritionCenter/
Body-CompositionTests_UCM_305883_Article.jsp

Methods of Body Composition Analysis Tutorials. Provides information about body composition assessment techniques, including underwater weighing, BIA, and DEXA.

http://nutrition.uvm.edu/bodycomp

National Heart, Lung, and Blood Institute: Obesity Education Initiative. Provides information on the latest federal obesity standards and a BMI calculator.

http://www.nhlbi.nih.gov/about/oei/index.htm

National Institute of Diabetes and Digestive and Kidney Diseases Weight-Control Information Network. Provides information about adult obesity: how it is defined and assessed, the risk factors associated with it, and its causes.

http://win.niddk.nih.gov

National Health and Nutrition Examination Survey (NHANES). Ongoing survey and assessment of health status and practices in the United States.

http://www.cdc.gov/nchs/nhanes/new_nhanes.htm

Robert Wood Johnson Foundation. Promotes the health and health care of Americans through research and distribution of information on healthy lifestyles. They publish an annual report on the status of the national obesity problem.

http://www.rwjf.org

USDA Food and Nutrition Information Center: Weight and Obesity. Provides links to recent reports and studies on the issue of obesity among Americans.

http://fnic.nal.usda.gov/weight-and-obesity

See also the listings for Chapters 2, 8, and 9.

SELECTED BIBLIOGRAPHY

Aatashak, S., et al. 2015. Cardiovascular risk factors adaptation to concurrent training in overweight sedentary middle- aged men. *Journal Sports Medicine Physical Fitness.* Published online February 12, 2015.

Acevedo, E., and M. Starks. 2011. *Exercise Testing and Prescription Lab Manual,* 2nd ed. Champaign, Ill.: Human Kinetics.

American College of Sports Medicine. 2009. *ACSM's Health Related Physical Fitness Assessment Manual,* 3rd ed. Philadelphia: Wolters Kluwer/Lippincott Williams & Wilkins Health.

American College of Sports Medicine. 2012. *ACSM's Health/Fitness Facility Standards and Guidelines,* 4th ed. Champaign, Ill. Human Kinetics.

American College of Sports Medicine. 2013. *ACSM's Guidelines for Exercise Testing and Prescription,* 9th ed. Philadelphia: Wolters Kluwer/Lippincott Williams & Wilkins Health.

American Diabetes Association. 2014. Economic Burden of Prediabetes Up 74 Percent Over Five Years, http://www.diabetes.org/newsroom/press-releases/2014/economic-burden-of-prediabetes-up-74-percent-over-five-years.html.

Ashwell, M., and S. Gibson. 2014. A proposal for a primary screening tool: "Keep your waist circumference to less than half your height." *BMC Medicine* 12: 207.

Baer, H. J., et al. 2011. Risk factors for mortality in the Nurses' Health Study: A competing risks analysis. *American Journal of Epidemiology* 173(3): 319–329.

Beam, W., and G. Adams. 2014. *Exercise Physiology Laboratory Manual,* 7th ed. New York: McGraw-Hill.

Berry, T. R., et al. 2014. Changing fit and fat bias using an implicit retraining task. *Psychological Health* 29(7): 796–812.

Bohm, A., and B. L. Heitmann. 2013. The use of bioelectrical impedance analysis for body composition in epidemiological studies. *European Journal Clinical Nutrition* 67(Suppl 1): S79–85.

Bosy-Westphal, A., and M. J. Muller. 2014. Measuring the impact of weight cycling on body composition: A methodological challenge. *Current Opinions in Clinical Nutrition & Metabolic Care* 17(5): 396–400.

Bray, G., and C. Bouchard, eds. 2014. *Handbook of Obesity,* vols. 1 and 2. Boca Raton, Fl.: CRC Press.

Buckinx, F., et al. 2015. Concordance between muscle mass assessed by bioelectrical impedance analysis and by dual energy X-ray absorptiometry: A cross-sectional study. *BMC Musculoskeletal Disorders* 16: 60.

Bye, A., et al. 2013. Circulating MicroRNAs and Aerobic Fitness—The HUNT-Study. *PLoS One* 8(2): e57496.

Campisi, J., et al. 2014. Sex and age-related differences in perceived, desired and measured percentage body fat among adults. *Journal Human Nutrition and Dietetics.* Published online June 30, 2014.

Cao, Z. B., et al. 2013. Prediction of maximal oxygen uptake from a 3-minute walk based on gender, age, and body composition. *Journal of Physical Activity and Health* 10(2): 280–287.

Centers for Disease Control and Prevention, National Center for Health Statistics. 2014. Health E-Stat: Prevalence of Overweight, Obesity, and Extreme Obesity Among Adults: United States, 1960–1962 Through 2011–2012, http://www.cdc.gov/nchs/data/hestat/obesity_adult_11_12/obesity_adult_11_12.htm.

Chuang, S. Y., et al. 2014. Skeletal muscle mass and risk of death in an elderly population. *Nutrition, Metabolism, and Cardiovascular Diseases* 24(7): 784–791.

Dagan, S. S., et al. 2013. Waist circumference vs body mass index in association with cardiorespiratory fitness in healthy men and women: A cross sectional analysis of 403 subjects. *Nutrition Journal* 12: 12.

Dixon, J. B., et al. 2015. Fat-free mass loss generated with weight loss in overweight and obese adults: What may we expect? *Diabetes, Obesity, and Metabolism* 17(1): 91–93.

Ellefsen, S., et al. 2014. Irisin and FNDC5: Effects of 12-week strength training, and relations to muscle phenotype and body mass composition in untrained women. *European Journal Applied Physiology* 114(9): 1875–1888.

Fahey, T., and M. Fahey. 2014. Nutrition, Physical Activity, and the Obesity Epidemic: Issues, Policies, and Solutions (1960s-Present). *The Guide to U.S. Health and Health Care Policy.* T. Oliver. New York: DWJ Books: 363–374.

Farrell, S. W., et al. 2010. Cardiorespiratory fitness, adiposity, and all-cause mortality in women. *Medicine and Science in Sports and Exercise* 42(11): 2006–2012.

Flegal, K. M., et al. 2013. Association of all-cause mortality with overweight and obesity using standard body mass index categories: A systematic review and meta-analysis. *Journal of the American Medical Association* 309(1): 71–82.

Ford, E. S., and W. H. Dietz. 2013. Trends in energy intake among adults in the United States: findings from NHANES. *American Journal of Clinical Nutrition* 97 (4): 848–853.

Ford, E. S., et al. 2011. Trends in obesity and abdominal obesity among adults in the United States from 1999–2008. *International Journal of Obesity* 35: 736–743.

Fosbol, M. O., and B. Zerahn. 2015. Contemporary methods of body composition measurement. *Clinical Physiology and Functional Imaging* 35(2): 81–97.

Fryar, C. D., Q. Gu, and C. L. Ogden. 2012. Anthropometric reference data for children and adults: United States, 2007–2010. *Vital Health and Statics* 11(252).

Gallagher, K. M., et al. 2011. When 'fit' leads to fit, and when 'fit' leads to fat: How message framing and intrinsic vs. extrinsic exercise outcomes interact in promoting physical activity. *Psychological Health* 26: (7): 819–834.

Geiss, L. S., et al. Increasing prevalence of diagnosed diabetes—United States and Puerto Rico, 1995–2010. *Morbidity and Mortality Weekly Report* 61(45): 918–921.

Gill, J. M., et al. 2014. Physical activity, ethnicity and cardio-metabolic health: Does one size fit all? *Atherosclerosis* 232(2): 319–333.

Goyal, A., et al. 2014. Is there a paradox in obesity? *Cardiology Reviews* 22(4): 163–170.

Graf, C. E., et al. 2015. Body composition and all-cause mortality in subjects older than 65 y. *American Journal Clinical Nutrition* 101(4): 760–767.

Heo, M., et al. 2012. Percentage of body fat cutoffs by sex, age, and race-ethnicity in the US adult population from NHANES, 1999–2004. *American Journal of Clinical Nutrition* 95(3): 594–602.

Heymsfield, S. B., and W. T. Cefalu. 2013. Does body mass index adequately convey a patient's mortality risk? *Journal of the American Medical Association* 309(1): 87–88.

Heymsfield, S. B., et al. 2014. Assessing skeletal muscle mass: Historical overview and state of the art. *Journal of Cachexia, Sarcopenia, and Muscle* 5(1): 9–18.

Heymsfield, S. B., et al. 2014. Weight loss composition is one-fourth fat-free mass: A critical review and critique of this widely cited rule. *Obesity Reviews* 15(4): 310–321.

Heymsfield, S. B., et al. 2015. Skeletal muscle mass and quality: Evolution of modern measurement concepts in the context of sarcopenia. *Proceedings of the Nutrition Society*. Published online April 8, 2015.

Heyward, V. H. 2014. *Advanced Fitness Assessment and Exercise Prescription,* 7th ed. Champaign, Ill.: Human Kinetics.

Hillier, S. E., et al. 2014. A comparison of body composition measurement techniques. *Journal Human Nutrition and Dietetics* 27(6): 626–631.

Hodgdon, J. A., and K. Friedl. 1998. Development of the DoD body composition estimation equations. Washington, D.C.: Bureau of Medicine and Surgery, Naval Health Research Center. Technical Document 99-2B.

Iemitsu, M., et al. 2014. Higher cardiorespiratory fitness attenuates the risk of atherosclerosis associated with ADRB3 Trp64Arg polymorphism. *European Journal Applied Physiology* 114(7): 1421–1428.

Jackson, A. A., et al. 2013. Body composition assessment in nutrition research: Value of BIA technology. *European of Clinical Nutrition* 67 (Suppl 1): S71–78.

Joy, E., et al. 2014. 2014 Female Athlete Triad coalition consensus statement on treatment and return to play of the Female Athlete Triad. *Current Sports Medicine Reports* 13(4): 219–232.

Katchunga, P. B., et al. 2015. Bioelectrical impedance outperforms waist circumference for predicting cardiometabolic risk in Congolese hypertensive subjects: A cross-sectional study. *BMC Cardiovascular Disorders* 15(1): 17.

Khalil, S. F., et al. 2014. The theory and fundamentals of bioimpedance analysis in clinical status monitoring and diagnosis of diseases. *Sensors* 14(6): 10895–10928.

Kim, S., et al. 2014. Combined impact of cardiorespiratory fitness and visceral adiposity on metabolic syndrome in overweight and obese adults in Korea *PLoS One.* 9(1): e85742.

Lang, P. O., et al. 2015. Markers of metabolic and cardiovascular health in adults: Comparative analysis of DEXA-based body composition components and BMI categories. *Journal Cardiology* 65(1): 42–49.

Levy, J. 2015. U.S. obesity rate inches up to 27.7% in 2014. Well-Being, Gallup. http://www.gallup.com/poll/181271/obesity-rate-inches-2014.aspx.

Loprinzi, P., et al. 2014. The "fit but fat" paradigm addressed using accelerometer-determined physical activity data. *North American Journal Medical Sciences* 6(7): 295–301.

Mallinson, R. J., and M. J. De Souza. 2014. Current perspectives on the etiology and manifestation of the "silent" component of the Female Athlete Triad. *International Journal Women's Health* 6: 451–467.

Mattsson, S., and B. J. Thomas. 2006. Development of methods for body composition studies. *Physics in Medicine and Biology* 51(13): R203–R228.

Min, K. B. and J. Y. Min. 2015. Android and gynoid fat percentages and serum lipid levels in United States adults. *Clinical Endocrinology* 82(3): 377–387.

Mountjoy, M., et al. 2014. The IOC consensus statement: Beyond the Female Athlete Triad–Relative Energy Deficiency in Sport (RED-S). *British Journal Sports Medicine* 48(7): 491–497.

Mozaffarian, D,. et al. 2015. *Heart Disease and Stroke Statistics–2015 Update.* 131(4):e29–e322.

Nana, A., et al. 2015. Methodology Review: Using dual-energy x-ray absorptiometry (DXA) for the assessment of body composition in athletes and active people. *International Journal Sports Nutrition and Exercise Metabolism* 25(2): 198–215.

Ogden, C. L., et al. 2012. Prevalence of obesity and trends in body mass index among U.S. children and adolescents, 1999–2010. *Journal of the American Medical Association* 307(5): 483–490.

Ortega, F. B., et al. 2014. Health inequalities in urban adolescents: Role of physical activity, diet, and genetics. *Pediatrics* 133(4): e884–895.

Peterson, D. D. 2015. History of the U.S. Navy Body Composition program. *Military Medicine* 180(1): 91–96.

Puterman, E., et al. 2010. The power of exercise: Buffering the effect of chronic stress on telomere length. *PLoS One* 5(5): e10837.

Roberts, C. K., et al. 2014. Strength fitness and body weight status on markers of cardiometabolic health. *Medicine Science Sports Exercise*. Published online September 23, 2014.

Sagayama, H., et al. 2014. Measurement of body composition in response to a short period of overfeeding. *Journal Physiological Anthropology* 33: 29.

Swain, D. P. 2013. *ACSM's Resource Manual for Guidelines for Exercise Testing and Prescription,* 7th ed. Philadelphia: Wolters Kluwer/Lippincott Williams & Wilkins Health.

Toss, F., et al. 2012. Body composition and mortality risk in later life. *Age and Ageing* 41(5): 677–681.

Vieira-Potter, V. J., et al. 2015. Exercise (and estrogen) make fat cells "fit." *Exercise Sport Sciences Reviews*. Published online April 26, 2015.

Wang, X., et al. 2008. Weight regain is related to decreases in physical activity during weight loss. *Medicine and Science in Sports and Exercise* 40(10): 1781–1788.

Widen, E. M. and D. Gallagher. 2014. Body composition changes in pregnancy: Measurement, predictors and outcomes. *European Journal Clinical Nutrition* 68(6): 643–652.

Wormser, D., et al. 2011. Separate and combined associations of body-mass index and abdominal adiposity with cardiovascular disease: Collaborative analysis of 58 prospective studies. *Lancet* 377(9771): 1085–1095.

Zhu, W., et al. 2014. Associations of cardiorespiratory fitness with cardiovascular disease risk factors in middle-aged Chinese women: A cross-sectional study *BMC Women's Health* 14: 62.

Zwierzchowska, A., et al. 2014. The body mass index and waist circumference as predictors of body composition in post CSCI wheelchair rugby players (preliminary investigations) *Journal of Human Kinetics.* 43: 191–198.

Name _____ Section _____ Date _____

LAB 6.1 Assessing Body Mass Index and Body Composition

Body Mass Index

Equipment

1. Weight scale

2. Tape measure or other means of measuring height

Instructions

Measure your height and weight, and record the results. Be sure to record the unit of measurement.

Height: _____ Weight: _____

Calculating BMI (see also the shortcut chart of BMI values in Lab 6.2)

1. Convert your body weight to kilograms by dividing your weight in pounds by 2.2.

   Body weight _____ lb ÷ 2.2 lb/kg = body weight _____ kg

2. Convert your height measurement to meters by multiplying your height in inches by 0.0254.

   Height _____ in. × 0.0254 m/in. = height _____ m

3. Square your height measurement.

   Height _____ m × height _____ m = height _____ m^2

4. BMI equals body weight in kilograms divided by height in meters squared (kg/m^2).

   Body weight _____ kg ÷ height _____ m^2 = BMI _____ kg/m^2
             (from step 1)   (from step 3)

Rating Your BMI

Refer to the table for a rating of your BMI. Record the results below and on the final page of this lab.

Classification	BMI(kg/m^2)
Underweight	<18.5
Normal	18.5–24.9
Overweight	25.0–29.9
Obesity (I)	30.0–34.9
Obesity (II)	35.0–39.9
Extreme obesity (III)	≥40.0

BMI _____ kg/m^2

Classification _____

Skinfold Measurements

Equipment

1. Skinfold caliper

2. Partner to take measurements

3. Marking pen (optional)

LABORATORY ACTIVITIES

Instructions

1. *Select and locate the correct sites for measurement.* All measurements should be taken on the right side of the body with the subject standing. Skinfolds are normally measured on the natural fold line of the skin, either vertically or at a slight angle. The skinfold measurement sites for males are chest, abdomen, and thigh; for females, triceps, suprailium, and thigh. If the person taking skinfold measurements is inexperienced, it may be helpful to mark the correct sites with a marking pen.

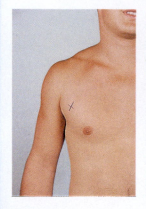 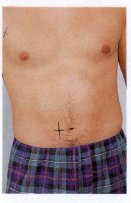 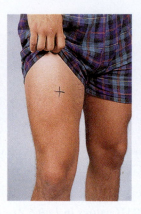 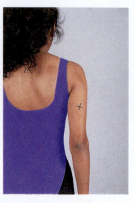 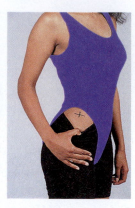

(a) Chest   (b) Abdomen   (c) Thigh   (d) Triceps   (e) Suprailium

(a) *Chest.* Pinch a diagonal fold halfway between the nipple and the shoulder crease. (b) *Abdomen.* Pinch a vertical fold about 1 inch to the right of the umbilicus (navel). (c) *Thigh.* Pinch a vertical fold midway between the top of the hipbone and the kneecap. (d) *Triceps.* Pinch a vertical skinfold on the back of the right arm midway between the shoulder and elbow. The arm should be straight and should hang naturally. (e) *Suprailium.* Pinch a fold at the top front of the right hipbone. The skinfold here is taken slightly diagonally according to the natural fold tendency of the skin.

2. *Measure the appropriate skinfolds.* Pinch a fold of skin between your thumb and forefinger. Pull the fold up so that no muscular tissue is included; don't pinch the skinfold too hard. Hold the calipers perpendicular to the fold and measure the skinfold about 0.25 inch away from your fingers. Allow the tips of the calipers to close on the skinfold and let the reading settle before marking it down. Take readings to the nearest half-millimeter. Continue to repeat the measurements until two consecutive measurements match, releasing and repinching the skinfold between each measurement. Make a note of the final measurement for each site.

Time of day of measurements: _____

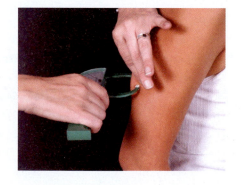

Men

Chest: _____ mm

Abdomen: _____ mm

Thigh: _____ mm

Women

Triceps: _____ mm

Suprailium: _____ mm

Thigh: _____ mm

Determining Percent Body Fat

Add the measurements of your three skinfolds. Use this sum as a point of comparison for future assessments and/or to find the percent body fat that corresponds to your total in the appropriate table. For example, a 20-year-old female with measurements of 17 mm, 21 mm, and 22 mm would have a skinfold sum of 60 mm; according to the following table her percent body fat is 23.5. The table lists ages in increments of five. If your age is not listed on the table, use the column for the age closest to your own.

Sum of three skinfolds: _____ mm   Percent body fat: _____ %

Prediction of Fat Percentage in Females from the Sum of Three Skinfolds

Sum of Skinfolds (mm)	Age (Years)								
	20	25	30	35	40	45	50	55	60 and over
20	9.3	9.6	9.9	10.2	10.5	10.8	11.1	11.4	11.7
25	11.2	11.5	11.8	12.1	12.4	12.7	13.0	13.3	13.6
30	13.1	13.4	13.7	14.0	14.3	14.6	14.9	15.2	15.5
35	14.9	15.2	15.5	15.8	16.1	16.4	16.7	17.0	17.3
40	16.7	17.0	17.3	17.6	17.9	18.2	18.5	18.8	19.1
45	18.4	18.8	19.1	19.4	19.7	20.0	20.3	20.6	20.9
50	20.2	20.5	20.8	21.1	21.4	21.7	22.0	22.4	22.7
55	21.9	22.2	22.5	22.8	23.1	23.4	23.7	24.1	24.4
60	23.5	23.8	24.1	24.4	24.8	25.1	25.4	25.7	26.0
65	25.1	25.4	25.7	26.1	26.4	26.7	27.0	27.3	27.7
70	26.7	27.0	27.3	27.6	27.9	28.3	28.6	28.9	29.2
75	28.2	28.5	28.8	29.1	29.5	29.8	30.1	30.4	30.8
80	29.7	30.0	30.3	30.6	31.0	31.3	31.6	31.9	32.3
85	31.1	31.4	31.7	32.1	32.4	32.7	33.0	33.4	33.7
90	32.5	32.8	33.1	33.5	33.8	34.1	34.4	34.8	35.1
95	33.8	34.1	34.5	34.8	35.1	35.5	35.8	36.1	36.5
100	35.1	35.4	35.8	36.1	36.4	36.8	37.1	37.4	37.8
105	36.3	36.7	37.0	37.3	37.7	38.0	38.3	38.7	39.0
110	37.5	37.9	38.2	38.5	38.9	39.2	39.5	39.9	40.2
115	38.7	39.0	39.3	39.7	40.0	40.4	40.7	41.0	41.4
120	39.8	40.1	40.4	40.8	41.1	41.5	41.8	42.1	42.5
125	40.8	41.2	41.5	41.8	42.2	42.5	42.9	43.2	43.5
130	41.8	42.1	42.5	42.8	43.2	43.5	43.9	44.2	44.5
135	42.7	43.1	43.4	43.8	44.1	44.5	44.8	45.1	45.5

NOTE: Find the value on the chart that most closely corresponds to your age and the sum of measurement skinfolds. To calculate the value more precisely, plug your age and sum of skinfolds into the appropriate formula:

Body Density = 1.0994921 − (0.0009929 × sum of skinfolds) + (0.0000023 × square of the sum of skinfolds) − (0.0001392 × age), where the skinfold sites (measured in mm) are triceps, suprailium, and thigh % Body Fat = (495 / Body Density) − 450

SOURCES: Table generated from equations in Jackson, A. S., M. L. Pollock, and A. Ward. 1980. Generalized equations for predicting body density in women, *Medicine and Science in Sports and Exercise* 12: 175–182; Siri, W. E. 1956. Gross composition of the body. In *Advances in Biological and Medical Physics*, IV, ed. J. H. Lawrence and C. A. Tobias. New York: Academic Press.

LABORATORY ACTIVITIES

Prediction of Fat Percentage in Males from the Sum of Three Skinfolds

Sum of Skinfolds (mm)	Age (Years)								
	20	25	30	35	40	45	50	55	60 and over
10	1.6	2.1	2.7	3.2	3.7	4.3	4.8	5.3	5.9
15	3.2	3.8	4.3	4.8	5.4	5.9	6.4	7.0	7.5
20	4.8	5.4	5.9	6.4	7.0	7.5	8.1	8.6	9.2
25	6.4	6.9	7.5	8.0	8.6	9.1	9.7	10.2	10.8
30	8.0	8.5	9.1	9.6	10.2	10.7	11.3	11.8	12.4
35	9.5	10.0	10.6	11.2	11.7	12.3	12.8	13.4	13.9
40	11.0	11.6	12.1	12.7	13.2	13.8	14.4	14.9	15.5
45	12.5	13.1	13.6	14.2	14.7	15.3	15.9	16.4	17.0
50	14.0	14.5	15.1	15.6	16.2	16.8	17.3	17.9	18.5
55	15.4	16.0	16.5	17.1	17.7	18.2	18.8	19.4	19.9
60	16.8	17.4	17.9	18.5	19.1	19.7	20.2	20.8	21.4
65	18.2	18.8	19.3	19.9	20.5	21.1	21.6	22.2	22.8
70	19.5	20.1	20.7	21.3	21.9	22.4	23.0	23.6	24.2
75	20.9	21.5	22.0	22.6	23.2	23.8	24.4	24.9	25.5
80	22.2	22.8	23.3	23.9	24.5	25.1	25.7	26.3	26.9
85	23.4	24.0	24.6	25.2	25.8	26.4	27.0	27.6	28.2
90	24.7	25.3	25.9	26.5	27.0	27.6	28.2	28.8	29.4
95	25.9	26.5	27.1	27.7	28.3	28.9	29.5	30.1	30.7
100	27.1	27.7	28.3	28.9	29.5	30.1	30.7	31.3	31.9
105	28.2	28.8	29.4	30.0	30.6	31.2	31.8	32.4	33.0
110	29.3	29.9	30.5	31.1	31.7	32.4	33.0	33.6	34.2
115	30.4	31.0	31.6	32.2	32.8	33.5	34.1	34.7	35.3
120	31.5	32.1	32.7	33.3	33.9	34.5	35.1	35.7	36.4
125	32.5	33.1	33.7	34.3	34.9	35.6	36.2	36.8	37.4

NOTE: Find the value on the chart that most closely corresponds to your age and the sum of measurement skinfolds. To calculate the value more precisely, plug your age and sum of skinfolds into the appropriate formula:

Body Density = 1.10938 − (0.0008267 × sum of skinfolds) + (0.0000016 × square of the sum of skinfolds) − (0.0002574 × age), where skinfold sites (measured in mm) are chest, abdomen, and thigh % Body Fat = (495 / Body Density) − 450

SOURCES: Table generated from equations in Jackson, A. S., and M. L. Pollock, 1978. Generalized equations for predicting body density in men. *British Journal of Nutrition* 40: 497–504; Jackson, A. S., M. L. Pollock, and A. Ward. 1980. Generalized equations for predicting body density in women, *Medicine and Science in Sports and Exercise* 12: 175–182; Siri, W. E. 1956. Gross composition of the body. In *Advances in Biological and Medical Physics,* IV, ed. J. H. Lawrence and C. A. Tobias. New York: Academic Press.

Bioelectrical Impedance Analysis (BIA)

Equipment

BIA analyzer such as Omron Body Fat Analyzer: The BIA device sends an extremely weak electrical current through your body to determine the amount of total body water. You will not feel the current during the test. The body fat percentage is calculated from a formula that uses body water, electric resistance, height, weight, age, and gender.

Instructions

1. Enter your height, weight, gender, and age into the BIA device.

2. Grasp the left and right handles and wrap your middle finger around the groove in the handle. With your thumbs facing up and resting on the unit, place the palms of your hands on the top and bottom electrodes.

3. Hold your arms straight out at a 90-degree angle to your body.

4. Confirm the ready to measure display and the **READY** indicator turns on. Push the start button and the display **START** turns on. The unit automatically detects that it is held and starts measurement. Do not move during measurement.

5. Record your fat, percent fat, and fat-free weight.

    Fat: _____

    Percent fat: _____

    Fat-free weight: _____

6. Compare the BIA measurements with other techniques of assessing body composition.

U.S. Navy Circumference Method of Measuring Percent Fat

This method measures fat percentage from abdominal circumference, neck circumference, and height in men and from abdominal circumference, hip circumference, neck circumference, and height in women.

Equipment

1. Measuring tape

2. Stadiometer or tape on wall to measure height

Instructions

1. Measure height without shoes using a stadiometer or tape measure. A stadiometer is a height-measuring device that is often part of a scale found in a gym or physician's office.

    Height (inches): _____

2. Measure neck circumference below the larynx (Adam's apple), with the tape sloping slightly downward at the front.

    Neck circumference (inches): _____

3. Measure waist circumference at navel level for men and at the smallest point for women.

    Waist circumference (inches): _____

4. Measure hip circumference (women only) at the largest point.

    Hip circumference (inches): _____

Calculating percent fat using charts developed by the U.S. Navy

Men:

Calculate circumference value: Abdominal circumference − neck circumference: _____

Read percent fat from the chart from where the circumference value intersects with height. Enter fat percentage: _____

Women:

Calculate circumference value: Abdominal circumference + hip circumference − neck circumference (in inches): _____

Read percent fat from the chart from where the circumference value intersects with height. Enter fat percentage: _____

LABORATORY ACTIVITIES

U.S. Navy Circumference Chart for Predicting Percent Fat in Men

Circumference	Height (inches)																				
	60	61	62	63	64	65	66	67	68	69	70	71	72	73	74	75	76	77	78	79	80
13	8	8	7	7	6	6	5	5	4	4	3	3									
14	11	10	10	9	9	8	8	7	7	7	6	6	5	5	4	4	4	3	3		
15	13	13	12	12	11	11	10	10	10	9	9	8	8	7	7	7	6	6	5	5	5
16	16	15	15	14	14	13	13	12	12	12	11	11	10	10	9	9	9	8	8	7	7
17	18	18	17	17	16	16	15	15	14	14	13	13	13	12	12	11	11	10	10	10	9
18	20	20	19	19	18	18	17	17	16	16	15	15	15	14	14	13	13	13	12	12	11
19	22	22	21	21	20	20	19	19	18	18	18	17	17	16	16	15	15	15	14	14	13
20	24	24	23	23	22	22	21	21	20	20	19	19	19	18	18	17	17	17	16	16	15
21	26	25	25	24	24	24	23	23	22	22	21	21	20	20	20	19	19	18	18	18	17
22	28	27	27	26	26	25	25	24	24	23	23	23	22	22	21	21	20	20	20	19	19
23	29	29	28	28	27	27	26	26	26	25	25	24	24	23	23	23	22	22	21	21	21
24	31	30	30	29	29	28	28	28	27	27	26	26	25	25	25	24	24	23	23	23	22
25	32	32	31	31	30	30	30	29	29	28	28	27	27	26	26	26	25	25	24	24	24
26	34	33	33	32	32	31	31	31	30	30	29	29	28	28	28	27	27	26	26	26	25
27	35	35	34	34	33	33	32	32	32	31	31	30	30	29	29	29	28	28	27	27	27
28	37	36	36	35	35	34	34	33	33	32	32	32	31	31	30	30	29	29	29	28	28
29	38	37	37	37	36	36	35	35	34	34	33	33	32	32	32	31	31	30	30	30	29
30	39	39	38	38	37	37	36	36	35	35	35	34	34	33	33	32	32	32	31	31	31
31	40	40	39	39	39	38	38	37	37	36	36	35	35	35	34	34	33	33	33	32	32
32	42	41	41	40	40	39	39	38	38	37	37	37	36	36	35	35	34	34	34	33	33
33	43	42	42	41	41	40	40	39	39	39	38	38	37	37	36	36	36	35	35	34	34
34	44	43	43	42	42	42	41	41	40	40	39	39	38	38	38	37	37	36	36	36	35
35	45	45	44	44	43	43	42	42	41	41	40	40	39	39	39	38	38	37	37	37	36

U.S. Navy Circumference Chart for Predicting Percent Fat in Women

Circumference	Height (inches)																				
	58	59	60	61	62	63	64	65	66	67	68	69	70	71	72	73	74	75	76	77	78
45	19	18	18	17	16	16	15	14	14	13	12	12	11	11	10	9	9	8	8		
46	21	20	19	19	18	17	17	16	15	15	14	13	13	12	12	11	10	10	9	9	8
47	22	22	21	20	19	19	18	17	17	16	16	15	14	14	13	12	12	11	11	10	10
48	24	23	22	22	21	20	20	19	18	18	17	16	16	15	15	14	13	13	12	12	11
49	25	24	24	23	22	22	21	20	20	19	18	18	17	17	16	15	15	14	14	13	13
50	27	26	25	24	24	23	22	22	21	21	20	19	19	18	17	17	16	16	15	15	14
51	28	27	27	26	25	25	24	23	23	22	21	21	20	19	19	18	18	17	17	16	15
52	29	29	28	27	27	26	25	25	24	23	23	22	21	21	20	20	19	19	18	17	17
53	31	30	29	29	28	27	27	26	25	25	24	23	23	22	22	21	20	20	19	19	18
54	32	31	31	30	29	29	28	27	27	26	25	25	24	24	23	22	22	21	21	20	20
55	33	33	32	31	31	30	29	29	28	27	27	26	25	25	24	24	23	22	22	21	21
56	35	34	33	33	32	31	30	30	29	29	28	27	27	26	25	25	24	24	23	23	22
57	36	35	34	34	33	32	32	31	30	30	29	29	28	27	27	26	26	25	24	24	23
58	37	36	36	35	34	34	33	32	32	31	30	30	29	29	28	27	27	26	26	25	25
59	38	38	37	36	36	35	34	34	33	32	32	31	30	30	29	29	28	27	27	26	26
60	40	39	38	37	37	36	35	35	34	33	33	32	32	31	30	30	29	29	28	28	27
61	41	40	39	39	38	37	37	36	35	35	34	33	33	32	32	31	30	30	29	29	28
62	42	41	40	40	39	38	38	37	36	36	35	35	34	33	33	32	32	31	30	30	29
63	43	42	42	41	40	40	39	38	38	37	36	36	35	34	34	33	33	32	32	31	30
64	44	43	43	42	41	41	40	39	39	38	37	37	36	36	35	34	34	33	33	32	32
65	45	45	44	43	42	42	41	40	40	39	38	38	37	37	36	35	35	34	34	33	33
66	46	46	45	44	43	43	42	41	41	40	40	39	38	38	37	37	36	35	35	34	34
67	47	47	46	45	45	44	43	43	42	41	41	40	39	39	38	38	37	36	36	35	35
68	48	48	47	46	46	45	44	44	43	42	42	41	40	40	39	39	38	38	37	36	36
69	49	49	48	47	47	46	45	45	44	43	43	42	41	41	40	40	39	39	38	37	37
70	50	50	49	48	48	47	46	46	45	44	44	43	43	42	41	41	40	40	39	38	38
71	51	51	50	49	49	48	47	47	46	45	45	44	44	43	42	42	41	41	40	39	39
72	52	52	51	50	50	49	48	48	47	46	46	45	45	44	43	43	42	42	41	40	40
73	53	53	52	51	51	50	49	49	48	47	47	46	45	45	44	44	43	43	42	41	41
74	54	54	53	52	52	51	50	50	49	48	48	47	46	46	45	45	44	44	43	42	42
75	55	55	54	53	53	52	51	51	50	49	49	48	47	47	46	46	45	44	44	43	43

SOURCES Adapted from Hodgdon, J. A., and K. Friedl. 1998. Development of the DoD body composition estimation equations. Washington, D.C.: Bureau of Medicine and Surgery, Naval Health Research Center. Technical Document 99-2B.

Rating Your Body Composition

Refer to the chart below to rate your percent body fat. Record it below and in the chart at the end of this lab.

Rating: _____

Percent Body Fat Classification

	Percent Body Fat (%)				Percent Body Fat (%)		
	20–39 Years	40–59 Years	60–79 Years		20–39 Years	40–59 Years	60–79 Years
Women				**Men**			
Essential*	8–12	8–12	8–12	Essential*	3–5	3–5	3–5
Low/athletic**	13–20	13–22	13–23	Low/athletic**	6–7	6–10	6–12
Recommended	21–32	23–33	24–35	Recommended	8–19	11–21	13–24
Overfat†	33–38	34–39	36–41	Overfat†	20–24	22–27	25–29
Obese†	≥39	≥40	≥42	Obese†	≥25	≥28	≥30

NOTE: The cutoffs for recommended, overfat, and obese ranges in this table are based on a study that linked body mass index classifications from the National Institutes of Health with predicted percent body fat (measured using dual-energy X-ray absorptiometry).

*Essential body fat is necessary for the basic functioning of the body.

**Percent body fat in the low/athletic range may be appropriate for some people as long as it is not the result of illness or disordered eating habits.

†Health risks increase as percent body fat exceeds the recommended range.

SOURCES: Gallagher, D., et al. 2009. Healthy percentage body fat ranges: An approach for developing guidelines based on body mass index. *American Journal of Clinical Nutrition* 72: 694–701; Swain, D. P. 2013. *ACSM's Resource Manual for Guidelines for Exercise Testing and Prescription,* 7th ed. Philadelphia: Wolters Kluwer/Lippincott Williams & Wilkins Health.

Other Methods of Assessing Percent Body Fat

If you use a different method, record the name of the method and the result below and in the chart at the end of this lab. Find your body composition rating on the chart above.

Method used: _____ Percent body fat: _____

% Rating (from chart above): _____

Body Fat Distribution

Waist Circumference and Waist-to-Hip Ratio

Equipment

1. Tape measure
2. Partner to take measurements

Preparation

Wear clothes that will not add significantly to your measurements.

Instructions

Stand with your feet together and your arms at your sides. Raise your arms only high enough to allow for taking the measurements. Your partner should make sure the tape is horizontal around the entire circumference and pulled snugly against your skin. The tape shouldn't be pulled so tight that it causes indentations in your skin. Record measurements to the nearest millimeter or one-sixteenth of an inch.

Waist. Measure at the smallest waist circumference. If you don't have a natural waist, measure at the level of your navel.

Waist measurement: _____

Hip. Measure at the largest hip circumference. Hip measurement: _____

Waist-to-Hip Ratio: You can use any unit of measurement (for example, inches or centimeters) as long as you are consistent. Waist-to-hip ratio equals waist measurement divided by hip measurement.

Waist-to-hip ratio: _____ ÷ _____ = _____
       (waist measurement)   (hip measurement)

LABORATORY ACTIVITIES

Determining Your Risk

The table below indicates values for waist circumference and waist-to-hip ratio above which the risk of health problems increases significantly. If your measurement or ratio is above either cutoff point, put a check on the appropriate line below and in the chart at the end of this lab.

Waist circumference: _____ (✔ high risk) Waist-to-hip ratio: _____ (✔ high risk)

Body Fat Distribution

Cutoff Points for High Risk

	Waist Circumference	Waist-to-Hip Ratio
Men	More than 40 in. (102 cm)	More than 0.94
Women	More than 35 in. (88 cm)	More than 0.82

SOURCE: National Heart, Lung, and Blood Institute. 1998. *Clinical Guidelines on the Identification, Evaluation, and Treatment of Overweight and Obesity in Adults: The Evidence Report.* Bethesda, Md.: National Institutes of Health; Heyward, V. H., and D. R. Wagner. 2004. *Applied Body Composition Assessment,* 2nd ed. Champaign, Ill.: Human Kinetics.

Rating Your Body Mass Index, Body Composition, and Body Fat Distribution

Assessment	Value	Classification
BMI	_____ kg/m^2	_____
Skinfold measurements or alternative method of determining percent body fat. Specify method: _____	_____ % body fat	_____
Bioelectrical Impedance Analysis (BIA)	_____ % body fat	_____
U.S. Navy Circumference Method	_____ % body fat	_____
Waist circumference Waist-to-hip ratio	_____ in. or cm _____ (ratio)	_____ (✔ high risk) _____ (✔ high risk)

Using Your Results

How did you score? Are you surprised by your ratings for body composition and body fat distribution? Are your current ratings in the range for good health? Are you satisfied with your current body composition? Why or why not?

If you're not satisfied, set a realistic goal for improvement:

What should you do next? Enter the results of this lab in the Preprogram Assessment column in Appendix C. If you've determined that you need to improve your body composition, set a specific goal by completing Lab 6.2, and then plan your program using the labs in Chapters 8 and 9. After several weeks or months of an exercise and/or dietary change program, complete this lab again and enter the results in the Postprogram Assessment column of Appendix C. How do the results compare?

Name _____ **Section** _____ **Date** _____

LAB 6.2   Setting Goals for Target Body Weight

This lab is designed to help you set body weight goals based on a target BMI or percent body fat. If the results of Lab 6.1 indicate that a change in body composition would be beneficial for your health, you may want to complete this lab to help you set goals.

Remember, though, that a wellness lifestyle—including a balanced diet and regular exercise—is more important for your health than achieving any specific body weight, BMI, or percent body fat. You may want to set goals for improving your diet and increasing physical activity and let your body composition change as a result. If so, use the labs in Chapters 3, 4, 8, and 9 as your guides.

Equipment

Calculator (or pencil and paper for calculations)

Preparation

Determine percent body fat and/or calculate BMI as described in Lab 6.1. Keep track of height and weight as measured for these calculations.

Height: _____   Weight: _____

Instructions: Target Body Weight from Target BMI

Use the chart below to find the target body weight that corresponds to your target BMI. Find your height in the left column, and then move across the appropriate row until you find the weight that corresponds to your target BMI. Remember, BMI is only an indirect measurement of body composition. It is possible to improve body composition without any significant change in weight. For example, a weight training program may result in increased muscle mass and decreased fat mass without any change in overall weight. For this reason, you may want to set alternative or additional goals, such as improving the fit of your clothes or decreasing your waist measurement.

	<18.5 Underweight		18.5–24.9 Normal						25–29.9 Overweight					30–34.9 Obesity (Class I)					35–39.9 Obesity (Class II)					≥40 Extreme Obesity
BMI	17	18	19	20	21	22	23	24	25	26	27	28	29	30	31	32	33	34	35	36	37	38	39	40
Height									Body Weight (pounds)															
4' 10"	81	86	91	96	101	105	110	115	120	124	129	134	139	144	148	153	158	163	168	172	177	182	187	192
4' 11"	84	89	94	99	104	109	114	119	124	129	134	139	144	149	154	159	163	168	173	178	183	188	193	198
5'	87	92	97	102	108	113	118	123	128	133	138	143	149	154	159	164	169	174	179	184	190	195	200	205
5' 1"	90	95	101	106	111	117	122	127	132	138	143	148	154	159	164	169	175	180	185	191	196	201	207	212
5' 2"	93	98	104	109	115	120	126	131	137	142	148	153	159	164	170	175	181	186	191	197	202	208	213	219
5' 3"	96	102	107	113	119	124	130	136	141	147	153	158	164	169	175	181	186	192	198	203	209	215	220	226
5' 4"	99	105	111	117	122	128	134	140	146	152	157	163	169	175	181	187	192	198	204	210	216	222	227	233
5' 5"	102	108	114	120	126	132	138	144	150	156	162	168	174	180	186	192	198	204	210	216	222	229	235	241
5' 6"	105	112	118	124	130	136	143	149	155	161	167	174	180	186	192	198	205	211	217	223	229	236	242	248
5' 7"	109	115	121	128	134	141	147	153	160	166	173	179	185	192	198	204	211	217	224	230	236	243	249	256
5' 8"	112	118	125	132	138	145	151	158	165	171	178	184	191	197	204	211	217	224	230	237	244	250	257	263
5' 9"	115	122	129	136	142	149	156	163	169	176	183	190	197	203	210	217	224	230	237	244	251	258	264	271
5' 10"	119	126	133	139	146	153	160	167	174	181	188	195	202	209	216	223	230	237	244	251	258	265	272	279
5' 11"	122	129	136	143	151	158	165	172	179	187	194	201	208	215	222	230	237	244	251	258	265	273	280	287
6'	125	133	140	148	155	162	170	177	184	192	199	207	214	221	229	236	243	251	258	266	273	280	288	295
6' 1"	129	137	144	152	159	167	174	182	190	197	205	212	220	228	235	243	250	258	265	273	281	288	296	303
6' 2"	132	140	148	156	164	171	179	187	195	203	210	218	226	234	242	249	257	265	273	281	288	296	304	312
6' 3"	136	144	152	160	168	176	184	192	200	208	216	224	232	240	248	256	264	272	280	288	296	304	312	320
6' 4"	140	148	156	164	173	181	189	197	206	214	222	230	238	247	255	263	271	280	288	296	304	312	321	329

SOURCE: Ratings from the National Heart, Lung, and Blood Institute. 1998. *Clinical Guidelines on the Identification, Evaluation, and Treatment of Overweight and Obesity in Adults.* Bethesda, Md.: National Institutes of Health.

LABORATORY ACTIVITIES

Current BMI: _____ Target BMI: _____ Target body weight (from chart): _____

Alternative/additional goals: _____

_____

Note: You can calculate target body weight from target BMI more precisely by using the following formula: (1) convert your height measurement to meters, (2) square your height measurement, (3) multiply this number by your target BMI to get your target weight in kilograms, and (4) convert your target weight from kilograms to pounds:

1. Height _____ in. × 0.0254 m/in. = height _____ m

2. Height _____ m × height _____ m = _____ m^2

3. Target BMI _____ × height _____ m^2 = target weight _____ kg

4. Target weight _____ kg × 2.2 lb/kg = target weight _____ lb

Instructions: Target Body Weight from Target Body Fat Percentages

Use the formula below to determine the target body weight that corresponds to your target percent body fat.

Current percent body fat: _____ Target percent body fat: _____

Formula

Example: 180-lb male, current percent body fat of 24%, goal of 21%

1. To determine the fat weight in your body, multiply your current weight by percent body fat (determined through skinfold measurements and expressed as a decimal).

   180 lb × 0.24 = 43.2 lb

2. Subtract the fat weight from your current weight to get your current fat-free weight.

   180 lb − 43.2 lb = 136.8 lb

3. Subtract your target percent body fat from 1 to get target percent fat-free weight.

   1 − 0.21 = 0.79

4. To get your target body weight, divide your fat-free weight by your target percent fat-free weight.

   136.8 lb ÷ 0.79 = 173 lb

NOTE: You can express weight in either pounds or kilograms, as long as you use the unit of measurement consistently.

1. Current body weight _____ × percent body fat _____ = fat weight _____

2. Current body weight _____ − fat weight _____ = fat-free weight _____

3. 1 − target percent body fat _____ = target percent fat-free weight _____

4. Fat-free weight _____ ÷ target percent fat-free weight _____ = target body weight _____

Setting a Goal

Based on these calculations and other factors (including heredity, individual preference, and current health status), select a target weight or range of weights for yourself.

Target body weight: _____

Putting Together a Complete Fitness Program

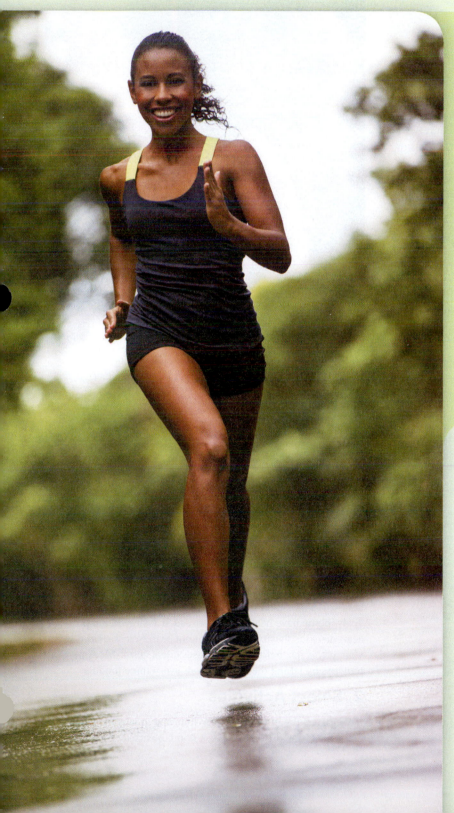

LOOKING AHEAD . . .

After reading this chapter, you should be able to

- List the steps you can follow to put together a successful personal fitness program.
- Describe strategies that can help you maintain a fitness program over the long term.
- Tailor a fitness program to accommodate different life stages.

TEST YOUR KNOWLEDGE

1. Which of the following physical activities is considered a high-intensity exercise?
   a. hiking uphill
   b. singles tennis
   c. jumping rope

2. Older adults should avoid exercise to protect themselves against falls and injuries. True or false?

3. Swimming is a total fitness activity that develops all the components of health-related fitness. True or false?

See answers on the next page.

U nderstanding the benefits of physical fitness, as explained in Chapters 1–6, is the first step toward creating a well-rounded exercise program. The next challenge is to choose activities and combine them into a program that develops all the components of fitness and helps you stay motivated. This chapter presents a step-by-step plan for creating and maintaining a well-rounded fitness program. At the end of this chapter, you'll find sample programs based on popular activities. These programs provide structure that can be helpful if you're beginning an exercise program for the first time.

DEVELOPING A PERSONAL FITNESS PLAN

If you're ready to create a complete fitness program based on the activities you enjoy most, begin by preparing the program plan and agreement in Lab 7.1. By carefully developing your plan and signing an agreement, you'll increase your chances of success. The step-by-step procedure outlined here will guide you through the steps of Lab 7.1 to create an exercise program that's right for you. (See Figure 7.1 for a sample personal fitness program plan and agreement.)

If you'd like additional help in setting up your program, choose one of the sample programs at the end of this chapter. Sample programs are provided for walking/jogging, cycling, swimming, and rowing. They include detailed instructions for starting a program and developing and maintaining fitness.

1. Set Goals

Ask yourself, "What do I want from my fitness program?" Develop different types of goals—general and specific, long term and short term. General or long-term goals might include lowering your risk for chronic disease, improving posture, having more energy, or improving the fit of your clothes.

It's also a good idea to develop some specific, short-term goals based on measurable factors. Specific goals might be:

- Raising cardiorespiratory capacity ($\dot{V}O_{2max}$) by 10%.
- Reducing the time it takes you to jog two miles from 22 minutes to 19 minutes.
- Increasing the number of push-ups you can do from 15 to 25.
- Lowering your BMI from 26 to 24.5.

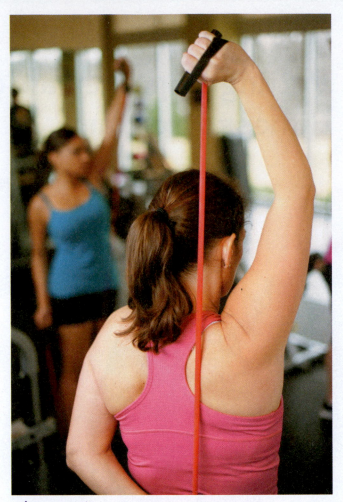

Fitness Tip An overall fitness program includes activities to develop all the components of physical fitness. Remember that you don't need to go to the gym for all your fitness activities. For example, research shows that, especially for young women, resistance bands are just as effective as weight machines or free weights for increasing muscular strength.

Having specific goals will allow you to track your progress and enjoy the measurable changes brought about by your fitness program. Break your specific goals into several smaller steps (mini-goals), such as those shown in Figure 7.1. For example, instead of dwelling on losing 20 or 30 pounds, try losing two pounds. Remember, yard by yard is hard; inch by inch is a cinch. (For detailed discussions of goals and goal setting in a behavior change or fitness program, refer back to Chapters 1 and 2.)

Physical fitness assessment tests—as described in Chapters 3–6—are essential to determining your goals. They help you decide which types of exercise you should emphasize, and they help you understand the relative difficulty of attaining specific goals. If you have health problems, such as high blood pressure, heart disease, obesity, or serious joint or muscle disabilities, see your physician before taking assessment tests. Measure your progress by taking these tests about every three months.

2. Select Activities

If you have already chosen activities and created separate program plans for different fitness components in Chapters 3–5,

A. I [Tracie Kaufman] am contracting with myself to follow a physical
           (name)
fitness program to work toward the following goals:

Specific or short-term goals

1. Improving cardiorespiratory fitness by raising my $\dot{V}O_{2max}$ from 34 to 37 ml/kg/min
2. Improving upper body muscular strength and endurance rating from fair to good
3. Improving body composition (from 28% to 25% body fat)
4. Improving my tennis game (hitting 20 playable shots in a row against the ball machine)

General or long-term goals

1. Developing a more positive attitude about myself
2. Improving the fit of my clothes
3. Building and maintaining bone mass to reduce my risk of osteoporosis
4. Increasing my life expectancy and reducing my risk for diabetes and heart disease

B. **My program plan is as follows:**

Activities	Components (Check X) CRE	MS	ME	F	BC	Time	Frequency (Check X) M	Tu	W	Th	F	S	S	Intensity*
Swimming	X	X	X	X	X	35min	X		X		X			140–170 bpm
Tennis	X	X	X	X	X	90min					X			RPE 13–16
Weight training		X	X	X	X	30min		X		X		X		see Lab 4.3
Stretching				X		25min	X		X		X	X		—

*List your target heart rate range or an RPE value if appropriate.

C. My program will begin on [Sept.] [21] My program includes the following schedule of mini-goals. For each step in my program, I will give myself the reward listed.

Completing 2 full weeks of program (mini-goal 1)	Oct.	5	movie with friends (reward)
$\dot{V}O_{2max}$ of 35 ml/kg/min (mini-goal 2)	Nov.	2	new app or game (reward)
Completing 10 full weeks of program (mini-goal 3)	Nov.	30	new sweater (reward)
Percent body fat of 27% (mini-goal 4)	Dec.	22	weekend away (reward)
$\dot{V}O_{2max}$ of 36 ml/kg/min (mini-goal 5)	Jan.	18	new app or game (reward)

D. My program will include the addition of physical activity to my daily routine (such as climbing stairs or walking to class):

1. Walking to and from campus job
2. Taking the stairs to dorm room instead of elevator
3. Bicycling to the library instead of driving
4. Taking a drop-in fitness class at the campus recreation center

E. My program will include the following strategies for reducing sedentary time:

1. Setting "move" reminders on phone and laptop
2. Moving during television commercial breaks or between programs
3. Standing or walking during phone calls

F. I will use the following tools to monitor my program and my progress toward my goals:

I'll use a chart that lists the number of laps and minutes I swim and the charts for strength and flexibility from Labs 4.3 & 5.2.

I sign this contract as an indication of my personal commitment to reach my goal.

Tracie Kaufman   Sep. 10
(your signature)

I have recruited a helper who will witness my contract and
[swim with me three days per week]
(list any way your helper will participate in your program)

Russell Walker   Sep. 10
(witness's signature)

FIGURE 7.1 **A sample personal fitness program plan and agreement.**

Table 7.1 — Examples of Different Aerobic Activities and Their Intensities

MODERATE-INTENSITY ACTIVITIES	VIGOROUS-INTENSITY ACTIVITIES
• Walking briskly (3 miles per hour or faster, but not race-walking)	• Race-walking, jogging, or running
• Water aerobics	• Swimming laps
• Bicycling slower than 10 miles per hour	• Singles tennis
• Doubles tennis	• Cardio dance and other group fitness
• Social dancing	• Bicycling 10 miles per hour or faster
• General gardening	• Jumping rope
	• Heavy gardening (continuous digging or hoeing)
	• Hiking uphill or with a heavy backpack

SOURCE: Adapted from the Centers for Disease Control and Prevention, 2014, "http://www.cdc.gov/nccdphp/dnpa/physical/pdf/PA_Intensity_table_2_1.pdf.

you can put those plans together into a single program. It's usually best to include exercises to develop each of the health-related components of fitness. The components (with abbreviations used in Figure 7.1, section B) are as follows:

- Cardiorespiratory endurance (CRE) is developed by activities that use continuous rhythmic movements of large-muscle groups, like those in the legs (see Chapter 3).
- Muscular strength and endurance (MS and ME) are developed by strength training against resistance (see Chapter 4).
- Flexibility (F) is developed by stretching the major muscle groups (see Chapter 5).
- Healthy body composition (BC) can be developed by combining a sensible diet and a program of regular exercise, including cardiorespiratory endurance exercise to burn calories and resistance training to build muscle mass (see Chapter 6).

Table 7.1 shows the intensity levels of several popular activities that promote health. Check the intensity levels of the activities you're considering to make sure the program you put together will help you achieve your goals.

If you select activities you enjoy and that support your commitment rather than activities that turn exercise into a chore, your program will provide plenty of incentive for continuing. Consider the following factors in making your choices:

- *Fun and interest.* Your fitness program is much more likely to be successful if you choose activities that you currently engage in and enjoy. Often you can modify your current activities to fit your fitness program. If you want to add a new activity to your program, try it for a while before committing to it.
- *Your current skill and fitness level.* Although many activities are appropriate for beginners, some sports and activities require a certain level of skill to obtain fitness benefits. For example, if you are a beginning tennis player, you will probably not be able to sustain rallies long enough to develop cardiorespiratory endurance. A better choice might be a walking program while you improve your tennis game. To build skill for a particular activity, consider taking a class or getting some instruction from a coach or fellow participant.
- *Time and convenience.* You are more likely to maintain a long-term exercise program if you can easily fit exercise into your daily routine. As you consider activities, think about whether a special location or facility is required. Can you participate in the activity close to your home, school, or job? Are the necessary facilities available at convenient times (see Lab 7.2)? Can you participate in the activity year-round, or will you need to find an alternative during the summer or winter? Would a home treadmill make you more likely to exercise regularly?

- *Cost.* Some sports and activities require equipment, fees, or some type of membership investment. If you are on a tight budget, limit your choices to free or inexpensive activities. Investigate the facilities on your campus, which you may be able to use at little or no cost. Many activities require no equipment beyond an appropriate pair of shoes. Chapter 4 provides examples of resistance exercises you can do at home without equipment.

- *Special health needs.* If you have a particular health problem, choose activities that will conform to your needs and enhance your ability to cope. Ask your physician how to tailor an exercise program to your needs and goals. Appendix B provides guidelines and safety tips for exercisers with common chronic conditions.

3. Set a Target Frequency, Intensity, and Time (Duration) for Each Activity

The next step is to apply the FITT principle and set a starting frequency, intensity, and time (duration) for each type of activity you've chosen (see the summary in Figure 7.2 and the sample in Figure 7.1).

Cardiorespiratory Endurance Exercise As noted in earlier chapters, based on more than 50 years of research on exercise and health, the U.S. Department of Health and Human Services concluded that most health benefits occur with at least 150 minutes per week of moderate-intensity physical activity (such as brisk walking) or 75 minutes per week of vigorous-intensity activity (such as jogging). Additional benefits occur with more exercise. An appropriate frequency for cardiorespiratory endurance exercise is three–five days per week. For intensity, note your target heart rate zone or RPE (rating of perceived exertion) value. Your target total workout time (duration) should

	Cardiorespiratory endurance training	Strength training	Flexibility training
Frequency	3–5 days per week	2–3 nonconsecutive days per week	2–3 days per week (minimum); 5–7 days per week (ideal)
Intensity	55/65–90% of maximum heart rate	Sufficient resistance to fatigue muscles	Stretch to the point of tension
Time	20–60 minutes in sessions lasting 10 minutes or more	8–12 repetitions of each exercise, 1 or more sets	2–4 repetitions of each exercise, held for 10–30 seconds, for a total of 60 seconds per stretch
Type	Continuous rhythmic activities using large muscle groups	Resistance exercises for all major muscle groups	Stretching exercises for all major joints

FIGURE 7.2 A summary of the FITT principle for the health-related components of fitness.

be about 20–60 minutes per day, depending on the intensity of the activity. You can exercise in a single session or in multiple sessions of 10 or more minutes. New research on high-intensity interval training suggests that you can exercise for shorter durations if you train at maximal intensities.

Muscular Strength and Endurance Training At least two nonconsecutive days per week of strength training is recommended. As described in Chapter 4, a general fitness strength training program includes one or more sets of 8–12 repetitions of 8–10 exercises that work all major muscle groups. For intensity, choose a weight that is heavy enough to fatigue your muscles but not so heavy that you cannot complete the full number of repetitions with proper form. Exercises that use body weight for resistance also build strength and muscle endurance. A note of caution: Years of weight training can lead to stiffer blood vessels. Some studies show that doing aerobics after weight training helps to prevent blood vessel stiffening.

Flexibility Training Stretches should be performed at least two–three days per week (five–seven days per week is ideal), when the muscles are warm. The stretches should work all major muscle groups. For each exercise, stretch to the point of slight tension or mild discomfort, and hold the stretch for 10–30 seconds; do 2–4 repetitions of each exercise.

4. Set Up a System of Mini-Goals and Rewards

To keep your program on track, set up a system of goals and rewards. Break your specific goals into several steps, and set a target date for each step. For example, if one of the goals of an 18-year-old male student's program is to improve upper-body strength and endurance, he could use the push-up test in Lab 4.2 to set intermediate goals. If he can currently perform 15 push-ups (for a rating of "very poor"), he might set intermediate goals of 17, 20, 25, and 30 push-ups (for a final rating of "fair"). By allowing several weeks between mini-goals and by specifying rewards, he'll be able to track his progress and reward himself as he moves toward his final goal. Reaching a

series of small goals is more satisfying than working toward a single, more challenging goal that may take months to achieve. For more on choosing appropriate rewards, see Chapter 1 and Activity 4 in the Behavior Change Workbook at the end of the text.

5. Include Lifestyle Physical Activity and Strategies to Reduce Sedentary Time in Your Program

Daily physical activity is a simple but important way to improve your overall wellness. As part of your fitness program plan, specify ways to be more active during your daily routine, say by taking the stairs up to class rather than taking an elevator. In addition, develop specific strategies to reduce the amount of time you spend being sedentary (see the box "The Importance of Reducing Sedentary Time"). You may find it helpful to first use a health journal to track your activities for several days. Review the records in your journal, identify routine opportunities to be more active, and add these to your program plan in Lab 7.1.

6. Develop Tools for Monitoring Your Progress

A record that tracks your daily progress will help remind you of your ongoing commitment to your program and give you a sense of accomplishment. Figure 7.3 shows you how to create a general program log and record the activity type, frequency, and times (durations). Or you can complete specific activity logs like those in Labs 3.2, 4.3, and 5.2 in addition to, or instead of, a general log. Post your log in a place where you'll see it often as a reminder and as an incentive for improvement. If you have specific, measurable goals, you can also graph your weekly or monthly progress toward each goal (Figure 7.4). To monitor the overall progress of your fitness program, you may choose to reassess your fitness every three months or so during the improvement phase of your program. Because the results of different fitness tests vary, be sure to compare results for the same assessments over time.

THE EVIDENCE FOR EXERCISE
The Importance of Reducing Sedentary Time

Does a 45-minute workout make up for the effects of 8 hours of sitting time? The answer to this question appears to be no. A complete exercise program focused on the health-related components of fitness provides many benefits. But researchers have found that too much sedentary time—sitting too much—is detrimental to health regardless of whether an individual meets the goals set by the Physical Activity Guidelines for Americans. A 2015 review found that sedentary time was associated with the following, independent of participation in physical activity:

- Deaths from all causes

- Cardiovascular disease

- Cancer (breast, colon, colorectal, endometrial, and certain types of ovarian cancers)

- Type 2 diabetes

The risk of negative outcomes from sedentary time was lower among people with higher levels of physical activity, but they were not eliminated.

How does sedentary time impact health? Although not completely understood, sedentary time is associated with markers of poor metabolic functioning, including unhealthy levels of blood glucose, insulin, and blood fats, as well as a large waist circumference. A study that looked at the impact of increased sedentary time in moderately active individuals found that sitting for more than 30 or 60 minutes at a time resulted in significantly elevated glucose and insulin levels. Sedentary time also affects blood fats and markers for inflammation. All these factors have the potential to contribute to the development of type 2 diabetes, metabolic syndrome, heart disease, and cancer.

What does this mean for an individual? Studies have found that the average American adult spends more that half her or his waking day in sedentary activities, such as using a computer or watching television. Luckily, evidence so far suggests that frequent breaks from sedentary time—2 minutes every 20 or 30 minutes, for example—are protective against some of the impacts of sedentary time. So, it is important to take frequent breaks when you are engaged in sedentary activities, whether at work or school or during leisure time. Try some of the strategies suggested in Chapter 2, "Move More, Sit Less" and invent your own. To help stick with your plan, include your strategies as part of your overall fitness program plan.

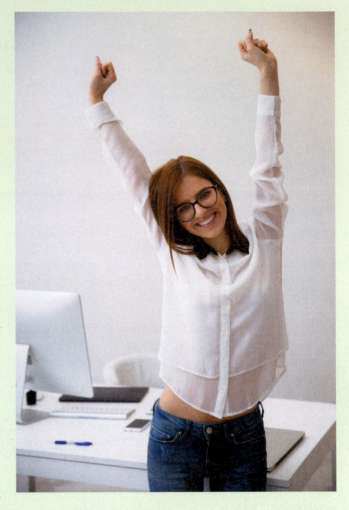

SOURCES: Biswas, A., et al. 2015. Sedentary time and its association with risk for disease incidence, mortality, and hospitalization in adults: A systematic review and meta-analysis. *Annals of Internal Medicine* 162: 123–132. Lyden, K., et al. 2015. Discrete features of sedentary behaviors impact cardiometabolic risk factors. *Medicine and Science in Sports and Exercise* 47(5): 1079–1086. President's Council on Fitness, Sports & Nutrition. 2012. Too much sitting: Health risks of sedentary behavior and opportunities for change. *Research Digest Series* 13, Number 3.

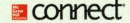

7. Make a Commitment

Your final step in planning your program is to make a commitment by signing an agreement. Find a witness for your agreement—preferably someone who will be actively involved in your program. Keep your agreement in a visible spot to remind you of your commitment.

PUTTING YOUR PLAN INTO ACTION

After you've developed a detailed plan and signed your agreement, you are ready to begin your fitness program. Refer to the specific training suggestions provided in Chapters 2–5 for advice on beginning and maintaining your program. Many

Enter time, distance, or another factor (such as heart rate or perceived exertion) to track your progress.

Activity/Date	M	Tu	W	Th	F	S	S	Weekly Total	M	Tu	W	Th	F	S	S	Weekly Total
1 Swimming	800 yd		725 yd		800 yd			2325 yd	800 yd		800 yd		850 yd			2450 yd
2 Tennis						90 min		90 min						95 min		95 min
3 Weight Training		X		X		X				X		X			X	
4 Stretching	X		X		X	X			X			X	X	X	X	

FIGURE 7.3 **A sample program log.**

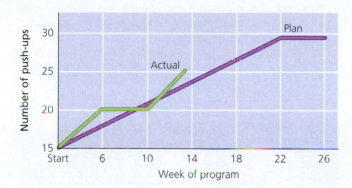

FIGURE 7.4 **A sample program progress chart.**

people find it easier to plan a program than to put their plan into action and stick with it over time. For that reason, adherence to healthy lifestyle programs has become an important area of study for psychologists and health researchers. The guidelines below and in the next section reflect research into strategies that help people stick with an exercise program.

- *Start slowly and increase fitness gradually.* Overzealous exercising can result in discouraging discomforts and injuries. Your program is meant to last a lifetime. The important first step is to break your established pattern of inactivity. Be patient and realistic. After your body has adjusted to your starting level of exercise, slowly increase the amount of overload. Small increases are the key— achieving a large number of small improvements will eventually result in substantial gains in fitness. It's usually best to increase duration and frequency before increasing intensity.

- *Find an exercise buddy.* The social side of exercise is an important factor for many regular exercisers. Working out with a friend will make exercise more enjoyable and increase your chances of sticking with your program. Find an exercise partner who shares your goals and general fitness level. On days when a partner isn't available, a smartphone or MP3 player can be your workout buddy; see the box "Digital Motivation" for more information.

- *Ask for support from others.* Consistent exercise requires the support of important people in your life, such as parents, spouse, partner, and friends. Talk with them about your program, and let them know the importance of exercise and wellness in your life. Exercise needs to be a critical component of your day (just like sleeping and eating). Good communication will help others become more supportive of and enthusiastic about the time you spend on your wellness program.

- *Vary your activities.* You can make your program more fun over the long term if you participate in a variety of activities that you enjoy. You can also add interest by varying the routes you take when walking, playing with different tennis partners, or switching to a new volleyball or basketball court. Varying your activities, a strategy known as *cross-training,* has other benefits. It can help you develop balanced, total-body fitness. For example, by alternating running with swimming, you build both upper- and lower-body strength. Cross-training can reduce the risk of injury and overtraining because the same muscles, bones, and joints are not continuously subjected to the stresses of the same activity. You can cross-train either by choosing different activities on different days or by alternating activities within a single workout.

- *Cycle the duration and intensity of your workouts.* Olympic athletes use a technique called periodization of training, meaning that they vary the duration and intensity of their workouts. Sometimes they exercise very intensely; other times they train lightly or rest. You can use the same technique to improve fitness more quickly and make your training program more varied and enjoyable. For example, if your program consists of walking, weight training, and stretching, pick one day a week for each activity to train a little harder or longer than you normally do. If you usually walk two miles at 16 minutes per mile, increase the pace to 15 minutes per mile once a week. If you lift weights twice a week, train more intensely during one of the workouts by using more resistance or performing multiple sets.

- *Adapt to changing environments and schedules.* Most people are creatures of habit and have trouble adjusting to

If you ever have trouble getting inspired to work out, motivation may be as close as your smartphone.

Since the iPhone's advent, dozens of interactive motivational applications ("apps") have been developed for use on smart cell phones. Coaching and motivational recordings are available for use on MP3 players, as well. These apps and recordings can substitute for an exercise partner when your workout buddy isn't around and can inspire you to keep your program on track. Some smartphone apps can monitor your workouts, track your progress, and even provide on-the-spot coaching to help you keep going.

Here are just a few examples of low-cost or free smartphone apps that can help you keep exercising:

- **Nike Training Club.** This training app designs programs according to your goals and experience. Goals include "get lean"—high-intensity cardio exercise to promote weight loss; "get toned"—light weight training and interval training; "get strong"—weight training to build strength and muscle mass; and "get focused"—15-minute workouts that target specific areas of the body. The app shows specific exercises, paces, and repetitions for the person exercising. It also has tools for motivating you to exercise, such as workout music and a clock that keeps track of the workout time. It is a digital personal trainer at an affordable price.

- **The "Fu" series.** Featuring titles like "CrunchFu" and "PushupFu," each app in this series focuses on one type of exercise and motivates you to excel at it. Using the motion sensors built into your smartphone, these apps can count your reps and monitor your speed as you exercise. A built-in coach offers suggestions and can challenge you to improve your performance.

- **Cyclemeter.** Use this highly motivational app for cycling, running, and walking. It brings detailed statistics to your workouts by keeping track of peak and average speed, caloric expenditure, rest times, elevation changes, and environmental conditions. You can store the results on the cloud or email them to yourself, friends, or social media. You can also integrate the app with a heart rate monitor. The GPS function gives you a map or satellite view of your route.

- **Endomondo.** This app uses GPS to keep track of routes used during running, walking, cycling, skating, or cross-country skiing. It also helps people share their workouts with social media, which promotes social accountability as a way to stick with the program.

- **NexTrack.** Track exercise and weight loss with this app and win "mPoints" for completing workouts. Many apps award mPoints for using their products, and you can cash them in for gift cards to companies such as Amazon. Several studies have found that rewards such as money or gift cards are effective for helping people with their fitness or weight loss goals.

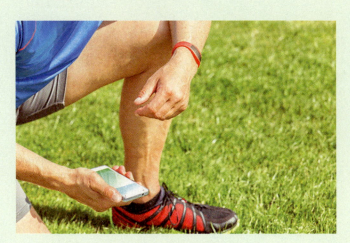

change. Don't use bad weather or a new job as an excuse to give up your exercise program. If you walk in the summer, put on a warm coat and walk in the winter as well. If you can't go out because of darkness, join a gym and walk on a treadmill. Review the results of Lab 2.2 on overcoming barriers to activity to develop additional strategies.

- *Expect fluctuations and lapses.* On some days, your progress will be excellent, but on others, you'll barely be able to drag yourself through your scheduled activities. Don't let off-days or lapses discourage you or make you feel guilty (see the box "Getting Your Fitness Program Back on Track").

- *Choose other healthy lifestyle behaviors.* Exercise provides huge benefits for your health, but other behaviors are also important. Choose a nutritious diet, and avoid harmful habits like smoking and overconsumption of alcohol. Be sure to stay hydrated with water or other healthy beverages (see the box "Choosing Healthy Beverages"). Don't skimp on sleep, which has a mutually beneficial relationship with exercise. Physical activity improves sleep, and adequate sleep can improve physical performance.

EXERCISE GUIDELINES FOR LIFE STAGES

A fitness program may need to be adjusted to accommodate the requirements of different life stages.

Children and Adolescents

Lack of physical activity has led to alarming increases in overweight and obesity in children and adolescents. If you have

Lapses are a normal part of any behavior change program. The important point is to move on and avoid becoming discouraged. Try again and keep trying. Know that continued effort will lead to success. Here are some tips to help you keep going:

• Don't judge yourself too harshly, especially in comparison with others. Some people make faster gains in fitness than others. Focus on the improvements you've already made from your program and how good you feel after exercise—both physically and mentally.

• Visualize what it will be like to reach your goals. Keep these images in mind as an incentive to stick with your program.

• Use your exercise journal to identify thoughts and behaviors that are causing noncompliance. Devise strategies to combat these problematic patterns. If needed, make additional changes in your environment or find more social support. For example, call a friend to walk with you, or keep exercise clothes in your car or backpack.

• Make changes in your plan and your reward system to help renew enthusiasm for and commitment to your program. Try changing fitness activities or your exercise schedule. Build in more opportunities to reward yourself.

• Plan ahead for difficult situations. Think about what circumstances might make it tough to keep up your fitness routine. Develop strategies to increase your chances of sticking with your program. For example, figure out ways to continue your program during vacation, travel, bad weather, and so on.

• If you're in a bad mood or just don't feel like exercising, remind yourself that physical activity is probably the one thing you can do that will make you feel better. Even if you can only do half your scheduled workout, you'll boost your energy, improve your mood, and help keep your program on track.

McGraw Hill Education **connect**

---

children or are in a position to influence children, keep these guidelines in mind:

• Provide opportunities for children and adolescents to exercise every day. Minimize sedentary activities, such as watching television. Children and adolescents should aim for at least 60 minutes of moderate activity every day. Less fit kids should start with 30 minutes a day until their fitness improves and they can exercise longer.

• During family outings, choose dynamic activities. For example, go for a walk or park away from a mall and then walk to the stores.

• For children younger than 12, emphasize skill development and fitness rather than excellence in competitive sports. For adolescents, combine participation and training in lifetime sports with traditional, competitive sports.

• Make sure children are developmentally capable of participating in an activity. For example, catching skills are difficult for young children because their nervous system is not developed enough to fully master the skill. Gradually increase the complexity of the skill once the child has mastered the simpler skill.

• Make sure children get plenty of water when exercising in the heat. Make sure they are dressed properly when exercising in the cold.

Pregnancy

Exercise is important during pregnancy, but women should be cautious because some types of exercise can pose increased risk to the mother and the unborn child. The following guidelines

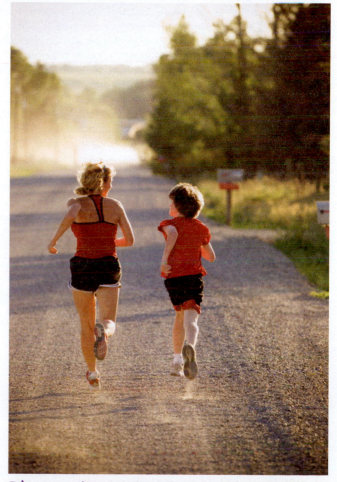

Fitness Tip People of all ages benefit from exercise. By including their children, parents not only set a positive example that can lead to a lifetime of physical activity, but both parent and child will have an exercise buddy.

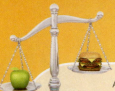

CRITICAL CONSUMER
Choosing Healthy Beverages

As discussed in other chapters, it's important to stay hydrated at all times, but especially when you are exercising. Too little water intake can leave you feeling fatigued, reduce your body's performance, and leave you vulnerable to heat-related sicknesses in hot weather. But *what* you drink is as significant as how much you drink, both when you are exercising and when you are going about your normal routine.

The Great Water Controversy

Wherever you see people exercising, you will see bottled water in abundance. For several years, a debate has been raging about the quality and safety of commercially bottled water. Recently, evidence has emerged showing that most bottled waters are no better for you than regular tap water, and some bottled waters may actually be bad for you. To make matters worse, bottled water costs up to 1,900 times more than tap water.

In a 2011 analysis of 173 bottled water products, the Environmental Working Group found 38 different contaminants in ten popular brands of bottled water. Contaminants included heavy metals such as arsenic, pharmaceutical residues and other pollutants commonly found in urban wastewater, and a variety of industrial chemicals. Bottled-water companies are notoriously secretive about their products. Overall, 18% of bottled waters failed to list the location of their source, and 32% disclosed nothing about the treatment or purity of the water.

Many commercially bottled water products are, in fact, tap water drawn from municipal water systems. Such revelations have caused the Food and Drug Administration (FDA) to require bottlers to put statements on their products' labels, identifying them as having been drawn from a standard water supply. These products, priced many times higher than water from a residential tap, provide no benefit over standard tap water.

An even bigger issue is that plastic water bottles have become a huge environmental problem: Billions of bottles now pile up in landfills and float in the world's oceans. Some types of plastic take years to biodegrade, and many kinds of plastic bottles will never decompose at all. Newer types of plastic bottles can decompose significantly faster than older bottles, but fast-degrading plastics have not yet come into widespread use in the bottled-water industry.

Experts say that when you're exercising, the cheapest and safest way to stay hydrated is to drink filtered tap water. If you need to carry water with you, buy a reusable container (preferably made of stainless steel) that you can clean after each use. If you drink from plastic bottles, be sure they are recyclable and dispose of them by recycling.

Other Choices

Instead of water, many people choose to drink sodas, juice, tea, or flavored water. While these kinds of beverages have their place, it's important not to drink them too often or in large amounts, especially if they are high in sugar or caffeine. Sugary drinks add empty calories to your diet, and caffeine is a psychoactive drug with a variety of side effects.

Regular (nondiet) sodas are now the leading source of calories in the American diet; most people don't count the calories from beverages as part of their daily caloric intake, leading them to underestimate their total intake. For this reason and others, many experts believe that soda consumption is a major factor in the increasing levels of obesity, metabolic syndrome, diabetes, and other chronic diseases among Americans.

If you're concerned that the liquid portion of your diet is not as healthy as it should be, choose water, fat-free milk, or unsweetened herbal tea more often. Avoid regular soda, sweetened bottled iced tea, flavored water, and fruit beverages made with little fruit juice. To make water more appealing, try adding slices of citrus fruit with sparkling water. With some imagination, you can make sure you stay hydrated without consuming excess calories, spending money unnecessarily, or hurting the environment.

SOURCE: Leiba, N., et. al. 2011. *The Environmental Working Group's 2011 Bottled Water Scorecard* (http://www.ewg.org/bottled-water-2011-home;5).

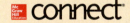

---

are consistent with the recommendations of the American College of Obstetrics and Gynecology:

- See your physician about possible modifications needed for your particular pregnancy.

- Continue mild to moderate exercise routines at least three times a week. (For most women, this means maintaining an exercise heart rate of 100–160 beats per minute.) Avoid exercising vigorously or to exhaustion, especially in the third trimester. Monitor exercise intensity by assessing how you feel rather than by monitoring your heart rate; RPE levels of 11–13 are appropriate.

- Favor non- or low-weight-bearing exercises such as swimming or cycling over weight-bearing exercises, which can carry increased risk of injury.

- Avoid exercise in a supine position—lying on your back—after the first trimester. This position restricts blood flow to the uterus. Also avoid prolonged periods of motionless standing.

- Avoid exercise that could cause loss of balance, especially in the third trimester, and exercise that might injure the abdomen, stress the joints, or carry a risk of falling (such as contact sports, vigorous racquet sports, skiing, and in-line skating).

- Avoid activities involving extremes in barometric pressure, such as scuba diving and mountain climbing.

- Especially during the first trimester, drink plenty of fluids and exercise in well-ventilated areas to avoid heat stress.

COMMON QUESTIONS ANSWERED

Q **Should I exercise every day?**

A Some daily exercise is beneficial, but if you train intensely every day without giving yourself a rest, you will likely injure yourself or overtrain. When strength training, for example, rest at least 48 hours between workouts before exercising the same muscle group. For cardiorespiratory endurance exercise, rest or exercise lightly the day after an intense or lengthy workout. Balancing the proper amount of rest and exercise will help you feel better and improve your fitness faster.

Q **If exercise is so good for my health, why hasn't my physician ever mentioned it to me?**

A A recent study by the American College of Sports Medicine (ACSM) suggests that most people would benefit from getting a physician's advice about exercising. According to the study, 65% of patients said they would be more interested in exercising if their physicians suggested it. About 40% of physicians said they talk to their patients about exercise.

To encourage physicians and patients to talk more often about exercise and its benefits, the ACSM and the American Medical Association have launched the Exercise Is Medicine program. The program advises physicians to give more guidance to patients about exercise and suggests that everyone try to exercise at least five days each week. For more information on the program, visit www.exerciseismedicine.org.

- Do three–five sets of 10 Kegel exercises daily. These exercises call for tightening the muscles of the pelvic floor for 5–15 seconds per repetition. Kegel exercises are thought to help prevent incontinence (involuntary loss of urine) and speed recovery after giving birth.

- After giving birth, resume prepregnancy exercise routines gradually, based on how you feel.

Older Adults

Older people readily adapt to endurance exercise and strength training. Exercise principles are the same as for younger people, but some specific guidelines apply:

- Follow the same guidelines for aerobic exercise as younger adults, but judge intensity on a 10-point scale of perceived exertion rather than by heart rate.

- For strength training, use a lighter weight and perform more (10–15) repetitions than young adults.

- Perform flexibility exercises at least two days per week for at least 10 minutes. Exercises that improve balance should also be performed two days per week.

- Drink plenty of water and avoid exercising in excessively hot or cold environments. Wear clothes that speed heat loss in warm environments and prevent heat loss in cold environments.

- Warm up slowly and carefully. Increase intensity and duration of exercise gradually.

- Cool down slowly, continuing very light exercise until the heart rate is below 100.

- If you have physical disabilities or limitations and cannot meet the recommendation of at least 150 minutes per week of moderate-intensity exercise, do as much exercise as you can.

SUMMARY

- Steps for putting together a complete fitness program include (1) setting realistic goals; (2) selecting activities to develop all the health-related components of fitness; (3) setting a target frequency, intensity, and time (duration) for each activity; (4) setting up a system of mini-goals and rewards; (5) making lifestyle physical activity and strategies to reduce sedentary time a part of the daily routine; (6) developing tools for monitoring progress; and (7) making a commitment.

- In selecting activities, consider fun and interest, your current skill and fitness levels, time and convenience, cost, and any special health concerns.

- Keys to beginning and maintaining a successful program include starting slowly, increasing intensity and duration gradually, finding a buddy, varying the activities and intensity of the program, and expecting fluctuations and lapses.

- Regular exercise is appropriate and beneficial for people in all stages of life, although program modifications may be necessary for safety.

FOR FURTHER EXPLORATION

American Academy of Orthopaedic Surgeons. Provides information about injuries, treatment, and rehabilitation along with exercise guidelines for people with bone, muscle, and joint pain.
http://www.aaos.org

American Congress of Obstetricians and Gynecologists. Provides guidelines for promoting a healthy pregnancy and postpartum recovery, including exercise during pregnancy.
http://www.acog.org

American Diabetes Association. Promotes diabetes education, research, and advocacy; includes guidelines for diet and exercise for people with diabetes.
http://www.diabetes.org

American Heart Association. Includes information on fitness for kids as well as diet, exercise, fitness, and weight management for adults.
http://www.americanheart.org

For additional listings, see Chapters 2–6.

SELECTED BIBLIOGRAPHY

American College of Sports Medicine, Pescatello, S., ed. 2013. *ACSM's Guidelines for Exercise Testing and Prescription,* 9th ed. Philadelphia: Wolters Kluwer/Lippincott Williams & Wilkins Health.

American College of Sports Medicine. 2013. *ACSM's Resource Manual for Guidelines for Exercise Testing and Prescription,* 7th ed. Philadelphia: Wolters Kluwer/Lippincott Williams & Wilkins Health.

Behm, D. G., et al. 2010. Canadian Society for Exercise Physiology position stand: The use of instability to train the core in athletic and nonathletic conditioning. *Applied Physiology, Nutrition and Metabolism* 35(1): 109–112.

Biswas, A., et al. 2015. Sedentary time and its association with risk for disease incidence, mortality, and hospitalization in adults: A systematic review and meta-analysis. *Annals of Internal Medicine* 162: 123–132.

Boarnet, M. G., et al. 2011. Retrofitting the suburbs to increase walking: Evidence from a land-use-travel study. *Urban Studies* 48(1): 129–159.

Canadian Society for Exercise Physiology. 2011. *Public Health Agency of Canada Physical Activity Guidelines* (www.publichealth.gc.ca5).

Carlson, S. A., et al. 2015. Inadequate physical activity and health care expenditures in the United States. *Progress in Cardiovascular Diseases* 57(4): 315–323.

Centers for Disease Control and Prevention. 2014. State Indicator Report on Physical Activity, 2014. Atlanta, GA: U.S. Department of Health and Human Services.

DeFina, L. F., et al. 2015. Physical activity versus cardiorespiratory fitness: Two (partly) distinct components of cardiovascular health? *Progress in Cardiovascular Diseases* 57(4): 324–329.

Duvall, J., and R. De Young. 2013. Some strategies for sustaining a walking routine: Insights from experienced walkers. *Journal of Physical Activity and Health* 10(1): 10–18.

Fahey, T., and M. Fahey. 2014. Nutrition, physical activity, and the obesity epidemic: Issues, policies, and solutions (1960s-present). *The Guide to U.S. Health and Health Care Policy.* T. Oliver, ed. New York: DWJ Books: 363–374.

Ferry, B., et al. 2013. Bone health during late adolescence: Effects of an 8-month training program on bone geometry in female athletes. *Joint Bone Spine* 80(1): 57–63.

Granacher, U., et al. 2013. Effects of core instability strength training on trunk muscle strength, spinal mobility, dynamic balance and functional mobility in older adults. *Gerontology* 59(2): 105–113.

Harrington, R. A., et al. 2015. More than 10 million steps in the right direction: Results from the first American Heart Association scientific sessions walking challenge. *Progress in Cardiovascular Diseases.* 57(4): 296–298.

Heinrich, K. M., et al. 2014. High-intensity compared to moderate-intensity training for exercise initiation, enjoyment, adherence, and intentions: An intervention study. *BMC Public Health* 14: 789.

Hills, A. P., et al. 2015. Supporting public health priorities: Recommendations for physical education and physical activity promotion in schools. *Progress in Cardiovascular Diseases* 57(4): 368–374.

Kaminsky, L. A., and A. H. Montoye. 2014. Physical activity and health: What is the best dose? *Journal American Heart Association* 3(5): e001430.

Koohsari, M. J., et al. 2015. Public open space, physical activity, urban design and public health: Concepts, methods and research agenda. *Health & Place* 33: 75–82.

Leskinen, T. and U. M. Kujala. 2015. Health-Related Findings among Twin Pairs Discordant for Leisure-Time Physical Activity for 32 Years: The TWINACTIVE Study Synopsis. *Twin Research in Human Genetics.* Published online April 27, 2015.

Lyden, K., et al. 2015. Discrete features of sedentary behaviors impact cardio-metabolic risk factors. *Medicine and Science in Sports and Exercise* 47(5): 1079–1086.

Malina, R. M. 2015. Physical activity, health and nutrition. *World Review of Nutrition and Dietetics* 113: 68–71.

Marques, A., et al. 2015. Do students know the physical activity recommendations for health promotion? *Journal Physical Activity and Health* 12(2): 253–256.

McGuire, S. 2014. CDC state indicator report on physical activity, 2014. *Advances in Nutrition* 5(6): 762–763.

Moholdt, T., et al. 2014. Current physical activity guidelines for health are insufficient to mitigate long-term weight gain: More data in the fitness versus fatness debate (The HUNT study, Norway). *British Journal Sports Medicine* 48(20): 1489–1496.

Myers, J., et al. 2015. Physical activity and cardiorespiratory fitness as major markers of cardiovascular risk: Their independent and interwoven importance to health status. *Progress Cardiovascular Diseases* 57(4): 306–314.

Park, J. W., et al. 2013. Maternal exercise during pregnancy affects mitochondrial enzymatic activity and biogenesis in offspring brain. *International Journal of Neuroscience* 123(4): 253–264.

Picorelli, A. M., et al. 2014. Adherence to exercise programs for older people is influenced by program characteristics and personal factors: A systematic review. *Journal of Physiotherapy* 60(3): 151–156.

Puett, R., et al. 2014. Physical activity: Does environment make a difference for tension, stress, emotional outlook, and perceptions of health status? *Journal Physical Activity and Health* 11(8): 1503–1511.

Rowlands, A. V. 2015. Physical activity, inactivity, and health. *Pediatric Exercise Science* 27(1): 21–25.

Saeterbakken, A. H., and M. S. Fimland. 2013. Electromyographic activity and 6RM strength in bench press on stable and unstable surfaces. *Journal of Strength and Conditioning Research* 27(4): 1101–1107.

Sjogren, P., et al. 2014. Stand up for health—Avoiding sedentary behaviour might lengthen your telomeres: Secondary outcomes from a physical activity RCT in older people. *British Journal Sports Medicine* 48(19): 1407–1409.

Soares-Miranda, L., et al. 2014. Physical activity and heart rate variability in older adults: The Cardiovascular Health Study. *Circulation* 129(21): 2100–2110.

Tschentscher, M., et al. 2013. Health benefits of Nordic walking: A systematic review. *American Journal Preventive Medicine* 44(1): 76–84.

U.S. Department of Health and Human Services. 2008. *Physical Activity Guidelines for Americans.* Washington, D.C.: U.S. Department of Health and Human Services.

Valle, C. G., et al. 2015. Physical activity in young adults: A signal detection analysis of Health Information National Trends Survey (HINTS) 2007 data. *Journal of Health Communication* 20(2): 134–146.

White, D. K., et al. 2015. Do short spurts of physical activity benefit cardiovascular health? The CARDIA Study. *Medicine & Science in Sports & Exercise.* Published online March 17, 2015.

Williams, P. T. 2013. Greater weight loss from running than walking during a 6.2-yr prospective follow-up. *Medicine and Science in Sports and Exercise* 45(4): 706–713.

SAMPLE PROGRAMS FOR POPULAR ACTIVITIES

The following sections present four sample programs based on different types of cardiorespiratory activities—walking/jogging, bicycling, swimming, and rowing. Each sample program includes regular cardiorespiratory endurance exercise, resistance training, and stretching. Read the descriptions of the programs you're considering, and decide which will work best for you based on your present routine, the potential for enjoyment, and adaptability to your lifestyle. If you choose one of these programs, complete the personal fitness program plan in Lab 7.1, just as if you had created a program from scratch.

No program will produce enormous changes in your fitness level in the first few weeks. Follow the specifics of the program for three–four weeks. Then, if the exercise program doesn't seem suitable, make adjustments to adapt it to your particular needs. But retain the basic elements of the program that make it effective for developing fitness.

GENERAL GUIDELINES

The following guidelines can help make the activity programs more effective for you:

- **Frequency and time.** To improve physical fitness, exercise for 20–60 minutes at least three times a week.

- **Intensity.** To work effectively for cardiorespiratory endurance training or to improve body composition, raise your heart rate into its target zone. Monitor your pulse or use rates of perceived exertion to monitor your intensity. If you've been sedentary, begin very slowly. Give your muscles a chance to adjust to their increased workload. It's probably best to keep your heart rate below target until your body has had time to adjust to new demands. At first you may not need to work very hard to keep your heart rate in its target zone, but as your cardiorespiratory endurance improves, you will probably need to increase intensity.

- **Interval training.** Some of the sample programs involve continuous activity. Others rely on interval training, which calls for alternating a relief interval with exercise (walking after jogging, for example, or coasting after biking uphill). Interval training is an effective method of progressive overload and improves fitness rapidly (see Chapter 3).

- **Resistance training and stretching guidelines.** For the resistance training and stretching parts of the program, remember the general guidelines for safe and effective exercise. See the summary of guidelines in Figure 7.2.

- **Warm-up and cool-down.** Begin each exercise session with a 10-minute warm-up. Begin your activity at a slow pace, and work up gradually to your target heart rate. Always slow down gradually at the end of your exercise session to bring your system back to its normal state. It's a good idea to do stretching exercises to increase your flexibility *after* cardiorespiratory exercise or strength training because your muscles will be warm and ready to stretch.

Follow the guidelines presented in Chapter 3 for exercising in hot or cold weather. Drink enough liquids to stay adequately hydrated, particularly in hot weather.

- **Record keeping.** After each exercise session, record your daily distance or time on a progress chart.

WALKING/JOGGING SAMPLE PROGRAM

Walking is the perfect exercise. It increases longevity; builds fitness; expends calories; prevents weight gain; and protects against heart disease, stroke, and back pain. You don't need to join a gym, and you can walk almost anywhere. People who walk 30 minutes five times per week will lose an average of 5 pounds in 6–12 months—without dieting, watching what they eat, or exercising intensely.

Jogging takes walking to the next level. Jogging only 75 minutes per week will increase fitness, promote weight control, and provide health benefits that will prevent disease and increase longevity. Your ultimate goal for promoting wellness is to walk at a moderate intensity for 150–300 minutes per week or jog at 70% effort or more for 75–150 minutes per week.

It isn't always easy to distinguish among walking, jogging, and running. For clarity and consistency, we'll consider walking to be any on-foot exercise of less than 5 miles per hour, jogging any pace between 5 and 7.5 miles per hour, and running any pace faster than that. The faster your pace or the longer you exercise, the more calories you burn (Table 1). The greater the number of calories burned, the higher the potential training effects of these activities. Table 2 contains a sample walking/jogging program.

Equipment and Technique

These activities require no special skills, expensive equipment, or unusual facilities. Comfortable clothing, well-fitted walking or running shoes (see Chapter 3), and a stopwatch or ordinary watch with a second hand are all you need.

When you advance to jogging, use proper technique:

- Run with your back straight and your head up. Look straight ahead, not at your feet. Shift your pelvis forward and tuck your buttocks in.

- Hold your arms slightly away from your body. Your elbows should be bent so that your forearms are parallel to the ground. You may cup your hands, but do not clench your fists. Allow your arms to swing loosely and rhythmically with each stride.

- Let your heel hit the ground first in each stride. Then roll forward onto the ball of your foot and push off for the next stride. If you find this difficult, you can try a more flat-footed style, but don't land on the balls of your feet. More of a forefoot landing is recommended in barefoot running or with minimal footwear.

Table 1

Estimated Calories Expended by a 165-Pound Adult at Different Intensities of Walking and Jogging for 150 and 300 Minutes per Week (min/wk)

	SPEED (MILES PER HOUR)	SPEED (MINUTES PER MILE)	CALORIES EXPENDED EXERCISING 150 MIN/WK	CALORIES EXPENDED EXERCISING 300 MIN/WK
	Rest	—	190	380
Walking	2.5	24	565	1130
	3.0	20	620	1240
	4.0	15	940	1880
	4.3	14	1125	2250
Jogging	5.0	12	1500	3000
	6.0	10	1875	3750
	7.0	8.6	2155	4310
	8.0	6.7	2530	5060
	10.0	6	3000	6000

NOTE: Heavier people will expend slightly more calories, while lighter people will expend slightly fewer.

SOURCE: Adapted from Physical Activity Guidelines Advisory Committee. 2008. *Physical Activity Guidelines Advisory Committee Report, 2008.* Washington, D. C.: U.S. Department of Health and Human Services.

Table 2

Sample Walking/Jogging Fitness Program

DAY	ACTIVITIES
Monday	• **Walking/Jogging:** Walk briskly for 30 minutes or jog for 25 minutes. • **Stretching:** Stretch major muscle groups for 10 minutes after exercise. Do each exercise two times; hold stretch for 10–30 seconds.
Tuesday	• **Resistance workout:** Using body weight for resistance, perform the following exercises: • Push-ups: 2 sets, 20 reps per set • Pull-ups: 2 sets, 5 reps per set • Unloaded squats: 2 sets, 10 reps per set • Curl-ups: 2 sets, 20 reps per set • Side bridges: 3 sets, 10-second hold (left and right sides) • Spine extensions: 3 sets, 10-second hold (left and right sides)
Wednesday	• Repeat Monday activities.
Thursday	• Repeat Tuesday activities.
Friday	• Repeat Monday activities.
Saturday	• **Rest.**
Sunday	• **Rest.**

• Keep your steps short by allowing your foot to strike the ground in line with your knee. Keep your knees bent at all times.

• Breathe deeply through your mouth. Try to use your abdominal muscles rather than just your chest muscles to take deep breaths.

• Stay relaxed.

Find a safe, convenient place to walk or jog. Exercise on a trail, path, or sidewalk to stay clear of bicycles and cars. Make sure your clothes are brightly colored so others can see you easily.

Beginning a Walking/Jogging Program

Start slowly if you have not been exercising, are overweight, or are recovering from an illness or surgery. At first, walk for 15 minutes at a slow pace, below your target heart rate zone. Gradually increase to 30-minute sessions. You will probably cover 1 to 2 miles. At the beginning, walk every other day.

You can gradually increase to walking five days per week or more if you want to expend more calories (which is helpful if you want to change body composition). Depending on your weight, you will expend ("burn") 90–135 calories during each 30-minute walking session. To increase the calories that you expend, walk for a longer time or for a longer distance instead of sharply increasing speed.

Start at the level of effort that is most comfortable for you. Maintain a normal, easy pace and stop to rest as often as you need to. Never prolong a walk past the point of comfort. When walking with a friend (a good motivator), let a comfortable conversation be your guide to pace. If you find that you cannot carry on a conversation without getting out of breath, you are walking too quickly.

Once your muscles have become adjusted to the exercise program, increase the duration of your sessions by no more than 10% each week. Keep your heart rate just below your target zone. Don't be discouraged by a lack of immediate progress, and don't try to speed things up by overdoing it. Remember that pace and heart rate can vary with the terrain, the weather, and other factors.

Advanced Walking

Advanced walking involves walking more quickly for longer times. You should feel an increased perception of effort, but the exercise intensity should not be too stressful. Vary your pace to allow for intervals of slow, medium, and fast walking. Keep your heart rate toward the lower end of your target zone with brief periods in the upper levels. At first, walk for 30 minutes and increase your walking time gradually until eventually you reach 60 minutes at a brisk pace and can walk 2–4 miles. Try to walk at least five days per week. Vary your program by changing the pace and distance or by walking routes with different terrains and views. You can expect to burn 200–350 calories or more during each advanced walking session.

Making the Transition to Jogging

Increase the intensity of exercise by gradually introducing jogging into your walking program. During a 2-mile walk, for example, periodically jog for 100 yards and then resume walking. Increase the number and distance of your jogging segments until you can jog continuously for the entire distance. More physically fit people may be capable of jogging without walking first. However, people unaccustomed to jogging should initially combine walking with short bouts of jogging.

A good strategy is to exercise on a 400-meter track at a local high school or college. Begin by covering 800 meters—jogging the straightaways and walking the turns. Progress to walking 200 meters (half lap) and jogging 200 meters; jogging 400 meters and walking 200 meters; jogging 800 meters, walking 200 meters; and jogging 1200 meters, walking 200 meters. Continue until you can jog 2 miles without stopping.

During the transition to jogging, adjust the ratio of walking to jogging to keep within your target heart rate zone as much as possible. Most people who sustain a continuous jogging or running program will find that they can stay within their target heart rate zone with a speed of 5.5–7.5 miles per hour (8–11 minutes per mile). Exercise at least every other day. Increasing frequency by doing other activities on alternate days will place less stress on the weight-bearing parts of your lower body than will a daily program of walking/jogging.

Developing Muscular Strength and Endurance and Flexibility

Walking, jogging, and running provide muscular endurance workouts for your lower body; they also develop muscular

strength of the lower body to a lesser degree. If you'd like to increase your speed and performance, you might want to focus your program on lower-body exercises. (Don't neglect upper-body strength. It is important for overall wellness.) For flexibility, pay special attention to the hamstrings and quadriceps, which are not worked through their complete range of motion during walking or jogging. Strength training, particularly body-building, can sometimes decrease flexibility, so stretching is particularly important for people who lift weights.

Staying with Your Walking/Jogging Program

Health experts have found that simple motivators such as using a pedometer, walking a dog, parking farther from the office or grocery store, or training for a fun run help people stay with their programs. Use a pedometer or GPS exercise device to track your progress and help motivate you to increase distance and speed. Accurate pedometers for walking, such as those made by Omron, Yamax, and New Lifestyles, cost $20–$40 and are accurate to about 5%. Sophisticated GPS-based devices and apps made by Polar, Garmin, and Nike keep track of your exercise speed and distance via satellite, monitor heart rate, and store data that can be downloaded wirelessly to your computer or their own websites. Several of these units can be plugged into programs such as Google Earth, which give you a satellite view of your walking or jogging route.

A pedometer can also help you increase the number of steps you walk each day. Most sedentary people take only 2000 to 3000 steps per day. Adding 1000 steps per day and increasing gradually until you reach 10,000 steps can increase fitness and help you manage your weight. The nonprofit organization Shape Up America! has developed the 10,000 Steps program to promote walking as a fitness activity (www.shapeup.org).

BICYCLING SAMPLE PROGRAM

Bicycling can also lead to large gains in physical fitness. For many people, cycling is a pleasant and economical alternative to driving and a convenient way to build fitness.

Equipment and Technique

Cycling has its own special array of equipment, including helmets, lights, safety gear, and biking shoes. The bike is the most expensive item, ranging from about $100 to $1000 or more. Avoid making a large investment until you're sure you'll use your bike regularly. While investigating what the marketplace has to offer, rent or borrow a bike. Consider your intended use of the bike. Most cyclists who are interested primarily in fitness are best served by a sturdy 10-speed rather than a mountain bike or sport bike. Stationary cycles are good for rainy days and areas that have harsh winters.

Clothing for bike riding shouldn't be restrictive or binding; nor should it be so loose that it catches the wind and slows you down. Shirts that wick moisture away from your skin and padded biking shorts make a ride more comfortable. Wear glasses or goggles to protect your eyes from dirt, small objects, and irritation from wind. Wear a pair of well-padded gloves if your hands tend to become numb while riding or if you begin to develop blisters or calluses.

To avoid saddle soreness and injury, choose a soft or padded saddle, and adjust it to a height that allows your legs to almost reach full extension while pedaling. To prevent backache and neck strain, warm up thoroughly and periodically shift the position of your hands on the handlebars and your body in the saddle. Keep your arms relaxed and don't lock your elbows. To protect your knees from strain, pedal with your feet pointed straight ahead or very slightly inward, and don't pedal in high gear for long periods.

Bike riding requires a number of precise skills that practice makes automatic. If you've never ridden before, consider taking a course. In fact, many courses are not just for beginners. They'll help you develop skills in braking, shifting, and handling emergencies, as well as teach you ways of caring for and repairing your bike. For safe cycling, follow these rules:

- Always wear a helmet.
- Keep on the correct side of the road. Bicycling against traffic is usually illegal and always dangerous.
- Obey all the same traffic signs and signals that apply to autos.
- On public roads, ride in single file, except in low-traffic areas (if the law permits). Ride in a straight line; don't swerve or weave in traffic.
- Be alert; anticipate the movements of other traffic and pedestrians. Listen for approaching traffic that is out of your line of vision.
- Slow down at street crossings. Check both ways before crossing.
- Use hand signals—the same as for automobile drivers—if you intend to stop or turn. Use audible signals to warn those in your path.
- Maintain full control. Avoid anything that interferes with your vision. Don't jeopardize your ability to steer by carrying anything (including people) on the handlebars.
- Keep your bicycle in good shape. Brakes, gears, saddle, wheels, and tires should always be in good condition.
- See and be seen. Use a headlight at night and equip your bike with rear reflectors. Use side reflectors on pedals, front and rear. Wear light-colored clothing or use reflective tape at night; wear bright colors or use fluorescent tape by day.
- Be courteous to other road users. Anticipate the worst and practice preventive cycling.
- Use a rear-view mirror.

Developing Cardiorespiratory Endurance

Cycling is an excellent way to develop and maintain cardiorespiratory endurance and a healthy body composition.

FIT—frequency, intensity, and time:

If you've been inactive for a long time, begin your cycling program at a heart rate that is 10–20% below your target zone.

Beginning cyclists should pedal at about 80–100 revolutions per minute; adjust the gear so you can pedal at that rate easily. You can equip your bicycle with a cycling computer that displays different types of useful information, such as speed, distance traveled, heart rate, altitude, and revolutions per minute.

Once you feel at home on your bike, try cycling 1 mile at a comfortable speed, and then stop and check your heart rate. Increase your speed gradually until you can cycle at 12–15 miles per hour (4–5 minutes per mile), a speed fast enough to bring most new cyclists' heart rate into their target zone. Allow your pulse rate to be your guide: More highly fit individuals may need to ride faster to achieve their target heart rate. Cycling for at least 20 minutes three days per week will improve your fitness.

At the beginning:

It may require several outings to get the muscles and joints of your legs and hips adjusted to this new activity. Begin each outing with a 10-minute warm-up. When your muscles are warm, stretch your hamstrings and your back and neck muscles. Until you become a skilled cyclist, select routes with the fewest hazards and avoid heavy automobile traffic.

As you progress:

Interval training is also effective with bicycling. Simply increase your speed for periods of 4–8 minutes or for specific distances, such as 1–2 miles. Then coast for 2–3 minutes. Alternate the speed intervals and slow intervals for a total of 20–60 minutes, depending on your level of fitness. Biking over hilly terrain is also a form of interval training.

Developing Muscular Strength and Endurance and Flexibility

Bicycling develops a high level of endurance and a moderate level of strength in the muscles of the lower body. If one of your goals is to increase your cycling speed and performance, be sure to include exercises for the quadriceps, hamstrings, and buttocks muscles in your strength training program. For flexibility, pay special attention to the hamstrings and quadriceps, which are not worked through their complete range of motion during bike riding, and to the muscles in your lower back, shoulders, and neck.

SWIMMING SAMPLE PROGRAM

Swimming works every major muscle group in the body. It increases upper- and lower-body strength, promotes cardiovascular fitness, and is excellent for rehabilitating athletic injuries and preventing day-to-day aches and pains. It promotes weight control; builds powerful lungs, heart, and blood vessels; and promotes metabolic health. People weigh only 6–10 pounds in the water, so swimming places less stress on the knees, hips, and back than jogging, hiking, volleyball, or basketball.

Swimming is one of the most popular recreational and competitive sports in the world. More than 120 million Americans swim regularly. More than 165,000 of these are competitive age-group swimmers (ages 5–18), and more than 30,000 competitors are over 19 years of age. You don't need a backyard pool to swim. Almost every town and city in America has a public pool. Pools are standard in many health clubs, YMCAs, and schools. Ocean and lake swimming may be options in the summer. High-tech wet suits make it possible to swim outdoors even in the middle of winter in many parts of the country.

Training Methods

Improved fitness from swimming depends on the quantity, quality, and frequency of training. Most swimmers use interval training to increase swimming fitness, speed, and endurance. Interval training calls for repeated fast swims at fixed distances followed by rest. Continuous distance or endurance training builds stamina and mental toughness. Interval and distance training each play important and different roles in improving fitness for swimming. Interval training improves overall swimming speed and the ability to swim fast at the beginning of a swim. Endurance training helps to maintain a faster average pace during a swim without becoming overly fatigued. Endurance training becomes more important when you want to compete in long, open-water swims or triathlons.

In swimming workouts, however, quality is better than quantity. Thirty years ago, elite swimmers from East Germany sometimes swam as much as 20,000 meters in a single workout (more than 12 miles). Recent studies found that competitive athletes who swam 4000 to 6000 meters per workout produced results similar to those who swam much farther. Likewise, recreational swimmers can improve fitness, strength, and power by swimming 1000–2000 meters (approximately 1100–2200 yards) per workout. Swim fast to get maximum benefits, but maintain good technique to maximize efficiency and minimize the risk of injury.

Interval training:

Interval training increases sprinting speed so you can accelerate faster at the beginning of a swim. It also helps the body cope with metabolic waste products so you can maintain your speed during the workout. To increase speed, swim intervals between 25 and 200 meters (or yards) at 80–90% effort. An example of a beginning program might be to swim 4 sets of 50 meters using the sidestroke at 70% of maximum effort, with a 1-minute rest between sets. A more advanced program would be to swim 10 sets of 100 meters using the freestyle stroke at 85–95% maximum effort with 30 seconds of rest between sets.

Endurance training:

Include longer swims—1000 meters or more at a time—to build general stamina for swimming. Endurance training will improve aerobic capacity and help your cells use fuels and clear metabolic wastes. This will allow you to swim faster and longer. Longer swims promote metabolic health and build physical fitness.

Cross-training:

Cross-training combines more than one type of endurance exercise, such as swimming and jogging, in your program at a time.

It also includes exercises that build strength, power, and skill. It is a good training method for people who prefer swimming but don't have daily access to a swimming pool or open water. Including multiple exercises, such as swimming and running, stair stepping, cycling, weight training exercises, and calisthenics, adds variety to the program. It also prepares you for a greater variety of physical challenges. See Chapter 3 for a discussion of cross-training and a description of typical workouts.

Technique: The Basic Swimming Strokes for General Conditioning

The best strokes for conditioning are the freestyle and sidestroke. Competitive athletes also swim the breaststroke, butterfly, and backstroke (but not the sidestroke). Learning efficient swimming strokes helps increase enjoyment and results in better workouts. Take a class from the Red Cross, local recreation department, or private coach if you are not a strong swimmer or need help with the basic strokes.

Freestyle:

While freestyle technically includes any unregulated stroke (such as the sidestroke), it generally refers to the front (Australian) crawl or overhand stroke. Freestyle is the fastest stroke and is best for general conditioning. Swim this stroke in a prone (face-down) position with arms stretched out in front and legs extended to the back. Move through the water by pulling first with the right arm and then with the left, while performing a kicking motion generated from the hips. During the stroke, rotate the thumb and palm 45 degrees toward the bottom of the pool. Pull in a semicircle downward toward the center of the body with the elbow higher than the hand. When the hand reaches the beginning of the ribcage, push the palm backward underneath the body as far as possible. Don't begin to stroke with the other hand until the first stroke is completed. Maximize the distance with each stroke by pulling fully and maintaining good posture.

The crawl uses a flutter kick, which involves moving the legs alternately with the force generated from the hips and a slight bend of the knees. Maintain a neutral spine during the stroke. A strong kick is important to minimize body roll during the stroke. For this reason, some of your training should include kicking without using the arms.

Breathing is almost always a problem for novice swimmers. Don't hold your breath! You will fatigue rapidly if you have poor air exchange during swimming. Breathe by turning the head to the side of a recovering stroke. Do not lift the head out of the water. Exhale continuously through the nose and mouth between breaths. Beginners should breathe on the same side following each stroke cycle (left and right arm strokes).

Sidestroke:

Even novices can get a good workout with minimal skill using the sidestroke. This is a good choice for beginners because you keep your head out of water and can swim great distances without fatigue. Lie in the water on your right side and stretch your right arm and hand in front of you in the direction you want to swim and place your left hand across your chest. Draw your right arm toward you, pulling at the water until your hand reaches your waist. At the same time, make a scissors kick with your legs. Repeat the stroke as your forward speed slows. Swim half the distance on your right side and the rest on your left side.

Beginning Swim Program

Take swimming lessons from a certified teacher or coach if you are a nonswimmer or have not used swimming as your primary form of exercise. A swim teacher can help you develop good technique, make more rapid progress, and avoid injuries.

To assess your starting fitness, take the 12-minute swim test described in Lab 3.1. Use the swim test table to help you measure progress in your program. Take the test every one or two months to help establish short-term goals.

Start your program by swimming one length (one-half lap) at a time, using either freestyle or sidestroke. If you can't swim the length of a standard pool (25 meters or yards), begin by swimming the width. As soon as you can, swim one length of the pool, rest for 30 seconds, and then repeat. Build up your capacity until you can swim 20 lengths with a short rest interval between each length. If you start your program with the sidestroke, try to switch to the freestyle stroke as quickly as you can.

Increase the distance of each swim to a full lap (50 meters or yards) with 30–60 seconds of rest between laps. Build up until you can swim 20 sets of 50-meter swims with 30 seconds of rest between sets. Gradually increase the distance of each set to 100-meter swims. You are ready for the next level when you can swim 10 sets of 100 meters with 30 seconds of rest between sets.

Swimming Program for Higher Levels of Fitness

This program includes a warm-up, specific conditioning drills for strokes and kicking, and a cool-down. It involves interval training three days a week and distance training two days per week.

Warm up before each workout by swimming 2–4 laps at an easy pace. It is also a good idea to warm up your legs and hips by holding on to the side of the pool and gently moving your legs using a flutter-kick motion. At the end of the workout, cool down by swimming 100–200 meters at a slow pace.

On Monday, Wednesday, and Friday, do interval training. Your goal is to swim intervals totaling 2000 meters per workout (20 sets of 100 meters each) at a fast pace with 30 seconds of rest between each set, or interval. (i.e., swim 100 meters, rest, swim 100 meters, rest, etc.) Every fifth interval, swim 25 meters using your legs alone, with your arms extended in front of you. Have someone watch you during the legs-only swims to make sure you are kicking mainly from the hips and maintaining a neutral spine. Add variety to your interval training workouts by using gloves, swim paddles, or fins.

If you are unable to do the interval workout at first, modify it by increasing rest intervals, decreasing speed, or decreasing the number of sets as you gradually increase the volume and intensity.

On Tuesday and Thursday, do distance training. Swim 1000–2000 meters continuously at a comfortable pace. Although distance days will help develop endurance, they are used mainly to help you recover from intense interval training days.

Rest on Saturday and Sunday. Rest is very important to help your muscles and metabolism recover and build fitness. Rest will also prevent overtraining and overuse injuries. Include two rest days per week. Rest days can be consecutive (such as Saturday and Sunday) or interspersed during the normal workout schedule.

Integrating Swimming into a Total Fitness Program

You will develop fitness best and maintain interest in continuing your exercise program by varying the structure of your workouts. Incorporate kick boards, pull-buoys, hand paddles, and fins into some of your training sessions. Cross-training is a good option for developing well-rounded fitness. Swimming results in moderate gains in strength and large gains in endurance.

Because swimming is not a weight-bearing activity and is not done in an upright position, it elicits a lower heart rate per minute. Therefore, swimmers need to adjust their target heart rate zone. To calculate your target heart rate for swimming, use this formula:

Maximum swimming heart rate (MSHR) = 205 − age

Target heart rate zone = 65–90% of MSHR

For example, a 19-year-old swimmer would calculate his or her target heart rate zone for swimming as follows:

MSHR: 205 − 19 = 186 bpm

65% intensity: 0.65 × 186 = 121 bpm

90% intensity: 0.90 × 186 = 167 bpm

Swimming does not preserve bone density as you age, so swimmers are advised to include weight training in their exercise program. Perform at least one set of 10 repetitions for 8–10 exercises that use the major muscle groups in the body. To improve swimming performance, include exercises that work key muscles. For example, if you primarily swim the freestyle stroke, include exercises to increase strength in your shoulders, arms, upper back, and hips. Training the muscles you use during swimming can also help prevent injuries. In your flexibility training, pay special attention to the muscles you use during swimming, particularly the shoulders, hips, and back. Table 3 shows a basic sample swimming program that incorporates all these types of exercises.

ROWING MACHINE SAMPLE PROGRAM

Rowing is a whole-body exercise that overloads the cardiorespiratory system and strengthens the major muscles of the body. The beauty and serenity of rowing on flat water in the morning is indescribable, but few people have access to a lake and rowing shell. Fortunately, sophisticated rowing machines simulate the rowing motion and make it possible to do this exercise at the fitness center or at a health club.

Modern rowing machines are very much like the real thing. They provide resistance with hydraulic pistons, magnets, air, or

Table 3	Sample Swimming Program	
DAY	**ACTIVITIES**	
Monday	• **Warm-up:** Swim 100–200 meters (2–4 laps of a standard pool) at an easy pace.	
	• **Intervals:** Swim 10–20 sets of 100-meter swims at 90% effort, with 30 seconds of rest between sets. After every 5 sets, swim 25 meters using your legs alone.	
	• **Cool-down:** Swim 100–200 meters at a slow pace.	
	• **Weight training:** Do at least 1 set of 10 repetitions of 8–10 exercises that work the body's major muscle groups.	
	• **Flexibility:** Do standard stretching exercises for the shoulders, chest, back, hips, and thighs.	
Tuesday	• **Distance:** Swim 1000–2000 meters continuously at a comfortable pace.	
Wednesday	• Repeat Monday activities.	
Thursday	• Repeat Tuesday activities.	
Friday	• Repeat Monday activities.	
Saturday	• **Rest.**	
Sunday	• **Rest.**	

water. The best machines are solid and comfortable, provide a steady stroke, and allow you to maintain a neutral spine so you don't injure your back. Many rowing machines come with LCD displays that show heart rate, stroke rate, power output, and estimated caloric expenditure. They are also preprogrammed with workouts for interval training, cardiovascular conditioning, and moderate-intensity physical activity. Good rowing mechanics are essential because, if done incorrectly, rowing can cause severe overuse injuries that can damage the back, hips, knees, elbows, and shoulders.

Technique: Basic Rowing Movement

Most of the power for rowing comes from the thigh and hip muscles and finishes with a pulling motion with the upper body. Maintain a neutral spine (that is, with normal curves) during the movement. Hinge at the hips and not at the back during the rowing motion.

The rowing movement includes the following phases:

• *The catch.* The catch involves sliding the seat forward on the track with arms straight as far as you can while keeping the spine neutral.

• *The drive.* The drive begins by pushing with the legs and keeping your arms straight.

• *The finish.* Finish by leaning back slightly (still maintaining a neutral spine) and pulling the handle to your abdomen.

• *The recovery.* Recover by extending your arms forward, hinging forward at the hips with a neutral spine, and sliding forward again on the seat for another "catch."

Training Methods

Your rowing program should include both continuous training and interval training. Continuous training calls for rowing for a specific amount of time—typically 20–90 minutes without

stopping. Most people enjoy rowing at about 70% of maximum heart rate.

Interval training involves a series of exercise bouts followed by rest. The method manipulates distance, intensity, repetitions, and rest. An example of an interval workout would be to row for 8 sets of 4-minute exercise bouts at 85% effort with 2 minutes of rest between intervals, or sets. During interval training, changing one factor affects the others. For example, if you increase the intensity of exercise, you will need more rest between intervals and won't be able to do as many repetitions. High-intensity exercise builds fitness best but also increases the risk of injury and loss of motivation. Make intervals challenging but not so difficult that you get injured or discouraged.

Beginning Rowing Program

During the first few workouts, start conservatively by rowing for 10 minutes at a rate of about 20 strokes per minute with a moderate resistance. Exercise at about 60% effort. Do this workout three times during the first week. The movement is deceptively easy and invigorating. You are, however, using all the major muscle groups in the body and are probably not ready for a more intense exercise program.

After the first workout, do a series of 5-minute intervals during the first few weeks of training. For example, row for 5 minutes, rest 3 minutes, row 5 minutes, then rest 3 minutes. Build up until you can do 4–6 repetitions of 5-minute exercise intervals, resting only 1 minute between sets. Gradually, increase the time for each interval to 15 minutes and vary the rowing cadence from 20 to 25 strokes per minute. Your first short-term goal is to complete 30 minutes of continuous rowing without stopping.

Rowing Program for Higher Levels of Fitness

Vary your training methods after you can row continuously for 30 minutes, gain some fitness, and are used to the technique.

Alternate between interval training and distance training. Doing both will help you develop fitness rapidly and improve rowing efficiency. A good strategy is to row continuously at about 70% effort for 30–60 minutes three days per week and practice interval training at 80–90% effort for two days per week. Do resistance and flexibility training two–three days per week. A basic but complete rowing machine program that includes continuous and interval training as well as resistance and flexibility exercises is shown in Table 4.

Table 4	Sample Rowing Machine Fitness Program

DAY	ACTIVITIES
Monday	• **Warm-up:** Row at low intensity for 2 minutes. • **Continuous rowing:** Row for 30 minutes at 70% effort (20–22 strokes per minute). • **Weight training (1–2 sets of 10 repetitions):** Squats, leg curls, bench press, lat pulls, raises, biceps curls, triceps extensions, curl-ups, side bridge (10 seconds per side), spine extensions (10 seconds per side). • **Stretching:** Do static stretching exercises for the shoulders, chest, back, hips, and thighs. Hold each stretch for 10–30 seconds.
Tuesday	• **Warm-up:** Row at low intensity for 2 minutes. • **Continuous rowing:** Row at 60–70% of maximum effort for 5 minutes. Rest for 3 minutes. • **Interval rowing:** Row 6 sets, for 5 minutes per set, at 25 strokes per minute (90% effort). Rest for 3 minutes between intervals.
Wednesday	• **Warm-up:** Row at low intensity for 2 minutes. • **Continuous rowing:** Row for 45 minutes at 70% effort (20–22 strokes per minute). • **Stretching:** Repeat Monday stretches.
Thursday	• **Warm-up:** Row at low intensity for 2 minutes. • **Continuous rowing:** Row for 30 minutes at 70% effort (20–22 strokes per minute). • **Weight training (1–2 sets of 10 repetitions):** Repeat Monday weight training exercises.
Friday	• **Warm-up:** Row at low intensity for 2 minutes. • **Continuous rowing:** Row for 30 minutes at 70% effort (20–22 strokes per minute). • **Stretching:** Repeat Monday stretches.
Saturday	• **Rest.**
Sunday	• **Rest.**

Name _____ Section _____ Date _____

LAB 7.1 A Personal Fitness Program Plan and Agreement

A. I, _____, am making an agreement with myself to follow a physical fitness program to
   (name)

work toward the following goals:

Specific or short-term goals (include current status for each):

1. _____
2. _____
3. _____
4. _____

General or long-term goals:

1. _____
2. _____
3. _____
4. _____

B. My program plan is as follows:

Activities	Components (Check ✓)					Frequency (Check ✓)							Intensity*	Time (duration)
	CRE	MS	ME	F	BC	M	Tu	W	Th	F	Sa	Su		

*Conduct activities for achieving CRE goals in your target range for heart rate or RPE.

C. My program will begin on _____. My program includes the following schedule of mini-goals. For each step in my program,
   (date)

I will give myself the reward listed.

_____	_____	_____
(mini-goal 1)	(date)	(reward)

_____	_____	_____
(mini-goal 2)	(date)	(reward)

_____	_____	_____
(mini-goal 3)	(date)	(reward)

_____	_____	_____
(mini-goal 4)	(date)	(reward)

_____	_____	_____
(mini-goal 5)	(date)	(reward)

LABORATORY ACTIVITIES

D. My program will include the addition of physical activity to my daily routine (such as climbing stairs or walking to class):

1. _____
2. _____
3. _____
4. _____

E. My program will include the following strategies for reducing sedentary time:

1. _____
2. _____
3. _____
4. _____

F. I will use the following tools to monitor my program and my progress toward my goals:

_____

(list any charts, graphs, or journals you plan to use)

_____

_____

I sign this agreement as an indication of my personal commitment to reach my goal.

_____   _____

(your signature)   (date)

I have recruited a helper who will witness my agreement and _____

_____

(list any way your helper will participate in your program)

_____

_____   _____

(witness's signature)   (date)

Name _____ Section _____ Date _____

LAB 7.2   Getting to Know Your Fitness Facility

To help create a successful training program, take time to learn more about the fitness facility you plan to use.

Basic Information

Name and location of facility: _____

Hours of operation: _____

Times available for general use: _____

Times most convenient for your schedule: _____

Can you obtain an initial session or consultation with a trainer to help you create a program? _____ yes _____ no

If so, what does the initial planning session involve? _____
_____

Are any of the staff certified? Do any have special training? If yes, list/describe: _____
_____

What types of equipment are available for the development of cardiorespiratory endurance? Briefly list/describe: _____
_____
_____
_____

Are any group activities or classes available? If so, briefly describe: _____
_____
_____

What types of weight training equipment are available for use? _____
_____

Yes	No	
_____	_____	Is there a fee for using the facility? If so, how much? $ _____
_____	_____	Is a student ID required for access to the facility?
_____	_____	Do you need to sign up in advance to use the facility or any of the equipment?
_____	_____	Is there typically a line or wait to use the equipment during the times you use the facility?
_____	_____	Is there a separate area with mats for stretching and/or cool-down?
_____	_____	Do you need to bring your own towel?
_____	_____	Are lockers available? If so, do you need to bring your own lock? _____ yes _____ no
_____	_____	Are showers available? If so, do you need to bring your own soap and shampoo? _____ yes _____ no
_____	_____	Is drinking water available? (If not, be sure to bring your own bottle of water.)

LABORATORY ACTIVITIES

What other amenities, such as vending machines or saunas, are available at the facility? Briefly list/describe: _____

_____

_____

Information about Equipment

Fill in the specific equipment and exercise(s) that you can use to develop cardiorespiratory endurance and each of the major muscle groups. For cardiorespiratory endurance, list the type(s) of equipment and a sample starting workout: frequency, intensity, time, and other pertinent information (such as a setting for resistance or speed). For muscular strength and endurance, list the equipment and exercises, and indicate the order in which you'll complete them during a workout session. Remember, you don't have to use equipment—you can use body weight or elastic bands as resistance.

Cardiorespiratory Endurance Equipment

Equipment	Sample Starting Workout

Muscular Strength and Endurance Equipment

Order	Muscle Groups	Equipment	Exercise(s)
	Neck		
	Chest		
	Shoulders		
	Upper back		
	Front of arms		
	Back of arms		
	Buttocks		
	Abdomen		
	Lower back		
	Front of thighs		
	Back of thighs		
	Calves		
	Other:		
	Other:		

Nutrition

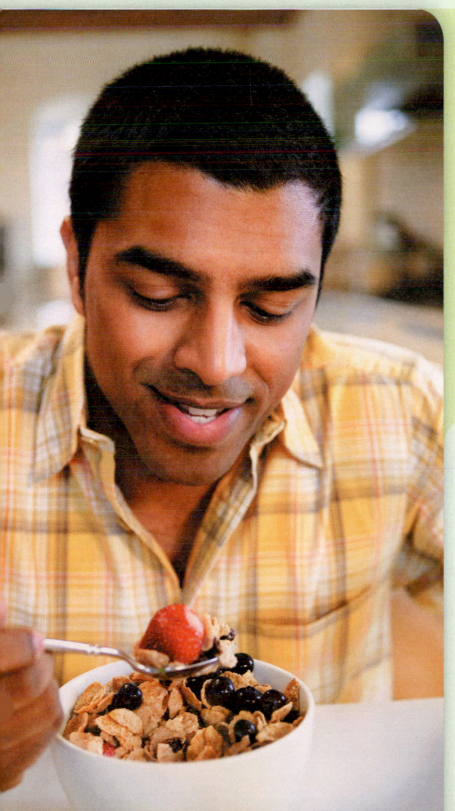

LOOKING AHEAD...

After reading this chapter, you should be able to

- List the essential nutrients and describe the functions they perform in the body.

- Describe the guidelines that have been developed to help people choose a healthy diet, avoid nutritional deficiencies, and reduce their risk of diet-related chronic diseases.

- Describe guidelines for vegetarians and special population groups.

- Explain how to use food labels and other consumer tools to make informed choices about foods.

- Create a personal food plan based on affordable foods that you enjoy and that will promote wellness, today and in the future.

TEST YOUR KNOWLEDGE

1. It is recommended that all adults consume one serving each of fruits and vegetables every day. True or false?

2. Candy is the leading source of added sugars in the American diet. True or false?

3. Which of the following is not a whole grain?
   a. brown rice
   b. wheat flour
   c. popcorn

See answers on the next page.

n your lifetime, you will spend about six years eating—about 70,000 meals and 60 tons of food. What you eat affects your energy level, well-being, and overall health. Your nutritional habits help determine your risk of major chronic diseases, including heart disease, cancer, stroke, and diabetes. Choosing a dietary pattern that provides the nutrients you need while limiting the substances linked to risk factors for disease should be an important part of your daily life.

Choosing a healthy diet is a two-part process. First, you have to know which nutrients you need and in what amounts. Second, you have to translate those requirements into a diet consisting of foods you like that are available, affordable, and fit into your lifestyle. After you know what constitutes a healthy diet for you, you can adjust your current diet to bring it into line with your goals.

This chapter explains the basic principles of **nutrition**. It introduces the six classes of essential nutrients, explaining their role in the functioning of the body. It also provides guidelines that you can use to design a healthy eating plan. Finally, it offers practical tools and advice to help you apply the guidelines to your life.

NUTRITIONAL REQUIREMENTS: COMPONENTS OF A HEALTHY DIET

You probably think about your diet in terms of the foods you like to eat. More important for your health, though, are the nutrients contained in those foods. Your body requires proteins, fats, carbohydrates, vitamins, minerals, and water—about 45 **essential nutrients**. In this context, the word *essential* means that you must get these substances from food because your body is unable to manufacture them, or at least not fast enough or in sufficient amounts to meet your physiological needs. The six classes of nutrients, along with their functions and major sources, are listed in Table 8.1

The body needs some essential nutrients in relatively large amounts; these **macronutrients** include protein, fat, carbohydrate, and water. **Micronutrients**, such as vitamins and minerals, are required in much smaller amounts. Your body obtains nutrients through the process of **digestion**, which breaks down food into compounds that the gastrointestinal tract can absorb and the body can use (Figure 8.1). A diet that provides enough essential nutrients is vital because they provide energy, help build and maintain body tissues, and help regulate body functions.

Food is partially broken down by being chewed and mixed with saliva in the mouth. After traveling to the stomach via the esophagus, food is broken down further by stomach acids and other secretions. As food moves through the digestive tract, it is mixed by muscular contractions and broken down by chemicals. Most absorption of nutrients occurs in the small intestine, aided by secretions from the pancreas, gallbladder, and intestinal lining. The large intestine reabsorbs excess water; the remaining solid wastes are collected in the rectum and excreted through the anus.

Calories

The energy in foods is expressed as **kilocalories**. One kilocalorie represents the amount of heat it takes to raise the temperature

Table 8.1	The Six Classes of Essential Nutrients	
NUTRIENT	**FUNCTION**	**MAJOR SOURCES**
Proteins (4 calories/gram)	Form important parts of muscles, bone, blood, enzymes, some hormones, and cell membranes; repair tissue; regulate water and acid-base balance; help in growth; supply energy	Meat, fish, poultry, eggs, milk, legumes, nuts
Carbohydrates (4 calories/gram)	Supply energy to cells in brain, nervous system, and blood; supply energy to muscles during exercise	Grains (breads and cereals), fruits, vegetables, milk
Fats (9 calories/gram)	Supply energy; insulate, support, and cushion organs; provide medium for absorption of fat-soluble vitamins	Animal foods, grains, nuts, seeds, fish, vegetables
Vitamins	Promote (initiate or speed up) specific chemical reactions within cells	Abundant in fruits, vegetables, and grains; also found in meat and dairy products
Minerals	Help regulate body functions; aid in growth and maintenance of body tissues; act as catalysts for release of energy	Found in most food groups
Water	Makes up 50–60% of body weight; provides medium for chemical reactions; transports chemicals; regulates temperature; removes waste products	Fruits, vegetables, liquids

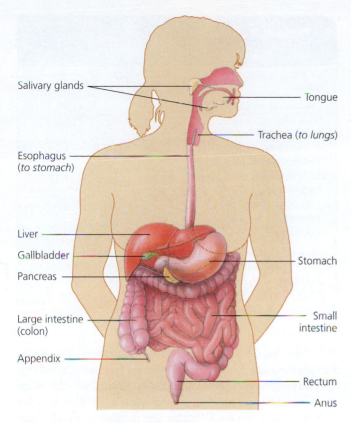

FIGURE 8.1 The digestive system.

Salivary glands
Tongue
Trachea (*to lungs*)
Esophagus
(*to stomach*)
Liver
Gallbladder
Pancreas
Stomach
Large intestine
(colon)
Small
intestine
Appendix
Rectum
Anus

of one liter of water 1°C. A person needs about 2,000 kilocalories a day to meet his or her energy needs. In common usage, people refer to kilocalories as *calories,* which is a much smaller energy unit: 1 kilocalorie contains 1,000 calories. This text uses the familiar word *calorie* to stand for the larger energy unit; you'll also find *calorie* used on food labels.

Of the six classes of essential nutrients, three supply energy:

- Fat = 9 calories per gram
- Protein = 4 calories per gram
- Carbohydrate = 4 calories per gram

Alcohol, though not an essential nutrient, also supplies energy, providing 7 calories per gram.

Just meeting energy needs is not enough. Our bodies need enough of the essential nutrients to function properly. Practically all foods contain combinations of nutrients, although foods are commonly classified according to their predominant nutrients. For example, spaghetti is considered a carbohydrate food, although it contains small amounts of other nutrients. The following sections discuss the functions and sources of each class of nutrients.

Proteins—The Basis of Body Structure

Proteins form important parts of the body's main structural components: muscles and bones. Proteins also form important parts of blood, enzymes, cell membranes, and some hormones.

When consumed, proteins also provide energy (4 calories per gram) for the body.

Amino Acids The building blocks of proteins are called **amino acids**. Twenty common amino acids are found in food. Nine of these are essential (or indispensable). As long as foods supply certain nutrients, the body can produce the other 11 amino acids.

Complete and Incomplete Proteins Individual protein sources are considered "complete" if they supply all the essential amino acids in adequate amounts and "incomplete" if they do not. Meat, fish, poultry, eggs, milk, cheese, and soy provide complete proteins. Incomplete proteins, which come from plant sources such as nuts and **legumes** (dried beans and peas), are good sources of most essential amino acids but are usually low in one or more.

Certain combinations of vegetable proteins, such as wheat and peanuts in a peanut butter sandwich or rice and beans, allow each vegetable protein to make up for the amino acids missing in the other protein. The combination yields a complete protein. It was once believed that vegetarians had to complement their proteins at each meal in order to receive the benefit of a complete protein. It is now known, however, that proteins consumed throughout the course of the day can complement each other to form a pool of amino acids the body can draw from to produce proteins. Vegetarians should include a variety of vegetable protein sources in their diets to make sure they get all the essential amino acids in adequate amounts. (Healthy vegetarian diets are discussed later in the chapter.)

Recommended Protein Intake The Food and Nutrition Board of the Institute of Medicine has established goals to help ensure adequate intake of protein as well as the other macronutrients (Table 8.2). For protein, adequate intake is set at 0.8 gram per kilogram (0.36 gram per pound) of body weight. So, if you weigh 125 pounds, you should eat 42 grams of protein per day. Someone who weighs 180 pounds would eat 65 grams. Table 8.3 lists some popular food items and the amount of protein each provides; labels on packaged foods show how much protein there is in each serving.

Most Americans meet or exceed the protein intake needed for adequate nutrition. A little extra protein is not harmful, but it can contribute excess energy and fat to the diet because protein-rich foods, especially those from animal sources, can be high in fat and calories.

The Food and Nutrition Board also recommends how much protein (and other nutrients) to consume as a percentage of total daily energy intake. These recommendations, called Acceptable Macronutrient Distribution Ranges (AMDRs), aim to ensure adequate intake of essential nutrients and to reduce the risk of chronic diseases. The Food and Nutrition Board recommends that the amount of protein adults age 19 and over eat should fall within the range of 10–35% of total daily calories. Because most people in the United States meet the recommendations for sufficient protein intake, nutrition experts recommend that Americans focus on a variety of low-fat protein choices to obtain adequate protein while reducing calorie intake. The recommended dietary patterns described later in the chapter, if followed, ensure adequate intake of all key nutrients.

Fats—Essential in Small Amounts

Fats, also known as *lipids,* are the most concentrated source of energy, at 9 calories per gram. The fats stored in your body represent usable energy, help insulate your body, and support and cushion your organs. Fats in the diet help your body absorb fat-soluble vitamins, and they add flavor and texture to foods. Fats are the major fuel for the body during rest and light activity.

Two fats—linoleic acid and alpha-linolenic acid—the essential fatty acids—are necessary components of the diet. They are used to make compounds that are key regulators of body functions such as the maintenance of blood pressure, vision, and the progress of a healthy pregnancy.

Types and Sources of Fats Food fats are usually composed of both **saturated** and **unsaturated** fatty acids (Table 8.4). The dominant type of fatty acid determines the fat's characteristics. Saturated fats come mostly from animal products—red meats (hamburger, steak, roasts), whole milk, cheese, hot dogs, and lunchmeats—but are also found in tropic oils (coconut and palm oils). They are usually solid at room

Table 8.3	Protein Content of Common Food Items

ITEM	PROTEIN (GRAMS)
3 ounces lean meat, poultry, or fish	20–27
½ cup tofu	20
1 cup baked/black cooked beans	13–15
1 container (6 oz) yogurt	6–8
1 ounce blue/camembert cheese	6
1/2–1 cup cereals	1–6
1 egg cooked	6
1 cup ricotta cheese	28
1 cup milk	9
1 ounce nuts	2–6

SOURCE: U.S. Department of Agriculture, Agricultural Research Service. 2015. *USDA National Nutrient Database for Standard Reference, Release 27. Nutrient Data Laboratory Home Page.* (http://www.ars.usda.gov/ba/bhnrc/ndl retrieved June 24, 2015).

Table 8.2	Goals for Protein, Fat, and Carbohydrate Intake for Adults		
	DAILY ADEQUATE INTAKES (GRAMS)		ACCEPTABLE MACRONUTRIENT DISTRIBUTION RANGES (PERCENT OF TOTAL DAILY CALORIES)
	MEN	WOMEN	
Protein*	56 g	46 g	10–35%
Fat (total)			20–35%
Linoleic acid	17 g	12 g	
Alpha-linolenic acid	1.6 g	1.1 g	
Carbohydrate	130 g	130 g	45–65%

*Protein intake goals can be calculated more specifically by multiplying your body weight in pounds by 0.36.

NOTE: Individuals can allocate total daily energy intake among the three classes of macronutrients to suit individual preferences. To translate percentage goals into daily intake goals expressed in calories and grams, multiply the appropriate percentages by total daily energy intake and then divide the results by the corresponding calories per gram. For example, a fat limit of 35% applied to a 2,200-calorie diet would be calculated as follows: 0.35 × 2200 = 770 calories of total fat; 770 ÷ 9 calories per gram = 86 grams of total fat.

SOURCE: Recommendations from *Dietary Reference Intakes for Energy, Carbohydrate, Fiber, Fat, Fatty Acids, Cholesterol, Protein, and Amino Acids* (2002/2005). The report may be accessed via www.nap.edu.

Table 8.4	Types of Fatty Acids

TYPE OF FATTY ACID	FOUND IN*
Saturated	• Animal fats (especially fatty meats and poultry fat and skin) • Butter, cheese, and other high-fat dairy products • Palm and coconut oils
Trans	• Some frozen pizza • Some types of popcorn • Deep-fried fast foods • Stick margarines, shortening • Packaged cookies and crackers • Processed snacks and sweets
Monounsaturated	• Olive, canola, and safflower oils • Avocados, olives • Peanut butter (without added fat) • Many nuts, including almonds, cashews, pecans, and pistachios
Polyunsaturated—Omega-3[†]	• Fatty fish, including salmon, white albacore tuna, mackerel, anchovies, and sardines • Compared to fish, lesser amounts are found in walnut, flaxseed, canola, and soybean oils; tofu; walnuts; flaxseeds; and dark green leafy vegetables
Polyunsaturated—Omega-6[†]	• Corn, soybean, and cottonseed oils (often used in margarine, mayonnaise, and salad dressings)

*Food fats contain a combination of types of fatty acids in various proportions. For example, canola oil is composed mainly of monounsaturated fatty acids (62%) but also contains polyunsaturated (32%) and saturated (6%) fatty acids.

[†]The essential fatty acids are polyunsaturated: linoleic acid is an omega-6 fatty acid and alpha-linolenic acid is an omega-3 fatty acid.

temperature. Most unsaturated fats in foods come from plant sources and are liquid at room temperature.

Depending on their structure, unsaturated fatty acids can be further divided into *monounsaturated* and *polyunsaturated* fats. Olive, canola, safflower, and peanut oils contain mostly monounsaturated fatty acids. Soybean, corn, and cottonseed oils contain mostly polyunsaturated fatty acids. You may sometimes also see polyunsaturated fats described more specifically by chemical structure as either omega-3 or omega-6 fats.

Hydrogenation When unsaturated vegetable oils undergo the process of **hydrogenation**, a mixture of saturated and unsaturated fatty acids is produced, creating a more solid fat from a liquid oil. Hydrogenation also changes some unsaturated fatty acids into **trans fatty acids (trans fats)**, unsaturated fatty acids with an atypical shape that affects their behavior in the body.

Food manufacturers use hydrogenation to increase the stability of an oil so that it can be reused for deep frying, to improve the texture of certain foods (to make pie crusts flakier, for example), and to extend the shelf life of foods made with oil. Hydrogenation is also used to transform liquid oil into margarine or vegetable shortening.

Small amounts of trans fats occur naturally in animal fat, particularly beef, lamb, and dairy products, but the majority of trans fats in the American diet are artificial, from partially hydrogenated oils. Many baked and fried foods are prepared with hydrogenated vegetable oils, so they can be relatively high in saturated and trans fatty acids. However, in 2013, the Food and Drug Administration (FDA) made a preliminary determination that trans fats were no longer generally recognized as

safe, because they are linked to a significant increase in coronary heart disease. In 2015, the FDA required all food manufacturers to stop using trans fats, allowing a three-year compliance period. At this time, trans fats are still used in many processed foods, such as crackers, cookies, cakes, frozen baked goods, snack foods such as microwave popcorn, stick margarines, and coffee creamers. Even with the new law, it is important to check ingredient labels for partially hydrogenated oils: as long as a product has no more than half a gram of trans fats, the label may claim zero.

In general, the more solid a hydrogenated oil is, the more saturated or trans fats it contains. For example, stick margarines typically contain more saturated and trans fats than do tub or squeeze margarines.

TERMS

saturated fats Fatty acids found mostly in animal products and tropical oils; usually solid at room temperature.

unsaturated fats Fatty acids found primarily in plant foods; usually liquid at room temperature.

hydrogenation A process by which hydrogens are added to unsaturated fats, increasing the degree of saturation and turning liquid oils into solid fats. Hydrogenation produces a mixture of saturated fatty acids and standard and trans forms of unsaturated fatty acids.

trans fatty acid (trans fat) A type of unsaturated fatty acid produced during the process of hydrogenation; trans fats have an atypical shape that affects their chemical activity.

Hydrogenated vegetable oils are not the only plant fats that contain saturated fats. Palm and coconut oils, although derived from plants, are also highly saturated. Yet fish oils, derived from an animal source, are rich in polyunsaturated fats.

Fats and Health Scientists are still unraveling the complex effects that individual types of fats and overall dietary patterns have on health and the risk for specific diseases. Recently, most health experts have agreed on the dangers of artificial trans fats because of their double-negative effect on heart health—they raise levels of **low-density lipoprotein (LDL)**—"bad" cholesterol—and they also lower **high-density lipoprotein (HDL)**—"good" cholesterol. Consuming trans fats appears to increase the risk of both cardiovascular disease and type 2 diabetes. In recent years, as awareness of these health risks has grown, cities and states have banned the use of trans fats in restaurants and food prepared for retail sale, and food manufacturers have reduced the amount of trans fats they use. And the 2015 ban by the FDA signals that this type of dangerous fat will be removed from the food supply.

What about other types of fats? Many studies have examined the effects of dietary fat intake on blood **cholesterol** levels and the risk of heart disease. Longstanding advice has been to limit saturated fat; however, a 2014 analysis published in *Annals of Internal Medicine* challenged the widely accepted saturated fat hypothesis that butter and other sources of saturated fat cause coronary heart disease. A Cambridge University analysis looked at 27 prior clinical trials and 49 observational studies, consisting of more than 600,000 participants. It concluded that "current evidence does not clearly support cardiovascular guidelines that encourage high consumption of polyunsaturated fatty acids and low consumption of total saturated fats." Other scientists challenged the methods and findings of the study, and the recommendations from the American Heart Association and American College of

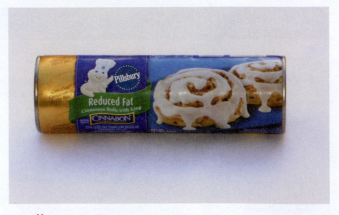

Wellness Tip An isolated focus on reducing dietary fat intake contributed to an explosion in the availability of processed foods promoted as being low in fat. Many of these choices, however, are high in refined grains and added sugars and are not healthy choices. Focus on your overall dietary pattern and limit your intake of both saturated fats and added sugars. Choose unsaturated fats, whole grains, and fruits and vegetables.

Cardiology strongly advise lowering saturated fat intake for reducing cardiovascular risk, especially for those people with risk factors for heart disease. Continued research on the health risks and benefits of individual fats is ongoing. For example, do saturated fats in beef, butter, milk, and chocolate all have the same effect on heart disease risk? And what are the health effects of shifts in the intake of particular fats within the overall context of the diet?

Dietary fat affects health in other ways besides heart disease risk. Diets high in fatty red meat are associated with an increased risk of certain forms of cancer, especially colon cancer. A high-fat diet can also make weight management more difficult, because fat is a concentrated source of calories. If you are trying to limit overall energy intake, consuming a high-fat diet can make it more difficult to consume all essential nutrients at your target calorie level.

What does all this mean for you? Although more research is needed on the precise effects of different types and amounts of fat on overall health, evidence suggests that most people benefit from keeping their overall fat and saturated fat intake at recommended levels. Dietary patterns are more important for health than a focus on a single nutrient. The fats in your diet are found in foods that contain other nutrients, and the foods you consume are in the context of your overall diet. Increased body weight, aging, and gender are more important for predicting negative health events than eating one kind of dietary fat rather than another. The U.S. Department of Agriculture recommends that Americans limit their intake of saturated fat to less than 10 percent of total calories per day—but that they do so in the context of a healthy dietary pattern that emphasizes vegetables, fruits, whole grains, low- or non-fat dairy, seafood, legumes, and nuts; is lower in red and processed meat; and is low in sugar-sweetened foods and drinks and refined grains. Don't replace one less-than-healthy choice with another. Healthy dietary patterns are described in detail later in the chapter.

TERMS

low-density lipoprotein (LDL) Blood fat that transports cholesterol to organs and tissues; excess amounts result in the accumulation of fatty deposits on artery walls.

cholesterol A waxy substance found in the blood and cells and needed for synthesis of cell membranes, vitamin D, and hormones.

high-density lipoprotein (HDL) Blood fat that helps transport cholesterol out of the arteries, thereby protecting against heart disease.

carbohydrate An essential nutrient; sugars, starches, and dietary fiber are all carbohydrates.

glucose A simple sugar that is the body's basic fuel.

glycogen A starch stored in the liver and muscles.

whole grain The entire edible portion of a grain (such as wheat, rice, or oats), including the germ, endosperm, and bran; processing removes parts of the grain, often leaving just the endosperm.

Table 8.5	Simple and Complex Carbohydrates in Foods

SIMPLE CARBOHYDRATES ("SUGARS")	COMPLEX CARBOHYDRATES
Single sugar molecules (monosaccharides)	Starches (long, complex chains of sugar molecules)
– Glucose (common in foods)	– grains (wheat, rye, rice, oats, barley, millet)
– Fructose (fruits)	– legumes (dry beans, peas, and lentils)
– Galactose (milk)	– tubers and other vegetables (potatoes, yams, corn)
Double sugar molecules (disaccharides; pairs of single sugars)	Fiber (nondigestible carbohydrates)
– Sucrose or table sugar (fructose + glucose)	– soluble (oats, barley, legumes, some fruits and vegetables)
– Maltose or malt sugar (glucose + glucose)	– insoluble (wheat bran, vegetables, whole grains)
– Lactose or milk sugar (galactose + glucose)	

Carbohydrates—A Key Source of Energy

Carbohydrates ("carbs") supply energy to body cells. Some cells, such as those in the brain and other parts of the nervous system and in the blood, use only the carbohydrate glucose for fuel. During high-intensity exercise, muscles use carbohydrates for fuel.

Simple and Complex Carbohydrates

Carbohydrates are classified into two groups: simple and complex (Table 8.5). *Simple carbohydrates* are the single sugar molecules (monosaccharides) and the double sugars (disaccharides). Three monosaccharides are glucose, fructose, and galactose. Glucose, the most common of the sugars, is used by both animals and plants for energy. Fructose is a very sweet sugar that is found in fruits, and galactose is the sugar in milk.

The disaccharides, pairs of single sugars, include sucrose (table sugar: fructose + glucose), maltose (malt sugar: glucose + glucose), and lactose (milk sugar: galactose + glucose). Simple carbohydrates add sweetness to foods. They are found naturally in fruits and milk and are added to soft drinks, fruit drinks, candy, and desserts. There is no evidence that any type of simple carbohydrate is more nutritious than others.

Complex carbohydrates include starches and most types of dietary fiber. Starches are found in a variety of plants, especially grains (wheat, rye, rice, oats, barley, and millet), legumes (dried beans, peas, and lentils), and tubers (potatoes and yams). Most other vegetables contain a mix of complex and simple carbohydrates. Fiber, which is discussed later in this chapter, is found in fruits, vegetables, and grains.

During digestion, your body breaks down carbohydrates into simple sugar molecules, such as **glucose**, for absorption. When glucose is in the bloodstream, the pancreas releases the hormone insulin, which allows cells to take up glucose and use it for energy. The liver and muscles also take up glucose and store it in the form of a starch called **glycogen**. The muscles use glucose from glycogen as fuel during endurance events or long workouts.

Refined Carbohydrates versus Whole Grains

Complex carbohydrates can be further divided into refined, or processed, carbohydrates and unrefined carbohydrates, or whole grains. Before they are processed, all grains are **whole grains**,

consisting of an inner layer of germ, a middle layer called the endosperm, and an outer layer of bran (Figure 8.2). During processing, the germ and bran are often removed, leaving just the starchy endosperm. The refinement of whole grains transforms whole-wheat flour into white flour, brown rice into white rice, and so on.

Refined carbohydrates usually retain all the calories of their unrefined counterparts, but they tend to be much lower in fiber, vitamins, minerals, and other beneficial compounds. Refined grain products are often enriched or fortified with vitamins and minerals, but many of the nutrients lost in processing are not replaced.

Unrefined carbohydrates tend to take longer to chew and digest than refined ones; they also generally enter the bloodstream more slowly. This slower digestive pace makes you feel full sooner and for a longer period. Also, a slower rise in blood glucose levels following consumption of complex carbohydrates may help in the management of diabetes. Whole grains are also high in dietary fiber (discussed later).

Consumption of whole grains has been linked to a reduced risk of heart disease, diabetes, and cancer, and plays an important role in gastrointestinal health and body weight management. For all these reasons, whole grains are recommended over those that have been refined. See the box "Choosing More Whole-Grain Foods" for tips on increasing your intake of whole grains.

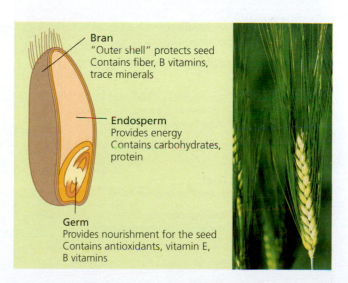

Bran
"Outer shell" protects seed
Contains fiber, B vitamins, trace minerals

Endosperm
Provides energy
Contains carbohydrates, protein

Germ
Provides nourishment for the seed
Contains antioxidants, vitamin E, B vitamins

FIGURE 8.2 The parts of a whole grain kernel.

TAKE CHARGE
Choosing More Whole-Grain Foods

What Are Whole Grains?

The first step in increasing your intake of whole grains is to correctly identify them. The following are whole grains:

- whole wheat
- whole rye
- whole oats
- oatmeal
- whole-grain corn
- popcorn
- brown rice
- whole-grain barley

Other choices include bulgur (cracked wheat), farro, millet, kasha (roasted buckwheat kernels), quinoa, wheat and rye berries, amaranth, wild rice, graham flour, whole-grain kamut, whole-grain spelt, and whole-grain triticale.

Wheat flour, unbleached flour, enriched flour, and degerminated corn meal are not whole grains. Wheat germ and wheat bran are also not whole grains, but they are the constituents of wheat typically left out when wheat is processed and so are healthier choices than regular wheat flour, which typically contains just the grain's endosperm.

Checking Packages for Whole Grains

To find packaged foods—such as bread or pasta—that are rich in whole grains, read the list of ingredients and check for special health claims related to whole grains. The *first* item in the list of ingredients should be one of the whole grains in the preceding list. Product names and food color can be misleading. *When in doubt, always check the list of ingredients and make sure "whole" is the first word in the list.*

The U.S. Food and Drug Administration (FDA) allows manufacturers to include special health claims for foods that contain 51% or more whole-grain ingredients. Such products may contain a statement such as the following on their packaging:

- "Rich in whole grain"
- "Made with 100% whole grain"
- "Diets rich in whole-grain foods may help reduce the risk of heart disease and certain cancers."

However, many whole-grain products will not carry such claims. This is one more reason to check the ingredient list to make sure you're buying a product made from one or more whole grains.

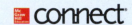

Glycemic Index and Glycemic Response Insulin and glucose levels rise following a meal or snack containing any type of carbohydrate. Some foods cause a quick and dramatic rise in glucose and insulin levels, while others have a slower, more moderate effect. A food that has a rapid effect on blood glucose levels is said to have a high **glycemic index**. The glycemic index of a food indicates the type of carbohydrate in that food. Unrefined complex carbohydrates, high-fiber foods, and high-fat foods tend to have a lower glycemic index.

Attempting to base food choices on glycemic index is a difficult task; however, for people with particular health concerns, such as diabetes, glycemic index may be an important consideration in choosing foods. In addition to the type of carbohydrate in the food, the total amount of carbohydrate in the diet is important for diabetes management. Your best bet, therefore, is to choose a variety of vegetables daily and limit refined grains as well as foods that are high in added sugars and low in other nutrients.

> **TERMS**
>
> **glycemic index** A measure of how a particular food affects blood glucose levels.
>
> **dietary fiber** Nondigestible carbohydrates and lignin that are intact in plants.
>
> **functional fiber** Nondigestible carbohydrates either isolated from natural sources or synthesized; these may be added to foods and dietary supplements.
>
> **total fiber** The total amount of dietary fiber and functional fiber in the diet.
>
> **soluble (viscous) fiber** Fiber that dissolves in water or is broken down by bacteria in the large intestine.
>
> **insoluble fiber** Fiber that does not dissolve in water and is not broken down by bacteria in the large intestine.
>
> **vitamins** Carbon-containing substances needed in small amounts to help promote and regulate chemical reactions and processes in the body.

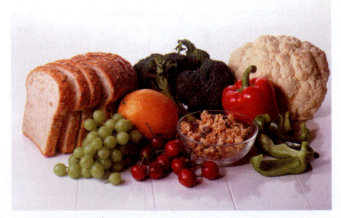

Wellness Tip To reduce the risk of chronic disease and maintain intestinal health, daily fiber intake of 38 grams for men and 25 grams for women is recommended. Americans currently consume about half this amount. Fruits, vegetables, and whole grains are excellent sources of carbohydrates and fiber. Drink plenty of water to get the most health benefits from the fiber you consume.

Added Sugars *Added sugars* are sugars that are added to foods by food manufacturers or individuals; they include white sugar, brown sugar, high-fructose corn syrup, and other sweeteners added to most processed foods. (Naturally occurring sugars in fruit and milk are not considered added sugars.) Foods high in added sugar are generally high in calories and low in nutrients and fiber, thus providing "empty calories." High intake of added sugars from foods and sugar-sweetened beverages is associated with dental caries ("cavities"), excess body weight, and increased risk of type 2 diabetes, and may also increase risk for hypertension, stroke, and heart disease.

Added sugars currently contribute about 250–300 calories in the typical daily American diet, representing about 13–17% of total energy intake. A limit of 10% is suggested by the USDA and other organizations; even lower intakes may be needed to meet all nutrient needs at a given level of calorie intake. Remember, added sugars are empty calories and do not supply any essential nutrients.

Sweetened beverages supply nearly half of all the added sugars consumed by Americans, followed by snacks and sweets. To decrease intake from added sugars, reduce your consumption of sugar-sweetened beverages (soft drinks, sweetened fruit drinks, sweetened sports beverages), sweet snacks, and desserts. In particular, choose water in place of sweetened beverages. Water is a readily available, low-cost, zero-calorie option. The sugars in your diet should be mostly those that are naturally occurring: from fruits, which are excellent sources of vitamins and minerals, and from low-fat or fat-free dairy products, which are high in protein, calcium, and other nutrients.

Fiber—A Closer Look

Fiber is the term given to nondigestible carbohydrates in plants. Instead of being digested, like starch, fiber moves through the intestinal tract and provides bulk for feces in the large intestine, which in turn facilitates elimination. In the large intestine, some types of fiber are broken down by bacteria into acids and gases, which explains why eating too much fiber-rich food can lead to intestinal gas. Even though humans don't digest fiber, it is necessary for good health.

Types of Fiber **Dietary fiber** refers to the nondigestible carbohydrates (and the noncarbohydrate substance *lignin*) that are naturally present in plants such as grains, fruits, legumes, and vegetables. There are two types of dietary fiber: soluble and insoluble. Both types are important for health.

- **Soluble (viscous) fiber**, such as that found in oat bran or legumes, can delay stomach emptying, slow the movement of glucose into the blood after eating, and reduce absorption of cholesterol.
- **Insoluble fiber**, such as that found in wheat bran or psyllium seed, increases fecal bulk and helps prevent constipation, hemorrhoids, and other digestive disorders.

Functional fiber refers to nondigestible carbohydrates that have been either isolated from natural sources or synthesized in

a laboratory and then added to a food product or dietary supplement. **Total fiber** is the sum of dietary and functional fiber in your diet.

A high-fiber diet can help reduce the risk of type 2 diabetes, heart disease, and pulmonary disease, as well as improve gastrointestinal health and aid in the management of metabolic syndrome and body weight. Some studies have linked high-fiber diets with a reduced risk of colon and rectal cancer.

Sources of Fiber All plant foods contain some dietary fiber. Fruits, legumes, oats (especially oat bran), and barley all contain the viscous types of fiber that help lower blood glucose and cholesterol levels. Wheat (especially wheat bran), cereals, grains, and vegetables are all good sources of cellulose and other fibers that help prevent constipation. Psyllium, which is often added to cereals or used in fiber supplements and laxatives, improves intestinal health and also helps control glucose and cholesterol levels. The processing of packaged foods can remove fiber, so it's important to depend on fresh fruits and vegetables and foods made from whole grains as your main sources of fiber.

Vitamins—Organic Micronutrients

Vitamins are organic (carbon-containing) substances required in small amounts to regulate various processes within living cells (Table 8.6). Humans need 13 vitamins; of these, four are fat-soluble (A, D, E, and K), and nine are water-soluble (C and the B vitamins; thiamin, riboflavin, niacin, vitamin B-6, folate, vitamin B-12, biotin, and pantothenic acid).

Solubility affects how a vitamin is absorbed, transported, and stored in the body. The water-soluble vitamins are absorbed directly into the bloodstream, where they travel freely. Excess amounts of water-soluble vitamins are generally removed by the kidneys and excreted in urine. Fat-soluble vitamins require a more complex absorptive process. They are usually carried in the blood by special proteins and are stored in the liver and in fat tissues rather than excreted.

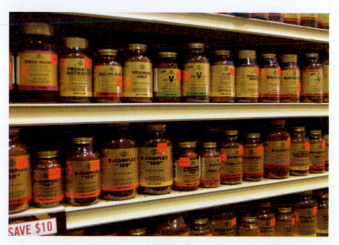

Wellness Tip Vitamin and mineral supplements are popular, but they are not usually necessary for healthy people who eat a balanced diet.

Table 8.6 — Facts about Vitamins

VITAMIN AND RECOMMENDED INTAKES*	IMPORTANT DIETARY SOURCES	MAJOR FUNCTIONS	SIGNS OF PROLONGED DEFICIENCY	TOXIC EFFECTS OF MEGADOSES
FAT-SOLUBLE				
Vitamin A Men: 900 µg Women: 700 µg	Liver, milk, butter, cheese, fortified margarine; carrots, spinach, and other orange and deep green vegetables and fruits	Maintenance of vision, skin, linings of the nose, mouth, digestive, and urinary tracts, immune function	Night blindness; dry, scaling skin; increased susceptibility to infection; loss of appetite; anemia; kidney stones	Liver damage, miscarriage and birth defects, headache, vomiting and diarrhea, vertigo, double vision, bone abnormalities
Vitamin D Men: 15 µg Women: 15 µg	Fortified milk and margarine, fish oils, butter, egg yolks (sunlight on skin also produces vitamin D)	Development and maintenance of bones and teeth; promotion of calcium absorption	Rickets (bone deformities) in children; bone softening, loss, fractures in adults	Kidney damage, calcium deposits in soft tissues, depression, death
Vitamin E Men: 15 mg Women: 15 mg	Vegetable oils, whole grains, nuts and seeds, green leafy vegetables, asparagus, peaches	Protection and maintenance of cellular membranes	Red blood cell breakage and anemia, weakness, neurological problems, muscle cramps	Relatively nontoxic but may cause excess bleeding or formation of blood clots
Vitamin K Men: 120 µg Women: 90 µg	Green leafy vegetables; smaller amounts widespread in other foods	Production of factors essential for blood clotting and bone metabolism	Hemorrhaging	None reported
WATER-SOLUBLE				
Biotin Men: 30 µg Women: 30 µg	Cereals, yeast, egg yolks, soy flour, liver; widespread in foods	Synthesis of fat, glycogen, and amino acids	Rash, nausea, vomiting, weight loss, depression, fatigue, hair loss	None reported
Folate Men: 400 µg Women: 400 µg	Green leafy vegetables, yeast, oranges, whole grains, legumes, liver	Amino acid metabolism, synthesis of RNA and DNA, new cell synthesis	Anemia, weakness, fatigue, irritability, shortness of breath, swollen tongue	Masking of vitamin B-12 deficiency
Niacin Men: 16 mg Women: 14 mg	Eggs, poultry, fish, milk, whole grains, nuts, enriched breads and cereals, meats, legumes	Conversion of carbohydrates, fats, and proteins into usable forms of energy	Pellagra (symptoms include diarrhea, dermatitis, inflammation of mucous membranes, dementia)	Flushing of skin, nausea, vomiting, diarrhea, liver dysfunction, glucose intolerance
Pantothenic acid Men: 5 mg Women: 5 mg	Animal foods, whole grains, broccoli, potatoes; widespread in foods	Metabolism of fats, carbohydrates, and proteins	Fatigue, numbness and tingling of hands and feet, gastrointestinal disturbances	None reported
Riboflavin Men: 1.3 mg Women: 1.1 mg	Dairy products, enriched breads and cereals, lean meats, poultry, fish, green vegetables	Energy metabolism; maintenance of skin, mucous membranes, nervous system structures	Cracks at corners of mouth, sore throat, skin rash, hypersensitivity to light, purple tongue	None reported
Thiamin Men: 1.2 mg Women: 1.1 mg	Whole-grain and enriched breads and cereals, organ meats, lean pork, nuts, legumes	Conversion of carbohydrates into usable forms of energy; maintenance of appetite and nervous system function	Beriberi (symptoms include muscle wasting, mental confusion, anorexia, enlarged heart, nerve changes)	None reported
Vitamin B-6 Men: 1.3 mg Women: 1.3 mg	Eggs, poultry, fish, whole grains, nuts, soybeans, liver, kidney, pork	Metabolism of amino acids and glycogen	Anemia, convulsions, cracks at corners of mouth, dermatitis, nausea, confusion	Neurological abnormalities and damage
Vitamin B-12 Men: 2.4 µg Women: 2.4 µg	Meat, fish, poultry, fortified cereals, cheese, eggs, milk	Synthesis of blood cells; other metabolic reactions	Anemia, fatigue, nervous system damage, sore tongue	None reported
Vitamin C Men: 90 mg Women: 75 mg	Peppers, broccoli, brussels sprouts, spinach, citrus fruits, strawberries, tomatoes, potatoes, cabbage, other fruits and vegetables	Maintenance and repair of connective tissue, bones, teeth, cartilage; promotion of healing; aid in iron absorption	Scurvy, anemia, reduced resistance to infection, loosened teeth, joint pain, poor wound healing, hair loss, poor iron absorption	Urinary stones in some people, acid stomach from ingesting supplements in pill form, nausea, diarrhea, headache, fatigue

*Recommended Intakes for adults ages 19–30; to calculate your personal DRIs based on age, sex, and other factors, visit the Interactive DRI website: http://fnic.nal.usda.gov/fnic/interactiveDRI.

SOURCES: Dietary Reference Intakes for Thiamin, Riboflavin, Niacin, Vitamin B6, Folate, Vitamin B12, Pantothenic Acid, Biotin and Choline (1998); Dietary Reference Intakes for Vitamin C, Vitamin E, Selenium, and Carotenoids (2000); Dietary Reference Intakes for Vitamin A, Vitamin K, Arsenic, Boron, Chromium, Copper, Iodine, Iron, Manganese, Molybdenum, Nickel, Silicon, Vanadium, and Zinc (2001); and Dietary Reference Intakes for Calcium and Vitamin D (2011). These reports may be accessed via www.nap.edu. Ross, A. C., et al., eds. 2012. *Modern Nutrition in Health and Disease,* 11th ed. Baltimore: Lippincott Williams and Wilkins.

Functions of Vitamins Many vitamins help chemical reactions take place. They provide no energy to the body directly but help release the energy stored in carbohydrates, proteins, and fats. Other vitamins are critical in the production of red blood cells and the maintenance of the nervous, skeletal, and immune systems. Some vitamins act as **antioxidants**, which help preserve the health of cells. Key vitamin antioxidants include vitamin E, vitamin C, and the vitamin A precursor beta-carotene. (Antioxidants are described later in the chapter.)

Sources of Vitamins The human body must obtain most of the vitamins it requires from foods. Vitamins are abundant in fruits, vegetables, and grains. In addition, many processed foods, such as flour and breakfast cereals, contain added vitamins. A few vitamins are made in the body: The skin makes vitamin D when it is exposed to sunlight, and intestinal bacteria make vitamin K. Nonetheless, you still need to get vitamin D and vitamin K from foods (see Table 8.6).

Vitamin Deficiencies and Excesses If your diet lacks a particular vitamin, characteristic symptoms of deficiency can develop (see Table 8.6). For example, vitamin A deficiency can cause night blindness, and people whose diets lack vitamin B-12 can develop anemia. Vitamin deficiency diseases are relatively rare in the United States because vitamins are readily available from our food supply. However, many Americans consume lower-than-recommended amounts of several vitamins. Nutrient intake that is consistently below recommended levels can have adverse effects on health even if it is not low enough to cause a deficiency disease. For example, low intake of folate increases a woman's chance of giving birth to a baby with a neural tube defect (a congenital malformation of the central nervous system). Low intake of folate and vitamins B-6 and B-12 has been linked to increased heart disease risk. Recent research suggests that vitamin D supplementation can reduce the risk of cardiovascular disease and of several cancers. As important as vitamins are, however, many Americans consume less-than-recommended amounts of some vitamins, especially vitamins A, D, E, and C, as well as folate.

Extra vitamins in the diet can be harmful, especially when taken as supplements. Megadoses of fat-soluble vitamins are particularly dangerous because the excess is stored in the body rather than excreted, increasing the risk of toxicity. Even when supplements are not taken in excess, relying on them for an adequate intake of vitamins can be problematic. There are many substances in foods other than vitamins and minerals that have important health effects. Later, this chapter discusses specific recommendations for vitamin intake and when a supplement is advisable. For now, keep in mind that it's best to get most of your vitamins from foods rather than supplements.

The vitamins and minerals in foods can be easily lost or destroyed during storage or cooking. To retain their value, eat or process vegetables immediately after buying them. If you can't do this, store them in a cool place, covered to retain moisture—either in the refrigerator (for a few days) or in the freezer (for a longer term). To reduce nutrient losses during food preparation, minimize the amount of water used and the total cooking time. Develop a taste for a crunchier texture in cooked vegetables. Baking, steaming, broiling, grilling, and microwaving are all good methods of preparing vegetables.

Minerals—Inorganic Micronutrients

Minerals are inorganic (non-carbon-containing) elements you need in relatively small amounts to help regulate body functions, aid in the growth and maintenance of body tissues, and help release energy (Table 8.7). There are about 17 essential minerals. The major minerals, those that the body needs in amounts exceeding 100 milligrams (mg) per day, include calcium, phosphorus, magnesium, sodium, potassium, and chloride. The essential trace minerals, which you need in minute amounts, include copper, fluoride, iodine, iron, selenium, and zinc.

Characteristic symptoms develop if an essential mineral is consumed in a quantity too small or too large for good health. The minerals commonly lacking in the American diet are iron, calcium, magnesium, and potassium. Low potassium intake is considered a public health concern because it is linked to high blood pressure and heart disease; you can improve your potassium intake by choosing a healthy dietary pattern rich in fruits, vegetables, and legumes. Iron-deficiency **anemia** is a problem in some age groups, and researchers fear poor calcium intakes in childhood are sowing the seeds for future **osteoporosis**, especially in women. See the box "Eating for Healthy Bones" to learn more.

Water—Vital but Often Ignored

Water is the major component in both foods and the human body: You are composed of about 50–60% water. Your need for other nutrients, in terms of weight, is much less than your need for water. You can live up to 50 days without food but only a few days without water.

Water is distributed all over the body, among lean and other tissues and in blood and other body fluids. Water is used in the digestion and absorption of food and is the medium in which most chemical reactions take place within the body. Some water-based fluids, such as blood, transport substances around the body; other fluids serve as lubricants or cushions. Water also helps regulate body temperature.

TERMS

antioxidant A substance that protects against the breakdown of food or body constituents by free radicals; antioxidants' actions include binding oxygen, donating electrons to free radicals, and repairing damage to molecules.

minerals Inorganic compounds needed in relatively small amounts for the regulation, growth, and maintenance of body tissues and functions.

anemia A deficiency in the oxygen-carrying material in the red blood cells.

osteoporosis A condition in which the bones become extremely thin and brittle and break easily; due largely to insufficient calcium intake.

Table 8.7   Facts about Selected Minerals

MINERAL AND RECOMMENDED INTAKES*	IMPORTANT DIETARY SOURCES	MAJOR FUNCTIONS	SIGNS OF PROLONGED DEFICIENCY	TOXIC EFFECTS OF MEGADOSES
Calcium Men: 1,000 mg Women: 1,000 mg	Milk and milk products, tofu, fortified orange juice and bread, green leafy vegetables, bones in fish	Formation of bones and teeth; control of nerve impulses, muscle contraction, blood clotting	Stunted growth in children, bone mineral loss in adults; urinary stones	Kidney stones, calcium deposits in soft tissues, inhibition of mineral absorption, constipation
Fluoride Men: 4 mg Women: 3 mg	Fluoridated water, tea, marine fish eaten with bones	Maintenance of tooth and bone structure	Higher frequency of tooth decay	Increased bone density, mottling of teeth, impaired kidney function
Iodine Men: 150 µg Women: 150 µg	Iodized salt, seafood, processed foods	Essential part of thyroid hormones, regulation of body metabolism	Goiter (enlarged thyroid), cretinism (birth defect)	Depression of thyroid activity, hyperthyroidism in susceptible people
Iron Men: 8 mg Women: 18 mg	Meat and poultry, fortified grain products, dark green vegetables, dried fruit	Component of hemoglobin, myoglobin, and enzymes	Iron-deficiency anemia, weakness, impaired immune function, gastrointestinal distress	Nausea, diarrhea, liver and kidney damage, joint pains, sterility, disruption of cardiac function, death
Magnesium Men: 400 mg Women: 310 mg	Widespread in foods and water (except soft water); especially found in grains, legumes, nuts, seeds, green vegetables, milk	Transmission of nerve impulses, energy transfer, activation of many enzymes	Neurological disturbances, cardiovascular problems, kidney disorders, nausea, growth failure in children	Nausea, vomiting, diarrhea, central nervous system depression, coma; death in people with impaired kidney function
Phosphorus Men: 700 mg Women: 700 mg	Present in nearly all foods, especially milk, cereal, peas, eggs, meat	Bone growth and maintenance, energy transfer in cells	Impaired growth, weakness, kidney disorders, cardio-respiratory and nervous system dysfunction	Drop in blood calcium levels, calcium deposits in soft tissues, bone loss
Potassium Men: 4,700 mg Women: 4,700 mg	Meats, milk, fruits, vegetables, grains, legumes	Nerve function and body water balance	Muscular weakness, nausea, drowsiness, paralysis, confusion, disruption of cardiac rhythm	Cardiac arrest
Selenium Men: 55 µg Women: 55 µg	Seafood, meat, eggs, whole grains	Defense against oxidative stress; regulation of thyroid hormone action	Muscle pain and weakness, heart disorders	Hair and nail loss, nausea and vomiting, weakness, irritability
Sodium Men: 1,500 mg Women: 1,500 mg	Salt, soy sauce, fast food, processed foods, especially lunch meats, canned soups and vegetables, salty snacks, processed cheese	Body water balance, acid-base balance, nerve function	Muscle weakness, loss of appetite, nausea, vomiting; deficiency rarely seen	Edema, hypertension in sensitive people
Zinc Men: 11 mg Women: 8 mg	Whole grains, meat, eggs, liver, seafood (especially oysters)	Synthesis of proteins, RNA, and DNA; wound healing; immune response; ability to taste	Growth failure, loss of appetite, impaired taste acuity, skin rash, impaired immune function, poor wound healing	Vomiting, impaired immune function, decline in blood HDL levels, impaired copper absorption

*Recommended Intakes for adults ages 19-30; to calculate your personal DRIs based on age, sex, and other factors, visit the Interactive DRI website: http://fnic.nal.usda.gov/fnic/interactiveDRI.

SOURCES: Dietary Reference Intakes for Calcium, Phosphorous, Magnesium, Vitamin D, and Fluoride (1997); Dietary Reference Intakes for Vitamin A, Vitamin K, Arsenic, Boron, Chromium, Copper, Iodine, Iron, Manganese, Molybdenum, Nickel, Silicon, Vanadium, and Zinc (2001); Dietary Reference Intakes for Water, Potassium, Sodium, Chloride, and Sulfate (2005); and Dietary Reference Intakes for Calcium and Vitamin D (2011). These reports may be accessed via www.nap.edu. Ross, A. C. et al., eds. 2012. *Modern Nutrition in Health and Disease,* 11th ed. Baltimore: Lippincott Williams and Wilkins.

Water is contained in almost all foods, particularly in liquids, fruits, and vegetables. The foods and beverages you consume provide 80–90% of your daily water intake; the remainder is generated through metabolism. You lose water in urine, feces, and sweat and through evaporation from your lungs.

Most people can maintain a healthy water balance by consuming beverages at meals and drinking fluids in response to thirst. The Food and Nutrition Board has set levels of adequate water intake to maintain hydration. All beverages, including those containing caffeine, can count toward your total daily fluid intake, although it is better to drink water than sweetened beverages. Under these guidelines, men need to consume about 3.7 total liters of water, with 3.0 liters (about 13 cups) coming from beverages; women need 2.7 total liters, with 2.2 liters (about 9 cups) coming from beverages. About 20% of daily water intake comes from food. If you exercise vigorously or live

Osteoporosis is a condition in which the bones become dangerously thin and fragile over time. An estimated 10 million Americans over age 50 have osteoporosis, and another 34 million are at risk. Women account for about 80% of osteoporosis cases.

Most of adult bone mass is built by age 18 in girls and 20 in boys. Bone density peaks between ages 25 and 35; after that, bone mass is lost over time. To prevent osteoporosis, the best strategy is to build as much bone as possible during your youth and do everything you can to maintain it as you age. Up to 50% of bone loss is determined by controllable lifestyle factors such as diet and exercise. Key nutrients for bone health include the following:

- **Calcium.** Getting enough calcium is important throughout life to build and maintain bone mass. Milk, yogurt, and calcium-fortified orange juice, bread, and cereals are all good sources.

- **Vitamin D.** Vitamin D is necessary for bones to absorb calcium; a daily intake of 600 IU (15 μg) is recommended for individuals ages 1–70. Vitamin D can be obtained from foods and is manufactured by the skin when exposed to sunlight. Candidates for vitamin D supplements include people who don't eat many foods rich in vitamin D; those who don't expose their face, arms, and hands to the sun for 5–15 minutes a few times each week; and those who live north of an imaginary line drawn across the United States from Boston to the Oregon-California border (where sunlight is weaker).

- **Vitamin K.** Vitamin K promotes the synthesis of proteins that help keep bones strong. Broccoli and leafy green vegetables are rich in vitamin K.

- **Other nutrients.** Other nutrients that may play an important role in bone health include vitamin C, magnesium, potassium, phosphorus, fluoride, manganese, zinc, copper, and boron.

Several dietary substances may have a *negative* effect on bone health, especially if consumed in excess. These include alcohol, sodium, caffeine, and retinol (a form of vitamin A). Drinking lots of soda, which often replaces milk in the diet, has been shown to increase the risk of bone fracture in teenage girls.

The effect of protein intake on bone mass depends on other nutrients: Protein helps build bone as long as calcium and vitamin D intake are adequate. But if intake of calcium and vitamin D is low, high protein intake can lead to bone loss.

Weight-bearing aerobic exercise helps maintain bone mass throughout life, and strength training improves bone density, muscle mass, strength, and balance. Drinking alcohol only in moderation, refraining from smoking, and managing depression and stress are also important for maintaining strong bones. For people who develop osteoporosis, a variety of medications are available to treat the condition.

SOURCE: Institute of Medicine of the National Academies. 2010. *Dietary reference intakes for calcium and vitamin D.* (http://www.iom.edu/~/media/Files/Report%20Files/2010/Dietary-Reference-Intakes-for-Calcium-and-Vitamin-D/Vitamin%20D%20and%20Calcium%202010%20Report%20Brief.pdf; retrieved April 17, 2015).

---

in a hot climate, you need to consume additional fluids to maintain a balance between water consumed and water lost. Severe dehydration causes weakness and can lead to death.

Other Substances in Food

Many substances in food are not essential nutrients but may influence health.

Antioxidants When the body uses oxygen or breaks down certain fats or proteins as a normal part of metabolism, substances called **free radicals** are produced. A free radical is a chemically unstable molecule that reacts with fats, proteins, and DNA, damaging cell membranes and mutating genes. Free radicals have been implicated in aging, cancer, cardiovascular disease, and other degenerative diseases like arthritis. Environmental factors such as cigarette smoke, exhaust fumes, radiation, excessive sunlight, certain drugs, and stress can increase free radical production.

Antioxidants found in foods can block the formation and action of free radicals and repair the damage they cause. Some antioxidants, such as vitamin C, vitamin E, and selenium, are also essential nutrients. Others—such as carotenoids, found in yellow, orange, and dark green leafy vegetables—are not. In general,

fruits and vegetables and foods that contain them have a high antioxidant value, as do herbs, spices, berries, nuts and chocolate.

Phytochemicals Antioxidants fall into the broader category of **phytochemicals**, substances found in plant foods that may help prevent chronic disease. For example, certain substances found in soy foods may help lower cholesterol levels. Sulforaphane, a compound isolated from broccoli and other **cruciferous vegetables**, may render some carcinogenic

TERMS

free radical An electron-seeking compound that can react with fats, proteins, and DNA, damaging cell membranes and mutating genes in its search for electrons; produced through chemical reactions in the body and by exposure to environmental factors such as sunlight and tobacco smoke.

phytochemical A naturally occurring substance found in plant foods that may help prevent and treat chronic diseases such as heart disease and cancer; *phyto* means "plant."

cruciferous vegetables Vegetables of the cabbage family, including cabbage, broccoli, brussels sprouts, kale, and cauliflower; the flower petals of these plants form the shape of a cross, hence the name.

Ask Yourself

QUESTIONS FOR CRITICAL THINKING AND REFLECTION

Experts say that two of the most important factors in a healthy diet are eating the "right" kinds of carbohydrates and eating the "right" kinds of fats. Based on what you've read so far in this chapter, which are the "right" carbohydrates and the "right" fats? How would you say your own diet stacks up when it comes to carbs and fats?

compounds harmless. Allyl sulfides, a group of chemicals found in garlic and onions, appear to boost the activity of immune cells. Phytochemicals found in whole grains are associated with a reduced risk of cardiovascular disease, diabetes, and cancer. Carotenoids found in green vegetables may help preserve eyesight with age. Further research on phytochemicals may extend the role of nutrition to the prevention and treatment of many chronic diseases.

To increase your intake of phytochemicals, eat a variety of fruits, vegetables, and grains rather than relying on supplements. Like many vitamins and minerals, isolated phytochemicals may be harmful if taken in high doses. In many cases, their health benefits may be the result of chemical substances working in combination. The role of phytochemicals in disease prevention is discussed further in Chapters 11 and 12.

NUTRITIONAL GUIDELINES: PLANNING YOUR DIET

Scientific and government groups have created a number of useful tools to help people design healthy diets:

- The **Dietary Reference Intakes (DRIs)** are standards for nutrient intake designed to prevent nutritional deficiencies and reduce the risk of chronic diseases.

- The **Dietary Guidelines for Americans** were established to promote health and reduce the risk of major chronic diseases through diet and physical activity.

Dietary Reference Intakes (DRIs) An umbrella term for four types of nutrient standards: Adequate Intake (AI), Estimated Average Requirement (EAR), and Recommended Dietary Allowance (RDA) are levels of intake considered adequate to prevent nutrient deficiencies and reduce the risk of chronic disease; Tolerable Upper Intake Level (UL) is the maximum daily intake that is unlikely to cause health problems.

Dietary Guidelines for Americans General principles of good nutrition intended to help prevent certain diet-related diseases.

MyPlate A food-group plan that provides practical advice to ensure a balanced intake of the essential nutrients.

Daily Values A simplified version of the RDAs used on food labels; also included are values for nutrients with no established RDA.

TERMS

- **MyPlate** is the USDA food guidance system developed to help Americans make healthy food choices consistent with the Dietary Guidelines for Americans.

- The **Daily Values** is a simplified version of the RDAs used on food labels.

Dietary Reference Intakes (DRIs)

The Food and Nutrition Board establishes dietary standards, or recommended intake levels, for Americans of all ages. The current set of standards, called Dietary Reference Intakes (DRIs), was introduced in 1997. The DRIs are frequently reviewed and are updated as substantial new nutrition-related information becomes available. The DRIs present different categories of nutrients in easy-to-read table format. The DRIs have a broad focus: They are based on research that looks not just at the prevention of nutrient deficiencies but also at the role of nutrients in promoting health and preventing chronic diseases such as cancer, osteoporosis, and heart disease.

The DRIs includes a set of four reference values used as standards for both recommended intakes and maximum safe intakes. The recommended intake of each nutrient is expressed as either a *Recommended Dietary Allowance* (RDA) or as *Adequate Intake* (AI). An AI is set when there is not enough information available to set an RDA value; regardless of the type of standard used, however, the DRI represents the best available estimate of intake for optimal health. Used primarily in nutrition policy and research, the *Estimated Average Requirement* (EAR) is the average daily nutrient intake level estimated to meet the requirement of half the healthy individuals in a particular life stage and gender group. The *Tolerable Upper Intake Level* (UL) is the maximum daily intake that is unlikely to cause health problems in a healthy person. For example, the RDA for calcium for an 18-year-old female is 1300 mg per day; the UL is 3000 mg per day.

Because of a lack of data, ULs have not been set for all nutrients. This does not mean that people can tolerate long-term intakes of these vitamins and minerals above recommended levels. Like all chemical agents, nutrients can produce adverse effects if intakes are excessive. There is no established benefit from consuming nutrients at levels above the RDA or AI. The DRIs for many nutrients are found in Tables 8.2, 8.6, and 8.7. For a personalized DRI report for your sex and life stage, visit the Interactive DRI website: http://fnic.nal.usda.gov/fnic/interactiveDRI.

Daily Values Because the DRIs are too cumbersome to use as a basis for food labels, the FDA developed another set of dietary standards, the **Daily Values**. The Daily Values are based on several different sets of guidelines and include standards for fat, cholesterol, carbohydrate, dietary fiber, and selected vitamins and minerals. The Daily Values represent appropriate intake levels for a 2000-calorie diet. The percent Daily Value shown on a food label shows how well that food contributes to your recommended daily intake. Food labels are described in detail later in the chapter.

Should You Take Supplements? The aim of the DRIs, the Dietary Guidelines for Americans, and MyPlate is to guide you in meeting your nutritional needs primarily with food, rather than with vitamin and mineral supplements. Supplements lack the potentially beneficial synergistic balance of nutrients, phytochemicals, and fiber that is found only in whole foods. Most Americans can get the vitamins and minerals they need by eating a varied, nutritionally balanced diet.

Over the past two decades, high-dose supplement use has been promoted as a way to prevent or delay the onset of many diseases, including heart disease and several forms of cancer. These claims remain controversial. According to the latest research, a balanced diet of whole foods—not high-dose supplementation—is the best way to promote health and prevent disease.

In setting the DRIs, the Food and Nutrition Board recommended supplements of particular nutrients for the following groups:

- Women who are capable of becoming pregnant should take 400 micrograms (µg) per day of folic acid (the synthetic form of the vitamin folate) from fortified foods and/or supplements in addition to folate from a varied diet. Research indicates that this level of folate intake will reduce the risk of neural tube defects. Enriched breads, flours, corn meals, rice, noodles, and other grain products are fortified with folic acid. Folate is found naturally in green leafy vegetables, legumes, oranges, and strawberries.

- People over age 50 should eat foods fortified with vitamin B-12, take B-12 supplements, or both to meet the majority of the DRI of 2.4 µg of B-12 daily. Up to 30% of people over 50 may have problems absorbing protein-bound B-12 in foods.

- Because of the oxidative stress caused by smoking, smokers should get 35 mg *more* vitamin C per day than the RDA set for their age and sex. However, supplements are not usually needed because this extra vitamin C can easily be found in foods. For example, an 8-ounce glass of orange juice has about 100 mg of vitamin C.

Supplements may also be recommended in other cases. Women with heavy menstrual flows may need extra iron. Older people, people with dark skin, and people exposed to little sunlight may need extra vitamin D. Some vegetarians may need supplemental calcium, iron, zinc, and vitamin B-12, depending on their food choices. Other people may benefit from supplementation based on their lifestyle, physical condition, medicines, or dietary habits.

Although dietary supplements are sold over the counter, the question of whether to take supplements is a serious one. Some vitamins and minerals are dangerous when ingested in excess, as described previously in Tables 8.4 and 8.5. Large doses of particular nutrients can also cause health problems by affecting the absorption of other vitamins and minerals or interacting with medications. For all these reasons, you should think carefully about whether to take high-dose supplements; and consult a physician or registered dietitian.

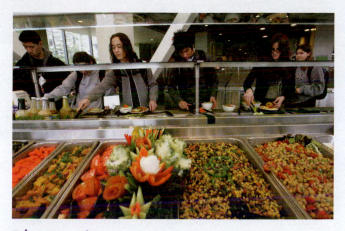

Fitness Tip A pound of body fat is equal to 3,500 calories. If you eat 100 calories more than you expend every day (36,500 extra calories), you will gain more than 10 pounds in a year. Food choices and portion control are key factors in weight management.

Dietary Guidelines for Americans

To provide general guidance for choosing a healthy diet, the USDA and the U.S. Department of Health and Human Services (DHHS) jointly issue the Dietary Guidelines for Americans, which are updated and revised every five years. The guidelines are supported by an extensive review of scientific and medical evidence. Following these guidelines promotes health and reduces the risk of chronic diseases, including heart disease, cancer, diabetes, stroke, osteoporosis, and obesity.

At the time this text was written, the final 2015 Guidelines were not yet released to the public. However, key findings from the 2015 Advisory Committee's Scientific Report, which is used to develop the Guidelines, included the following:

- About half of all American adults have one or more preventable chronic diseases that are related to poor eating habits and inactivity; these diseases include high blood pressure, type 2 diabetes, cardiovascular disease, and certain forms of cancer. Further increasing health risks is the fact that more than two-thirds of adults and nearly one-third of children and adolescents are overweight or obese.

- On average, Americans consume a dietary pattern that is too low in vegetables, fruits, and whole grains and too high in sodium, saturated fat, refined grains, added sugars, and calories. This dietary pattern is associated with increased risk for chronic diseases as well as underconsumption of essential nutrients.

- A healthy dietary pattern is higher in vegetables, fruits, whole grains, low-fat or fat-free dairy, seafood, legumes, and nuts; moderate in alcohol (for adults who consume alcohol); lower in red and processed meats; and low in refined grains and sugar-sweetened foods and drinks. There is no one best diet; people can combine foods in a variety of ways to create a healthy dietary pattern. Regular physical activity is also strongly recommended.

- People can make changes in eating and physical activity behaviors to help improve their lifestyles (see the box

Key recommendations for individuals and families from the 2015 Dietary Guidelines Advisory Committee Report include the following:

Take stock: Assess and monitor your health risks, set personal goals, and take action to promote positive lifestyle changes.

Focus on gradual and sustainable changes to achieve a healthy dietary pattern:

• Improve your food and menu choices, watch your portion sizes, and modify recipes and food preparation techniques.

• Include more vegetables, fruits, whole grains, seafood, nuts, legumes, low-fat or fat-free dairy or dairy alternatives. Choose foods without added sugars, fats, or salt.

• Reduce your consumption of red and processed meat, refined grains, added sugars, sodium, and saturated fat. Choose polyunsaturated fats, nontropical vegetable oils, and nuts in place of saturated fats and solid animal fats. Reduce added sugars by shifting beverage choices and limiting other sweetened processed foods. Limit saturated fat to 10% of total daily calories, added sugars to 10% of daily calories, and sodium to 2,400 mg per day (or 1,500 mg for those who would benefit from blood pressure lowering).

Move more and sit less: Achieve and maintain a healthy weight, and follow physical activity guidelines. Limit your sedentary activities, and get adequate sleep.

Be a positive force in your community: Help create and support community efforts and policy changes that promote healthy eating and activity patterns for all Americans—for example, creating safe places to exercise and making healthy food choices more widely available in low-income neighborhoods; changing food labeling and food manufacturing practices; and adding insurance coverage for nutritional counseling. Support efforts to reinforce healthy dietary and physical activity patterns for young children to help promote lifelong healthy habits.

SOURCE: Adapted from U.S. Department of Health and Human Services and U.S. Department of Agriculture. 2015. *Scientific Report of the 2015 Dietary Guidelines Advisory Committee.* Available from: http://www.health.gov/dietaryguidelines/2015-scientific-report.

"Making Positive Dietary Changes"). Individual changes should be supported by policies and programs targeting environmental factors that impact dietary choices—including things like nutrition standards, food labeling, and school lunch programs.

Healthy Dietary Patterns

The 2015 Dietary Guidelines Advisory Committee developed three general dietary patterns that can be used as the basis for creating a healthy diet (Table 8.8). All three dietary patterns are associated with reduced rates of chronic disease:

• Healthy U.S.-Style Pattern—an updated version of the existing USDA food pattern.

• Healthy Vegetarian Pattern—includes more legumes, processed soy products, nuts and seeds, and whole grains; it contains no meat, poultry, or seafood, but is close to the Healthy U.S.-Style Pattern in amounts of all other food groups.

• Healthy Mediterranean-Style Pattern—reflecting a dietary pattern associated with many cultures bordering the Mediterranean Sea, which includes more fruit and seafood and less dairy than the Healthy U.S.-Style Pattern.

All three patterns are based on amounts of food from different foods groups (and subgroups) according to energy intake. Also shared by all the patterns is the general principle that people should eat nutrient-dense foods—foods with significant amounts of vitamins, minerals, and other nutrients with relatively few calories, especially empty calories (solid fats and added sugars). See the Nutrition Resources section at the end of the chapter for a more detailed breakdown of the recommendations for the three healthy dietary patterns.

Too Little of This, Too Much of That

In addition to emphasizing dietary patterns, the Dietary Guidelines Advisory Committee identified nutrients that Americans tend to over- or under-consume. For example, we eat too much salt, added sugar, and saturated fat and too little of a number of vitamins and minerals. Selected nutrients of concern are described in the sections that follow.

ADDED SUGARS For the first time, the Advisory Committee recommended that Americans limit added sugars to no more than 10 percent of daily calories—roughly a quarter cup of sugar per day for someone consuming a 2,000-calorie diet (12 teaspoons = 1/4 c sugar = ~200 calories).

Americans consume 22 to 30 teaspoons (~1/2 to 5/8 cup) of added sugar daily, half of which comes from soda, juices, and other sugary drinks. The Committee suggested removing sugary drinks from schools and requiring a distinct line in food labels quantifying added sugars, a rule already proposed by the Food and Drug Administration that the food and sugar industries have aggressively fought. Individuals can choose to drink water in place of sugar-sweetened beverages.

FATS In keeping with the emphasis on overall dietary patterns, the Advisory Committee focused fat guidelines on limiting saturated and trans fats rather than reducing overall fat intake. Although saturated fats should be limited to less than 10% of total calories per day, individuals should focus on healthy replacements—unsaturated fats rather than refined carbohydrates and added sugars, which can worsen cardiovascular

Table 8.8 USDA Food Patterns at the 2000-Calorie Level

FOOD GROUP	HEALTHY U.S.-STYLE PATTERN	HEALTHY VEGETARIAN PATTERN	HEALTHY MEDITERRANEAN-STYLE PATTERN
Fruit	2 c per day	2 c per day	2-1/2 c per day
Vegetables	2-1/2 c per day	2-1/2 c per day	2-1/2 c per day
Legumes	1-1/2 c per wk	3 c per wk	1-1/2 c per wk
Grains	6 oz eq per day	6-1/2 oz eq per day	6 oz eq per day
Whole Grains	3 oz eq per day	3-1/2 oz eq per day	3 oz eq per day
Dairy	3 c per day	3 c per day	2 c per day
Protein Foods	5-1/2 oz eq per day	3-1/2 oz eq per day	6-1/2 oz eq per day
Meat	12-1/2 oz eq/wk	—	12-1/2 oz eq/wk
Poultry	10-1/2 oz eq/wk	—	10-1/2 oz eq/wk
Seafood	8 oz eq/wk	—	15 oz eq/wk
Eggs	3 oz eq/wk	3 oz eq/wk	3 oz eq/wk
Nuts/seeds	4 oz eq/wk	7 oz eq/wk	4 oz eq/wk
Processed soy	1/2 oz eq/wk	7 oz eq/wk	1/2 oz eq/wk
Oils	27 g per day	27 g per day	27 g per day

SOURCE: U.S. Department of Health and Human Services and U.S. Department of Agriculture. 2015. *Scientific Report of the 2015 Dietary Guidelines Advisory Committee*, Part D Chapter 1 Table D1.32; Appendix E-3, Tables E3.1.A1, A1, and A2. Available from: http://www.health.gov/dietaryguidelines/2015-scientific-report/.

health. Top sources of saturated fats in the American diet are regular cheese, pizza, grain- and dairy-based desserts, chicken, and meat products.

SODIUM The average daily American intake of sodium is about 3,400 mg, most of it coming from processed foods. Experts recommend that adults aim for no more than 2,300 mg of sodium a day, the amount in a teaspoon of salt, or the amount of salt you might consume if you ate a cup of soup with a turkey sandwich. Check food labels to identify foods high in sodium; limit the number and serving sizes of high-sodium foods to manage your overall sodium intake.

SHORTFALL NUTRIENTS Americans consume too few fruits, vegetables, whole grains, and low-fat dairy foods, which leads to lower-than-recommended intakes of a number of key nutrients. Deficits of calcium, vitamin D, potassium, and fiber are of particular concern because they are linked to adverse health outcomes. Iron is also of special concern for adolescent and premenopausal women because of the potential for iron deficiency. To increase intake of these nutrients, follow the recommendations in the healthy dietary patterns to consume a range of nutrient-dense choices within each food group.

Changing Perspectives The 2015 Advisory Committee Report retained many key recommendations from earlier Dietary Guidelines for Americans, especially the focus on fruits, vegetables, and whole grains. However, there were some differences from earlier Guidelines:

- *Dietary cholesterol:* The Committee chose to not bring forward a specific limit on dietary cholesterol, stating that there is no clear relationship between the amount of cholesterol in the diet and blood cholesterol levels. (Dietary

cholesterol is found only in animal foods, including eggs, chicken, beef, and dairy products.)

- *Caffeine:* The Committee looked at caffeine for the first time and stated that moderate amounts of coffee (3 to 5 cups per day or up to 400 mg caffeine) can be part of a healthy dietary pattern. Consistent evidence indicates that coffee consumption is associated with reduced risk of type 2 diabetes and cardiovascular disease in healthy adults, and possibly reduced risk of Parkinson's disease.

- *Sustainability:* The Committee also recommended consideration of sustainability in terms of environmental outcomes and food security. A healthy dietary pattern that is higher in plant-based foods and lower in calories and animal-based foods has a lower environmental impact—more favorable use of land, water, and energy and lower production of greenhouse gasses—than the current typical American dietary pattern.

A Culture of Health To support and encourage widespread healthy living in the United States, the Advisory Committee recommended the following actions:

- Establish local, state, and federal policies to make healthy foods accessible and affordable and to limit access to high-calorie, nutrient-poor foods and sugar-sweetened beverages in public buildings and facilities.

- Improve retail food environments and make healthy foods accessible and affordable in underserved neighborhoods and communities.

- Implement the comprehensive school meal guidelines (National School Lunch Program) from the USDA that increase intake of vegetables (without added salt), fruits (without added sugars), and whole grains.

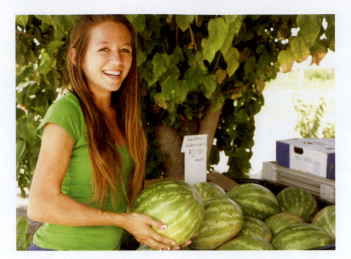

Wellness Tip Farmers' markets are an important way to bring healthy food choices to residents of inner cities. Support the establishment of farmers' markets in your community.

- Limit the marketing of unhealthy foods to children.
- Make drinking water freely available to students throughout the day.
- Ensure that competitive foods (i.e., vending machine foods and those sold on school grounds outside school meal programs) meet the Dietary Guidelines for Americans.
- Eliminate sugar-sweetened beverages from schools.
- Include amounts of added sugars in grams and tablespoons on Nutrition Facts labels.

USDA's MyPlate

To help consumers put the Dietary Guidelines for Americans into practice, the USDA also issues the food guidance system known as MyPlate. MyPlate is designed to allow individuals to take advantage of the customization made possible by the Internet (Figure 8.3).

Key Messages of MyPlate MyPlate reminds consumers to make healthy food choices and to be active every day. Key messages include the following:

- *Personalization* is an important element of the MyPlate program and the ChooseMyPlate.gov site, which includes individualized recommendations, interactive assessments of food intake and physical activity, weight-management tools, and tips for success.
- *Daily physical activity* is imperative for maintaining a healthy weight and reducing the risk of chronic disease.
- *Tracking and planning* are important tools to help find out what and how much to eat; track foods, physical activities, and weight; and personalize with goal setting, virtual coaching, and journaling. The *MyPlate SuperTracker* is

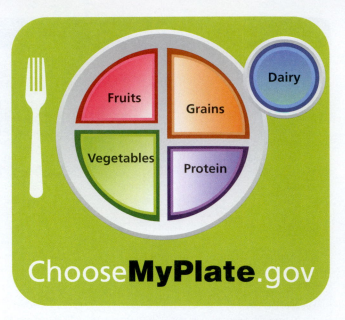

FIGURE 8.3 USDA's MyPlate. The USDA food guidance system, called MyPlate, can be personalized based on an individual's sex, age, and activity level; visit http://www.ChooseMyPlate.gov to obtain a food plan appropriate for you.
SOURCE: U.S. Department of Agriculture. 2011. *MyPlate.* (http://www.choosemyplate.gov; retrieved April 17, 2015).

a diet and physical activity planner that allows users to set personal calorie and physical activity goals and track progress.

Table 8.9 provides guidance for determining an appropriate calorie intake for weight maintenance. Use the table to identify an energy intake that is about right for you, and then refer to ChooseMyPlate.gov for personalized recommendations; healthy food patterns based on different calorie levels can also be found in the Nutrition Resources section at the end of the chapter. Each food group is described briefly in the following sections. Many Americans have trouble identifying serving sizes, so recommended daily intakes from each group are given in terms of cups and ounces; see the box "Judging Portion Sizes" for additional advice. MyPlate On Campus is an initiative to allow students to become ambassadors of healthy eating and healthy lifestyles. My Plate On Campus provides resources and practical guidelines for promoting health and wellness uniquely customized for students and campus lifestyle.

Whole and Refined Grains Grains are divided into two groups: *whole grains,* which contain the entire grain kernel, and *refined grains,* which have been milled to remove the bran and germ. Refining leaves a smoother texture and improves shelf life, but it also removes the dietary fiber, iron, and many B vitamins. Foods from this group are usually low in fat and rich in complex carbohydrates, dietary fiber (if grains are unrefined), and many vitamins and minerals. A 2,000-calorie diet should include 6-ounce-equivalent servings each day, and half of those servings should be whole grains, such as whole-grain bread,

Table 8.9	USDA Daily Calorie Intake Levels		
AGE (YEARS)	SEDENTARY*	MODERATELY ACTIVE**	ACTIVE†
FEMALE			
2–3	1000	1000–1200	1000–1400
4–8	1200–1400	1400–1600	1400–1800
9–13	1400–1600	1600–2000	1800–2200
14–18	1800	2000	2400
19–25	2000	2200	2400
26–30	1800	2000	2400
31–50	1800	2000	2200
51+	1600	1800	2000–2200
MALE			
2–3	1000	1000–1400	1000–1400
4–8	1200–1400	1400–1600	1600–2000
9–13	1600–2000	1800–2200	2000–2600
14–18	2000–2400	2400–2800	2800–3200
19–20	2600	2800	3000
21–25	2400	2800	3000
26–30	2400	2600	3000
31–35	2400	2600	3000
36–40	2400	2600	2800
41–45	2200	2600	2800
46–50	2200	2400	2800
51–55	2200	2400	2800
56+	2000–2200	2200–2400	2400–2600

*A lifestyle that includes only the light physical activity associated with typical day-to-day life.

**A lifestyle that includes physical activity equivalent to walking about 1.5–3 miles per day at 3–4 miles per hour (30–60 minutes a day of moderate physical activity), in addition to the light physical activity associated with typical day-to-day life.

†A lifestyle that includes physical activity equivalent to walking more than 3 miles per day at 3–4 miles per hour (60 or more minutes a day of moderate physical activity), in addition to the light physical activity associated with typical day-to-day life.

SOURCE: U.S. Department of Health and Human Services and U.S. Department of Agriculture. 2015. *Appendix E-3.1.A3. Energy levels used for assignment of individuals to USDA Food Patterns. Scientific Report of the 2015 Dietary Guidelines Advisory Committee.* (http://health.gov /dietaryguidelines/2015-scientific-report/15-appendix-e3/e3-1-a3.asp)

whole-wheat pasta, high-fiber cereal, or brown rice. The following count as 1-ounce-equivalent:

- 1 slice of bread
- 1 small (2½-inch diameter) muffin
- 1 cup ready-to-eat cereal flakes
- ½ cup cooked cereal, rice, grains, or pasta
- 1 6-inch tortilla

Choose foods that are typically made with little fat or added sugar (bread, rice, pasta) over those that are high in fat and added sugar (croissants, chips, cookies, doughnuts). The key message is to *make at least half your grains whole grains.*

Vegetables Vegetables contain carbohydrates, dietary fiber, and many other nutrients, and they are naturally low in fat. A 2,000-calorie diet should include 2½ cups of vegetables daily. Each of the following counts as ½ cup or equivalent of vegetables:

- ½ cup raw or cooked vegetables
- 1 cup raw leafy salad greens
- ½ cup vegetable juice

Because vegetables vary in the nutrients they provide, MyPlate recommends weekly servings from five different subgroups within the vegetables group. Choose vegetables from several subgroups each day. For clarity, MyPlate patterns show servings from the subgroups in terms of weekly consumption. For a 2,000-calorie diet:

- 1.5 cups per week *dark-green vegetables* (examples: broccoli, bok choy, romaine lettuce, spinach, collards, kale)
- 5.5 cups per week *red and orange vegetables* (tomatoes, carrots, sweet potatoes, red peppers, winter squash)
- 1.5 cups per week *legumes* (dried peas and beans—split and black-eyed peas; lentils; black, kidney, navy, pinto, white, and soy beans)
- 5 cups per week *starchy vegetables* (corn, potatoes, green peas)
- 4 cups per week *other vegetables* (artichokes, asparagus, beets, cauliflower, green beans, head lettuce, onions, mushrooms, zucchini)

The key message is to *fill half your plate with fruits and vegetables.*

Fruits Fruits are rich in carbohydrates, dietary fiber, and many vitamins, especially vitamin C. A 2,000-calorie diet should include 2 cups of fruits daily. Each of the following counts as ½ cup or equivalent of fruit:

- ½ cup fresh, canned, or frozen fruit
- ½ cup fruit juice (100% juice)
- ½ large (3½-inch diameter) whole fruit
- ¼ cup dried fruit

Choose whole fruits often; they are higher in fiber and often lower in calories than fruit juices. Fruit *juices* typically contain more nutrients and less added sugar than fruit *drinks.* Choose canned fruits packed in 100% fruit juice or water rather than in syrup. Again, MyPlate's key message for consumers is to *fill half your plate with fruits and vegetables.*

Dairy This group includes all milk and milk products such as yogurt and cheeses, as well as lactose-free and lactose-reduced products. Soymilk (calcium-fortified) is also part of the dairy group. Those consuming 2,000 calories per day should include 3 cups of milk or the equivalent daily. Each of the following counts as the equivalent of 1 cup:

- 1 cup milk or yogurt
- ½ cup ricotta cheese

Studies have shown that most people underestimate the size of their food portions, in many cases by as much as 50%. If you need to retrain your eye, try using measuring cups and spoons and an inexpensive kitchen scale when you eat at home. With a little practice, you'll learn the difference between 3 and 8 ounces of chicken or meat, and what a half-cup of rice really looks like. For quick estimates, use the following equivalents:

- 1 teaspoon of margarine = one die
- 1½ ounce of cheese = your thumb, four dice stacked together
- 3 ounces of chicken or meat = a deck of cards

- ½ cup of cooked rice, pasta, or potato = ½ baseball
- 1 cup of cereal flakes = a fist
- 2 tablespoons of peanut butter = a ping-pong ball
- 1 medium potato = a computer mouse
- 1–2-ounce muffin or roll = a plum or large egg
- 2-ounce bagel = a hockey puck or yo-yo
- 1 medium fruit (apple or orange) = a baseball
- ¼ cup nuts = a golf ball
- small cookie or cracker = a poker chip

- 1½ ounces natural cheese
- 2 ounces processed cheese

For the healthiest option and to limit calories and saturated fat in your diet, MyPlate's key message for consumers is to *switch to fat-free or low-fat (1%) milk* and dairy products.

Protein Foods (Meat and Beans) This group includes meat, poultry, fish, dried beans and peas, eggs, nuts, seeds, and processed soy products. A 2,000-calorie diet should include 5½ ounce-equivalents daily. Each of the following counts as equivalent to 1 ounce:

- 1 ounce cooked lean meat, poultry, or fish
- ¼ cup cooked beans (legumes) or tofu
- 1 egg
- 1 tablespoon peanut butter
- ½ ounce nuts or seeds

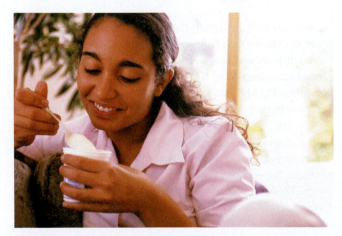

Wellness Tip Research shows that some protein-rich foods can give you a quick mental boost, which can be helpful before an exam.

Choose lean meats and skinless poultry, and watch your serving sizes carefully. Choose at least one serving of plant proteins, such as black beans, lentils, or tofu, every day. Include at least 8 ounces of cooked seafood per week and select a variety of protein foods to improve nutrient intake and health benefits.

Oils Oils and soft margarines include vegetable oils and soft vegetable oil table spreads that have no trans fats. These are major sources of vitamin E and unsaturated fatty acids, including the essential fatty acids. Oils and fats that are liquid at room temperature and come from many plants and fish sources are included in this list. A 2,000-calorie diet should include 6 teaspoons of oils per day. One teaspoon is the equivalent of the following:

- 1 teaspoon vegetable oil or soft margarine
- 1 tablespoon salad dressing or light mayonnaise

Foods that are mostly oils include nuts, olives, avocados, and some fish. The following portions include about 1 teaspoon of oil: 4 large olives, ½ medium avocado, 2 tablespoons peanut butter, and 1 ounce roasted nuts. Food labels can help you identify the type and amount of fat in various foods.

Solid Fats and Added Sugars If you consistently choose nutrient-dense foods that are fat-free or low-fat and that contain no added sugars, you can also have a small amount of additional calories in the form of solid fats and added sugars (SoFAS). For recommended limits on solid fats and added sugars for different calorie intakes, refer to your MyPlate program or to the dietary patterns in the Nutrition Resources section at the end of the chapter.

People who are trying to lose weight may choose not to use SoFAS calories. As described earlier, making better beverage choices is a key strategy for reducing intake of added sugars. Sodas, energy drinks, and sports drinks contribute added sugars but few nutrients to the American diet. The

Nutrient	Recommended Daily Intake* 2000 calories	Orange Juice 168 calories % Daily	Orange Juice Nutrient value	Low-Fat (1%) Milk 150 calories % Daily	Low-Fat (1%) Milk Nutrient value	Regular Cola 152 calories % Daily	Regular Cola Nutrient value	Bottled Iced Tea 150 calories % Daily	Bottled Iced Tea Nutrient value
Carbohydrate	300 g	14%	40.5 g	6%	18 g	13%	38 g	13%	37.5 g
Added sugars	32 g					119%	38 g	108%	34.5 g
Fat	65 g			6%	3.9 g				
Protein	55 g			22%	12 g				
Calcium	1000 mg	3%	33 mg	45%	450 mg	1%	11 mg		
Potassium	4700 mg	15%	710 mg	12%	570 mg	<1%	4 mg		
Vitamin A	700 µg	4%	30 µg	31%	216 µg				
Vitamin C	75 mg	193%	145.5 mg	5%	3.6 mg				
Vitamin D	5 µg			74%	3.7 µg				
Folate	400 µg	40%	160 µg	5%	20 µg				

Bars show percentage of recommended daily intake or limit

*Recommended intakes and limits appropriate for a 19-year-old woman consuming 2,000 calories per day.

FIGURE 8.4 Nutrient density of 12-ounce portions of selected beverages. Color bars represent percentage of recommended daily intake or limit for each nutrient.

differences in nutrients between soda and other beverages are shown in Figure 8.4. For those wanting to maintain weight, these calories may be used to increase the amount of food from a food group; to consume foods that are not in the lowest-fat form or that contain added sugars; to add oil, fat, or sugars to foods; or to consume alcohol.

The current American diet includes higher levels of calories in the form of solid fats and added sugars (SoFAS) than recommended.

Physical Activity Like the Dietary Guidelines and other plans, MyPlate encourages physical activity for improving health, preventing chronic diseases, and managing weight. If you meet the Department of Health and Human Services' guidelines of 150 minutes per week of moderate physical activity, you will meet the recommendations found in MyPlate. To get the most health benefits, choose moderate physical activity such as brisk walking, cycling, and dancing, or vigorous activity such as running, swimming, basketball, or aerobics.

DASH Eating Plan

Other food-group plans have been proposed by a variety of experts and organizations, some to address the needs of special populations. One well-studied alternative is DASH, which stands for Dietary Approaches to Stop Hypertension. As its name suggests, the DASH eating plan was developed to help people control high blood pressure and it is tailored with special attention to sodium, potassium, and other nutrients of concern for blood pressure. Refer to Figure 4 in the Nutrition Resources at the end of the chapter for more information on DASH.

The Vegetarian Alternative

Vegetarians choose a diet with one essential difference from the diets described previously—they eliminate or restrict foods of animal origin (meat, poultry, fish, eggs, milk). Many people choose such diets for health reasons; vegetarian diets tend to be lower in total calories and calories from fat, saturated fat, cholesterol, and animal protein and higher in complex carbohydrates, dietary fiber, potassium, folate, vitamins C and E, carotenoids, and phytochemicals. Some people adopt a vegetarian diet out of concern for the environment, for financial considerations, or for reasons related to ethics or religion. Individuals who follow a vegetarian diet generally have a lower body mass index than those who do not.

Types of Vegetarian Diets There are various vegetarian styles. The wider the variety of the diet eaten, the easier it is to meet nutritional needs.

- *Vegans* eat only plant foods.
- *Lacto-vegetarians* eat plant foods and dairy products.
- *Lacto-ovo-vegetarians* eat plant foods, dairy products, and eggs.

Others can be categorized as partial vegetarians, semivegetarians, or pescovegetarians. These people eat plant foods, dairy

> **vegetarian** Someone who follows a diet that restricts or eliminates foods of animal origin.
>
> **TERMS**

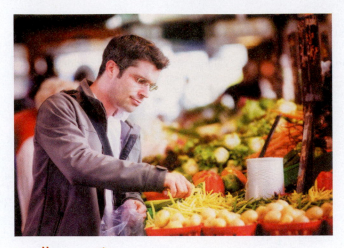

Wellness Tip Variety is the key to maintaining a healthy, balanced vegetarian diet. Choose nutrient dense foods rich in calcium, iron, zinc, and vitamins D and B-12.

products, eggs, and usually a small selection of poultry, fish, and other seafood. Many other people choose vegetarian meals frequently but are not strictly vegetarian. Including some animal protein (such as dairy products) in a mostly vegetarian diet makes meal planning easier, but it is not necessary.

A Food Plan for Vegetarians Table 8.8 outlines the USDA's Healthy Vegetarian diet plan. Also, MyPlate can be adapted for use by vegetarians with only a few key modifications (refer to Figure 2 in Nutrition Resources at the end of the chapter). For the meat and beans group, vegetarians can focus on the non-meat choices of dry beans and peas, nuts, seeds, eggs, and soy foods like tofu. Vegans and other vegetarians who do not eat or drink any dairy products must find other rich sources of calcium (see the following list). Fruits, vegetables, and whole grains are healthy choices for people following all types of vegetarian diets.

A healthy vegetarian diet, emphasizing a wide variety of plant foods, will supply all the essential amino acids. Choosing minimally processed and unrefined foods will maximize nutrient value and provide ample dietary fiber. Daily consumption of a variety of plant foods in amounts that meet total energy needs can provide all needed nutrients except vitamin B-12 and possibly vitamin D, calcium, iron, and zinc. Strategies for getting these and other nutrients include the following:

- *Vitamin B-12* is found naturally only in animal foods. If dairy products and eggs are limited or avoided, B-12 can be found in fortified foods such as ready-to-eat cereals, soy beverages, meat substitutes, special yeast products, and supplements.
- *Vitamin D* can be obtained by spending 5–15 minutes a day in the sun, by consuming vitamin D–fortified products like ready-to-eat cereals and soy or rice milk, or by taking a supplement.
- *Calcium* is found in legumes, tofu processed with calcium, dark-green leafy vegetables, nuts, tortillas made from lime-processed corn, fortified orange juice, soy milk, bread, and other foods.

- *Iron* is found in whole grains, fortified bread and breakfast cereals, dried fruits, leafy green vegetables, nuts and seeds, legumes, and soy foods. The iron in plant foods is more difficult for the body to absorb than the iron from animal sources. Eating or drinking a good source of vitamin C with most meals is helpful because vitamin C improves iron absorption.
- *Zinc* is found in whole grains, nuts, legumes, and soy foods.

If you are a vegetarian, remember that it's especially important to eat as wide a variety of foods as possible to ensure that all your nutritional needs are satisfied. Consulting with a registered dietitian will make your planning easier. Vegetarian diets for children, teens, and pregnant and lactating women warrant professional guidance.

Functional Foods

The American diet already contains numerous *functional foods.* Two of the earliest functional foods introduced in the United States were iodized salt and milk fortified with Vitamins A and D. More recently, manufacturers began fortifying breads and grains with folic acid to reduce the incidence of neural tube defects.

Although experts suggest that all foods are functional, functional foods are defined as foods to which health-promoting or disease-preventing components have been added. They include foods that are fortified, enriched, or enhanced or that contain dietary components with additional potential to benefit health. Some examples of functional foods are calcium-fortified orange juice, margarine enriched with sterols or stanols to lower the risk of heart disease, sports bars for energy and improved athletic performance, and vitamin B-12-enriched soy milk for vegetarians.

Dietary Challenges for Various Population Groups

MyPlate and the Dietary Guidelines for Americans provide a basis that nearly everyone can use to create a healthy diet. However, different population groups should be aware of special dietary challenges.

Children and Teenagers The best approach for parents with young children is to provide a variety of foods. For example, parents can add vegetables to casseroles and fruit to cereal, or they can offer fruit and vegetable juices or homemade yogurt or fruit shakes instead of sugary drinks. Many children and teenagers enjoy eating at fast-food restaurants, but they should be encouraged to select the healthiest menu choices and to balance the day's diet with low-fat, nutrient-rich foods. Allowing children to help prepare meals is another good way to encourage good eating habits.

College Students Foods that are convenient for college students are not always the healthiest choices. Students who

Eating Wherever

- Eat a colorful, varied diet. The more colorful your diet is, the more varied and rich in fruits and vegetables it will be. Fruits and vegetables are typically inexpensive, delicious, nutritious, and low in fat and calories.

- Eat breakfast. You'll have more energy in the morning and be less likely to grab an unhealthy snack later on.

- Choose healthy snacks—fruits, vegetables, whole grains, and cereals.

- Drink nonfat milk, water, mineral water, or 100% fruit juice more often than soft drinks or sweetened beverages.

- Pay attention to portion sizes.

- Combine physical activity with healthy eating.

Eating in the Dining Hall

- Choose a meal plan that includes breakfast.

- Decide what you want to eat before you get in line, and stick to your choices.

- Build your meals around whole grains and vegetables. Ask for small servings of meat and high-fat main dishes.

- Choose leaner poultry, fish, or bean dishes rather than high-fat meats and fried entrees.

- Ask that gravies and sauces be served on the side; limit your intake.

- Choose broth-based or vegetable soups rather than cream soups.

- At the salad bar, load up on leafy greens, beans, and fresh vegetables. Avoid mayonnaise-coated salads, bacon, croutons, and high-fat dressings. Put dressing on the side; dip your fork into it rather than pouring it over the salad.

- Choose fruit for dessert rather than cookies or cakes.

Eating in Fast-Food Restaurants

- Most fast-food chains can provide a brochure with the nutritional content of their menu items. Ask for it, or check the restaurant's website for nutritional information. Order small single burgers with no cheese instead of double burgers with many toppings. If possible, get them broiled instead of fried.

- Ask for items to be prepared without mayonnaise, tartar sauce, sour cream, or other high-fat sauces. Ketchup, mustard, and fat-free mayonnaise or sour cream are better choices and are available at many fast-food restaurants.

- Choose whole-grain buns or bread for sandwiches.

- Choose chicken items made from chicken breast, not processed chicken.

- Order vegetable pizzas without extra cheese.

- If you order french fries or onion rings, get the smallest size and/or share them with a friend. Better yet, get a salad or a fruit cup instead.

Eating on the Run

- When you need to eat in a hurry, remember that you can carry healthy foods in your backpack or a small insulated lunch sack (with a frozen gel pack to keep fresh food from spoiling).

- Carry items that are small and convenient but nutritious, such as fresh fruits or vegetables, whole-wheat buns or muffins, snack-size cereal boxes, and water.

- Make healthy choices at vending machines such as water or 100% fruit juice for beverages and whole grain crackers or pretzels, nuts, seeds, baked chips, low-fat popcorn, and low-fat granola bars as snacks.

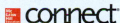

eat in buffet-style dining halls, cafeterias, and snack bars can easily overeat, and the foods offered are not necessarily high in nutrients or low in fat. The same is true of meals at fast-food restaurants. However, it is possible to make healthy eating both convenient and affordable. See the tips in the box "Eating Strategies for College Students."

Pregnant and Breastfeeding Women Good nutrition is essential to a healthy pregnancy. Nutrition counseling before conception can help a women establish a balanced eating plan and healthy body weight for a healthy pregnancy. During pregnancy and while breastfeeding, women have special nutritional needs. Pregnant or breastfeeding women are often advised to take a nutrient supplement in addition to following a special diet, as recommended by MyPlate's Daily Food Plan for Moms.

To reduce the risk of neural tube defects in the fetus, the U.S. Public Health Service recommends that all women of child-bearing age get 400 μg of folic acid daily from fortified foods or supplements.

Ask Yourself

QUESTIONS FOR CRITICAL THINKING AND REFLECTION

What factors influence your food choices—convenience, cost, availability, habit? Do you ever consider nutritional content or nutritional recommendations like those found in MyPlate? If not, how big a change would it be for you to think of nutritional content first when choosing food? Is it something you could do easily?

Older Adults Nutrient needs do not change much as people age, but because older adults tend to become less active, they don't need as many calories to maintain body weight. At the same time, the absorption of some nutrients tends to be lower in older adults because of age-related changes in the digestive tract. For these reasons, older adults should focus on eating nutrient-dense foods. For example, foods fortified with vitamin B-12 and/or B-12 supplements are recommended for people over age 50. Calcium and vitamin D intake can be inadequate; therefore, physicians may suggest supplementation to reduce bone loss and risk of osteoporosis. Antioxidants from fruits and vegetables are important in older adults to reduce age-related changes in vision and cognitive functioning. Because constipation is a common problem, consuming foods high in dietary fiber and drinking enough fluids are important goals.

Athletes Key dietary concerns for athletes are meeting increased energy and fluid requirements for training and making healthy food choices throughout the day. For more on this topic, see the box "Do Athletes Need a Different Diet?"

People with Special Health Concerns Many Americans have special health concerns that affect their dietary needs. For example, people with diabetes benefit from a well-balanced diet that is low in simple sugars, high in complex carbohydrates, and relatively rich in monounsaturated fats. People with high blood pressure need to limit their sodium consumption and control their weight. If you have a health problem or concern that may require a special diet, discuss your situation with a physician or registered dietitian.

NUTRITIONAL PLANNING: MAKING INFORMED CHOICES ABOUT FOOD

Knowing about nutrition is a good start to making sound choices about food. It also helps if you can interpret food labels, understand food additives, and avoid foodborne illnesses.

Food Labels

All processed foods regulated by either the FDA or the USDA include standardized nutrition information on their labels. Every food label shows serving sizes and the amount of many nutrients in each serving—including saturated fat, protein, dietary fiber, and sodium. In 2014, the FDA proposed significant changes to food labels, which may begin to take effect in 2016. See the box "Using Food Labels" for suggestions on what to look for on food labels, in both the current and proposed new formats.

Food label regulations also require that foods meet strict definitions if their packaging includes terms such as *light, low-fat,* or *high-fiber* (Table 8.10). Health claims such as "good source of dietary fiber" or "low in saturated fat" on packages are also regulated and can be signals that a product can be wisely included in your diet. Overall, the food label is an important tool to help you choose a healthy dietary pattern.

Food labels are not required on fresh meat, poultry, fish, fruits, and vegetables (many of these products are not packaged). You can get information on the nutrient content of these items from basic nutrition books, registered dietitians, nutrient analysis computer software, the Web, and the companies that

Table 8.10	Food Package Nutrient Claims
Healthy	A food that is low in fat, is low in saturated fat, has no more than 360–480 mg of sodium and 60 mg of cholesterol, and provides 10% or more of the Daily Value for vitamin A, vitamin C, protein, calcium, iron, or dietary fiber
Light or lite	33% fewer calories or 50% less fat than a similar product
Reduced or fewer	At least 25% less of a nutrient than a similar product; can be applied to fat ("reduced fat"), saturated fat, cholesterol, sodium, and calories
Extra or added	10% or more of the Daily Value per serving when compared to what a similar product has
Good source	10–19% of the Daily Value for a particular nutrient per serving
High, rich in, or excellent source of	20% or more of the Daily Value for a particular nutrient per serving
Low calorie	40 calories or less per serving
High fiber	5 grams or more of fiber per serving
Good source of fiber	2.5–4.9 grams of fiber per serving
Fat-free	Less than 0.5 gram of fat per serving
Low-fat	3 grams of fat or less per serving
Saturated or trans fat-free	Less than 0.5 gram of saturated fat and 0.5 gram of trans fatty acids per serving
Low saturated fat	1 gram or less of saturated fat per serving and no more than 15% of total calories
Low sodium	140 mg or less of sodium per serving
Very low sodium	35 mg or less of sodium per serving
Lean	Cooked seafood, meat, or poultry with less than 10 grams of fat, 4.5 grams or less of saturated fat, and less than 95 mg of cholesterol per serving
Extra lean	Cooked seafood, meat, or poultry with less than 5 grams of fat, 2 grams of saturated fat, and 95 mg of cholesterol per serving

NOTE: The FDA has not yet defined nutrient claims relating to carbohydrates, so foods labeled low- or reduced-carbohydrate do not conform to any approved standard.

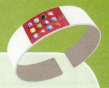

THE EVIDENCE FOR EXERCISE
Do Athletes Need a Different Diet?

If you exercise vigorously and frequently, or if you are an athlete in training, you likely have increased energy and fluid requirements. Research supports the following recommendations for athletes:

- **Energy intake:** Someone engaged in a vigorous training program may have energy needs as high as 6,000 calories per day—far greater than the energy needs of a moderately active person. For athletes, the Academy of Nutrition and Dietetics (formerly the American Dietetic Association) recommends a diet with 60–65% of calories coming from carbohydrates, 10–15% from protein, and no more than 30% from fat.

Athletes who need to maintain low body weight and fat (such as gymnasts, skaters, and wrestlers) need to get enough calories and nutrients while avoiding unhealthy eating patterns such as bulimia. The combination of low body fat, high physical activity, disordered eating habits—and, in women, amenorrhea—is associated with osteoporosis, stress fractures, and other injuries. If keeping your weight and body fat low for athletic reasons is important to you, seek dietary advice from a qualified dietitian and make sure your physician is aware of your eating habits.

- **Carbohydrates:** Endurance athletes involved in competitive events lasting longer than 90 minutes may benefit from increasing carbohydrate intake to 65–70% of their total calories. Specifically, the American College of Sports Medicine (ACSM) recommends that athletes consume 2.7–4.5 grams per pound of body weight daily, depending on their weight, sport, and other nutritional needs. This increase should come in the form of complex carbohydrates.

High carbohydrate intake builds and maintains glycogen stores in the muscles, resulting in greater endurance and delayed fatigue during competitive events. The ACSM recommends that before exercise an active adult or athlete eat a meal or snack that is relatively high in carbohydrates, moderate in protein, and low in fat and fiber. Eating carbohydrates 30 minutes, two hours, and four hours after exercise can help replenish glycogen stores in the liver and muscles.

- **Fat:** The ACSM recommends that all athletes get 20–35% of calories from fat in their diets. This is in line with the daily intake suggested by the Food and Nutrition Board. Reducing fat intake to less than 20% of daily calories can negatively affect performance and be harmful to health.

- **Protein:** For endurance and strength-trained athletes, the ACSM recommends eating 0.5–0.8 gram of protein per pound of body weight each day, which is considerably higher than the standard DRI of 0.36 gram per pound. This level of protein is easily obtainable from foods; in fact, most Americans eat more protein than they need every day. A balanced, moderate-protein diet can provide the protein most athletes need.

There is no evidence that consuming supplements containing vitamins, minerals, protein, or specific amino acids builds muscle or improves sports performance. Strength and muscle are built with exercise, not extra protein, and carbohydrates provide the fuel needed for muscle-building exercise.

- **Fluids:** If you exercise heavily or live in a hot climate, you should drink extra fluids to maximize performance and prevent heat illness. For a strenuous endurance event, prepare yourself the day before by drinking plenty of fluids. The ACSM recommends drinking 2–3 milliliters of fluid per pound of body weight about four hours before the event. During the event, take in enough fluids to compensate for fluid loss due to sweating; the amount required depends on the individual and his or her sweat rate. Afterward, drink enough to replace lost fluids—about 16–24 ounces for every pound of weight lost.

Water is a good choice for fluid replacement for events lasting 60–90 minutes. For longer workouts or events, a sports drink can be a good choice. These contain water, electrolytes, and carbohydrates and can provide some extra energy as well as replace electrolytes like sodium lost in sweat.

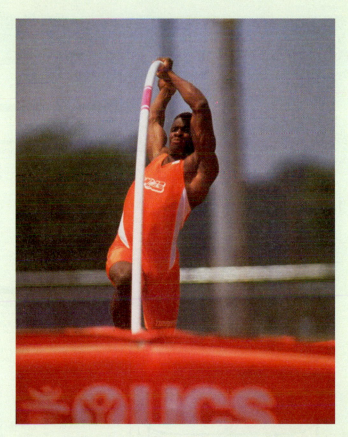

SOURCE: American College of Sports Medicine. 2009. *American College of Sports Medicine Position Stand: Nutrition and Athletic Performance.* (http://www.acsm-msse.org/pt/pt-core/template-journal/msse/media/0309nutrition.pdf, 2015 http://journals.lww.com/acsm-msse/Fulltext/2009/03000/Nutrition_and_Athletic_Performance.27.aspx).

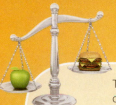

CRITICAL CONSUMER
Using Food Labels

The "Nutrition Facts" section of a food label is designed to help consumers make food choices based on the nutrients that are most important to good health. In addition to listing nutrient content by weight, the current label puts the information in the context of a daily diet of 2,000 calories that includes no more than 65 grams of fat (approximately 30% of total calories). For example, if a serving of a particular product has 13 grams of fat, the label will show that the serving represents 20% of the daily fat allowance. If your daily diet contains fewer or more than 2000 calories, you need to adjust these calculations accordingly.

Food labels use uniform serving sizes. This means that if you look at different brands of salad dressing, for example, you can compare calories and fat content based on the serving amount. Food label serving sizes may be larger or smaller than USDA serving size equivalents, however.

The current Nutrition Facts label has been in use since the 1990s. Based on research into how consumers use food labels as well as changes to the nutrients of most concern to Americans, the FDA has proposed changes to the look and content of the label. After it is finalized, you could begin to see the new style of labels on foods you purchase, but food manufacturers will have two years to change their labels. Some of the key proposed changes to the food label are the following:

- Requiring added sugars, vitamin D, and potassium on all labels
- Revising Daily Values for certain nutrients
- Updating serving size labeling for certain packages to be more realistic and to reflect amounts typically eaten at one time
- Refreshing the design to highlight calorie content and serving size and to make other parts of the label easier to read

SOURCES: U.S. Food and Drug Administration. 2015. Proposed Changes to the Nutrition Facts Label, http://www.fda.gov/Food/GuidanceRegulation/GuidanceDocumentsRegulatoryInformation/LabelingNutrition/ucm385663.htm. U.S. Food and Drug Administration. 2014. Factsheet on the New Proposed Nutrition Facts Label, http://www.fda.gov/Food/GuidanceRegulation/GuidanceDocumentsRegulatoryInformation/LabelingNutrition/ucm387533.htm.

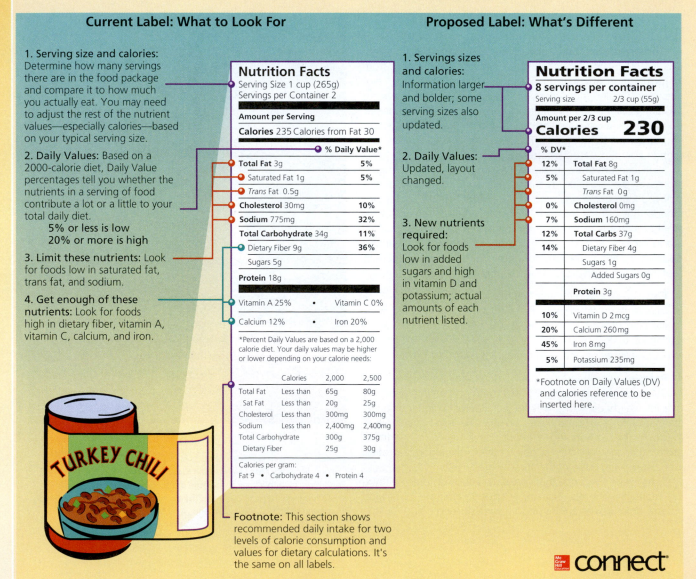

Current Label: What to Look For

1. Serving size and calories: Determine how many servings there are in the food package and compare it to how much you actually eat. You may need to adjust the rest of the nutrient values—especially calories—based on your typical serving size.

2. Daily Values: Based on a 2000-calorie diet, Daily Value percentages tell you whether the nutrients in a serving of food contribute a lot or a little to your total daily diet.
    5% or less is low
    20% or more is high

3. Limit these nutrients: Look for foods low in saturated fat, trans fat, and sodium.

4. Get enough of these nutrients: Look for foods high in dietary fiber, vitamin A, vitamin C, calcium, and iron.

Nutrition Facts
Serving Size 1 cup (265g)
Servings per Container 2

Amount per Serving

Calories 235 Calories from Fat 30

	% Daily Value*
Total Fat 3g	**5%**
Saturated Fat 1g	**5%**
Trans Fat 0.5g	
Cholesterol 30mg	**10%**
Sodium 775mg	**32%**
Total Carbohydrate 34g	**11%**
Dietary Fiber 9g	**36%**
Sugars 5g	
Protein 18g	

Vitamin A 25%	•	Vitamin C 0%	
Calcium 12%	•	Iron 20%	

*Percent Daily Values are based on a 2,000 calorie diet. Your daily values may be higher or lower depending on your calorie needs:

		Calories	2,000	2,500
Total Fat	Less than		65g	80g
Sat Fat	Less than		20g	25g
Cholesterol	Less than		300mg	300mg
Sodium	Less than		2,400mg	2,400mg
Total Carbohydrate			300g	375g
Dietary Fiber			25g	30g

Calories per gram:
Fat 9 • Carbohydrate 4 • Protein 4

Proposed Label: What's Different

1. Servings sizes and calories: Information larger and bolder; some serving sizes also updated.

2. Daily Values: Updated, layout changed.

3. New nutrients required: Look for foods low in added sugars and high in vitamin D and potassium; actual amounts of each nutrient listed.

Nutrition Facts
8 servings per container
Serving size   2/3 cup (55g)

Amount per 2/3 cup
Calories   **230**

% DV*	
12%	**Total Fat** 8g
5%	Saturated Fat 1g
	Trans Fat 0g
0%	**Cholesterol** 0mg
7%	**Sodium** 160mg
12%	**Total Carbs** 37g
14%	Dietary Fiber 4g
	Sugars 1g
	Added Sugars 0g
	Protein 3g
10%	Vitamin D 2mcg
20%	Calcium 260mg
45%	Iron 8mg
5%	Potassium 235mg

*Footnote on Daily Values (DV) and calories reference to be inserted here.

Footnote: This section shows recommended daily intake for two levels of calorie consumption and values for dietary calculations. It's the same on all labels.

TURKEY CHILI

McGraw Hill Education **connect**

produce or distribute these foods. Also, supermarkets may also have posters or pamphlets listing the nutrient contents of these foods. In Lab 8.3, you compare foods using the information on their labels.

Calorie Labeling: Restaurants and Vending Machines

In 2014, the FDA issued new regulations requiring that calorie information be provided on restaurant menus and vending machines; these new rules were required as part of the 2010 Affordable Care Act and are set to go into effect by December 2016. Calorie information is required on menus and menu boards in chain restaurants and similar retail food establishments (those with 20 or more locations). If no menus or boards are available, calories must be shown on signs near the foods. In addition, chain restaurants are also required to provide more detailed nutrition information on their menu items—on posters, tray liners, signs, handouts, or another similar location—so look for it!

Calorie labels are also now required for vending machine operators who own or operate 20 or more machines. Calories will be shown on a sign or digital display near the food items or selection button. Use the information to help consider your options and to monitor your calorie intake.

Dietary Supplements

Dietary supplements include vitamins, minerals, amino acids, herbs, enzymes, and other compounds. Although dietary supplements are sold over the counter and often thought of as safe and natural, they may contain powerful bioactive chemicals that have the potential for harm. About one-quarter of all pharmaceutical drugs are derived from botanical sources, and even essential vitamins and minerals can have toxic effects if consumed in excess.

In the United States, dietary supplements are not legally considered drugs and are not regulated like drugs. Before they are approved by the FDA and put on the market, drugs undergo clinical studies to determine safety, effectiveness, side effects and risks, possible interactions with other substances, and appropriate dosages. The FDA does not authorize or test dietary supplements, and manufacturers are not required to demonstrate either safety or effectiveness before they are marketed. Although dosage guidelines exist for some of the compounds in dietary supplements, dosages for many are not well established.

Large doses of some dietary supplements can cause health problems by affecting the absorption of certain vitamins or minerals or interacting with medications. Garlic supplements, for example, can cause bleeding if taken with anticoagulant (blood-thinning) medications. Some supplements can have side effects. St. John's wort, for example, increases the skin's sensitivity to sunlight and may decrease the effectiveness of oral contraceptives, drugs used to treat HIV infection, and many other medications. For this reason, ask your doctor or a dietitian before taking any high-dosage supplement.

There are also key differences in the way drugs and supplements are manufactured: FDA-approved medications are standardized for potency, and quality control and proof of purity are required. Dietary supplement manufacture is not as closely regulated, and there is no guarantee that a product contains a given ingredient at all, let alone in the appropriate amount. The potency of herbal supplements can vary widely due to differences in growing and harvesting conditions, preparation methods, and storage. Contamination and misidentification of plant compounds are also potential problems.

In an effort to provide consumers with more reliable and consistent information about supplements, the FDA has developed labeling regulations. Labels similar to those found on foods are now required for dietary supplements; for more information, see the box "Using Dietary Supplement Labels."

Food Additives

Today, approximately 3000 substances are intentionally added to foods to maintain or improve nutritional quality, to maintain freshness, to help in processing or preparation, or to alter taste or appearance. The most widely used additives in foods are sugar, salt, and corn syrup; these three, plus citric acid, baking soda, vegetable colors, mustard, and pepper, account for 98% by weight of all food additives used in the United States.

Food additives pose no significant health hazard to most people because the levels used are well below any that could produce toxic effects. Two additives of potential concern for some people are sulfites, used to keep vegetables from turning brown, and monosodium glutamate (MSG), used as a flavor enhancer. Sulfites can cause severe reactions in some people, and the FDA strictly limits their use and requires clear labeling on any food containing them. MSG may cause some people to experience episodes of sweating and increased blood pressure. If you have any sensitivity to an additive, check food labels when you shop and ask questions when you eat out.

Foodborne Illness

Many people worry about additives or pesticide residues in their food, but a greater threat comes from microorganisms that cause foodborne illnesses. Raw or undercooked animal products, such as chicken, hamburger, and oysters, pose the greatest risk, although in recent years contaminated fruits and vegetables have been catching up.

The Centers for Disease Control and Prevention (CDC) estimates that 48 million illnesses, 128,000 hospitalizations, and 3,000 deaths occur each year in the United States due to foodborne contaminants. One out of six people contract a foodborne disease each year. Symptoms include diarrhea, vomiting, fever, pain, headache, and weakness. Although the effects of foodborne illness are usually not serious, some groups, such as children, pregnant women, and elderly people, are more at risk for severe complications such as rheumatic diseases, seizures, blood poisoning, and death. Young children and older adults are more likely to have severe complications or to die

CRITICAL CONSUMER
Using Dietary Supplement Labels

Since 1999, specific types of information have been required on the labels of dietary supplements. In addition to basic information about the product, labels include a "Supplement Facts" panel, modeled after the "Nutrition Facts" panel used on food labels (see the figure below). Under the Dietary Supplement Health and Education Act (DSHEA) and food labeling laws, supplement labels can make three types of health-related claims:

- *Nutrient-content claims,* such as "high in calcium," "excellent source of vitamin C," or "high potency." The claims "high in" and "excellent source of" mean the same as they do on food labels. A "high potency" single-ingredient supplement must contain 100% of its Daily Value; a "high potency" multi-ingredient product must contain 100% or more of the Daily Value of at least two-thirds of the nutrients present for which Daily Values have been established.

- *Health claims,* if they have been authorized by the FDA or another authoritative scientific body. The association between adequate calcium intake and lower risk of osteoporosis is an example of an approved health claim. The FDA also allows so-called *qualified health claims* for situations in which there is emerging but as yet inconclusive evidence for a particular claim. Such claims must include qualifying language such as "scientific evidence suggests but does not prove" the claim.

- *Structure-function claims,* such as "antioxidants maintain cellular integrity" or "this product enhances energy levels." Because these claims are not reviewed by the FDA, they must carry a disclaimer (see the sample label).

Tips for Choosing and Using Dietary Supplements

- Check with your physician before taking a supplement. Many are not meant for children, older people, women who are pregnant or breastfeeding, people with chronic illnesses or upcoming surgery, or people taking prescription or over-the-counter medications. When you visit your doctor, bring a list of all dietary supplements you are taking. Do not take megadoses (more than double the daily recommended intake) without your doctor's approval.

- Follow the cautions, instructions for use, and dosage given on the label.

- Look for the United States Pharmacopeia (USP) verification mark on the label, indicating that the product meets minimum safety and purity standards developed under the Dietary Supplement Verification Program by the USP. The USP mark means that the product (1) contains the ingredients stated on the label, (2) has the declared amount and strength of ingredients, (3) will dissolve effectively, (4) has been screened for harmful contaminants, and (5) has been manufactured using safe, sanitary, and well-controlled procedures. The National Nutritional Foods Association has a self-regulatory testing program for its members; other, smaller associations and labs, including http://www.ConsumerLab.com, also test and rate dietary supplements.

- Choose brands made by nationally known food and drug manufacturers or "house brands" from large retail chains. Due to their size and visibility, such sources are likely to have high manufacturing standards.

- If you experience side effects, stop using the product and contact your physician. Report any serious reactions to the FDA's MedWatch monitoring program (1-800-FDA-1088 or online at http://www.fda.gov/Safety/MedWatch/default.htm).

For More Information about Dietary Supplements

ConsumerLab.Com: http://www.consumerlab.com

Food and Drug Administration: http://www.fda.gov/Food/DietarySupplements/default.htm

National Institutes of Health, Office of Dietary Supplements: http://ods.od.nih.gov

Natural Products Association: http://www.npainfo.org

U.S. Department of Agriculture: http://fnic.nal.usda.gov/nal_display/index.php?info_center=4&tax_level=1&tax_subject=274

U.S. Pharmacopeia: http://www.usp.org/USPVerified/DietarySupplements

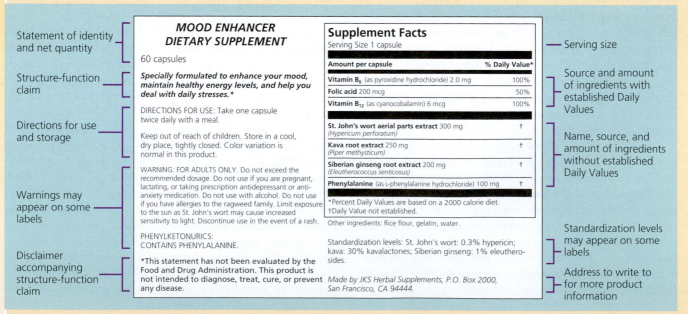

from foodborne illnesses. Thirteen percent of infections, 24% of hospitalizations, and 57% of deaths due to food-borne illnesses occurred among adults age 65 and over.

Causes of Foodborne Illnesses Most cases of food-borne illness are caused by **pathogens**, disease-causing micro-organisms that contaminate food, usually from improper handling. According to the CDC, 31 pathogens are known to cause foodborne illness, and the majority of illnesses, hospital-izations, and deaths are due to 8 pathogens, notably *Salmonella* (most often found in eggs, on vegetables, and on poultry); norovirus (most often found in salad ingredients and shellfish); *Campylobacter jejuni* (most often found in meat and poultry); *Toxoplasma* (most often found in meat); *Escherichia coli (E. coli)* O157:H7 (most often found in meat and water); *Listeria monocytogenes* (most often found in lunch meats, sausages, and hot dogs); and *Clostridium perfringens* (most often found in meat and gravy). The most frequent cause of infection was *Salmonella*, which accounted for 38% of reported infections. The second most frequent cause was *Campylobacter* (35%). *Vibrio* accounted for 1.3% of reported infections. Although the incidence of disease caused by food-borne bacteria, especially *Salmonella*, is slowly declining, approximately 80 people died as a result of food-borne illness in the United States in 2013.

Although pathogens are usually destroyed during cooking, the U.S. government is taking steps to bring down levels of contamination by improving national testing and surveillance. Raw meat and poultry products are now sold with safe-handling and cooking instructions, and all packaged, unpasteurized fresh fruit and vegetable juices carry warnings about poten-tial contamination. To ensure that the U.S. food supply is safe, the FDA Food Safety Modernization Act (FSMA) was signed into law on January 4, 2011, to reform the food safety system. The FSMA enables the FDA to focus more on preventing food safety problems rather than primarily on reacting to problems after they occur.

Although foodborne illness outbreaks associated with food-processing plants make headlines, most cases of illness trace back to poor food handling in the home or in restaurants. The FDA encourages people to follow four basic food safety principles:

- *Clean* hands, food contact surfaces, and vegetables and fruits.
- *Separate* raw, cooked, and ready-to-eat foods while shop-ping, storing, and preparing foods.
- *Cook* foods to a safe temperature.
- *Chill* (refrigerate) perishable foods promptly.

The FDA also advises people to avoid certain high-risk foods, including raw (unpasteurized) milk, cheeses, and juices; raw or undercooked animal foods, such as seafood, meat, poul-try, and eggs; and raw sprouts. These precautions are especially important for pregnant women, young children, older adults, and people with weakened immune systems or certain chronic diseases. For more information on food safety, see the box "Safe Food Handling."

Treating Foodborne Illness If you think you may be having a bout of foodborne illness, drink plenty of clear fluids to prevent dehydration, and rest to speed recovery. To pre-vent further contamination, wash your hands often and always before handling food until you recover. A fever higher than 102°F, blood in the stool, or dehydration deserves a physician's evaluation, especially if the symptoms persist for more than 2 to 3 days. In cases of suspected botulism—characterized by symptoms such as double vision, paralysis, dizziness, and vomiting—consult a physician immediately.

Irradiated Foods

Food irradiation is the treatment of foods with gamma rays, X-rays, or high-voltage electrons to kill potentially harmful pathogens, including bacteria, parasites, insects, and fungi that cause foodborne illness. It also reduces spoilage and extends shelf life. Even though irradiation has been generally endorsed by agencies such as the World Health Organization, the CDC, and the American Medical Association, few irradiated foods are currently on the market due to consumer resistance and skepticism. Studies indicate that when consumers are given information about the process of irradiation and the benefits of irradiated foods, most want to purchase them.

All primary irradiated foods (meat, vegetables, and so on) are labeled with the flowerlike radura symbol and a brief information label; spices and foods that are merely ingredients do not have to be labeled. Proper handling of irradiated foods is still critical for preventing foodborne illness.

Environmental Contaminants and Organic Foods

Contaminants are present in the food-growing environment. Environmental contaminants include various minerals, antibiotics, hormones, pesticides, and industrial chemicals. Safety regulations attempt to keep our exposure to contaminants at safe levels, but monitoring is difficult, and many substances (such as pesticides) persist in the environment long after being banned from use.

Organic Foods Some people who are concerned about pesticides and other environmental contaminants choose to buy foods that are **organic**. To be certified as organic, foods must meet strict production, pro-cessing, handling, and labeling criteria. Organic crops must meet limits on pesticide residues.

---

pathogen A microorganism that causes disease. **TERMS**

food irradiation The treatment of foods with gamma rays, X-rays, or high-voltage electrons to kill potentially harmful pathogens and increase shelf life.

organic A designation applied to foods grown and produced according to strict guidelines limiting the use of pesticides, nonorganic ingredients, hormones, antibiotics, genetic engineering, irradiation, and other practices.

TAKE CHARGE
Safe Food Handling

Shopping

- Don't buy food in containers that leak, bulge, or are severely dented. Refrigerated foods should be cold, and frozen foods should be solid.

- Check the food label for an expiration date and for safe-handling instructions.

- Place meat, poultry, and seafood in plastic bags, and separate foods in your grocery cart.

- Select cold and frozen foods last to ensure they stay refrigerated until just before checkout.

Storing Food

- Store raw meat, poultry, fish, and shellfish in containers in the refrigerator so the juices don't drip onto other foods. Keep these items away from other foods, surfaces, utensils, and serving dishes to prevent cross-contamination.

- Store eggs in the coldest part of the refrigerator, not in the door, and use them within three–five weeks.

- Keep hot foods hot (140°F or above) and cold foods cold (40°F or below); harmful bacteria can grow rapidly between these two temperatures. Refrigerate foods within two hours of purchase or preparation and within one hour if the air temperature is above 90°F. Freeze foods at or below 0°F. Use or freeze fresh meats within three–five days and fresh poultry, fish, and ground meat within one–two days. Use refrigerated leftovers within three–four days.

Preparing Food

- Thoroughly wash your hands with warm soapy water for 20 seconds before and after handling food, especially raw meat, fish, shellfish, poultry, or eggs.

- Make sure counters, cutting boards, dishes, utensils, and other equipment are thoroughly cleaned with hot soapy water before and after use. Wash dishcloths and kitchen towels frequently.

- Use separate cutting boards for meat, poultry, and seafood and for foods that will be eaten raw, such as fruits and vegetables. Replace cutting boards once they become worn or develop hard-to-clean grooves.

- Thoroughly rinse and scrub fruits and vegetables with a brush (but not with soap or detergent), or peel off the skin.

- Don't eat raw animal products, including raw eggs in homemade hollandaise sauce, eggnog, or cookie dough.

- Thaw frozen food in the refrigerator, in cold water, or in the microwave, not on the kitchen counter. Cook foods immediately after thawing.

Cooking

- Cook foods thoroughly, especially beef, poultry, fish, pork, and eggs; cooking kills most microorganisms. Use a food thermometer to ensure that foods are cooked to a safe temperature. Hamburgers should be cooked to 160°F. Turn or stir microwaved food to make sure it is heated evenly throughout.

- Cook stuffing separately from poultry; or wash poultry thoroughly, stuff immediately before cooking, and transfer the stuffing to a clean bowl immediately after cooking. The temperature of cooked stuffing should reach 165°F.

- Cook eggs until they're firm, and fully cook foods containing eggs.

- To protect against *Listeria,* reheat ready-to-eat foods like hot dogs and cold cuts until steaming hot.

- Because of possible contamination with *E. coli* 0157:H7 and *Salmonella,* avoid raw sprouts.

According to the USDA, "When in doubt, throw it out." Even if a food looks and smells fine, it may not be safe. If you aren't sure that a food has been prepared, served, and stored safely, don't eat it. For more information, visit Foodsafety.gov.

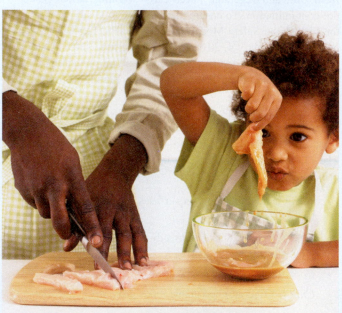

For meat, milk, eggs, and other animal products to be certified organic, animals must be given organic feed and access to the outdoors and may not be given antibiotics or growth hormones. The use of genetic engineering, ionizing radiation, and sewage sludge is prohibited. Products can be labeled "100% organic" if they contain all organic ingredients and "organic" if they contain at least 95% organic ingredients; all such products may carry the USDA organic seal. A product with at least 70% organic ingredients can be labeled "made with organic ingredients" but cannot use the USDA seal.

Organic foods, however, are not necessarily free of chemicals. They may be contaminated with pesticides used on neighboring lands or on foods transported in the same train or truck. However, they tend to have lower levels of pesticide residues than conventionally grown crops. Some experts recommend that consumers who want to buy organic fruits and vegetables spend their money on those that carry lower pesticide residues than their conventional counterparts (the "dirty dozen"): apples, bell peppers, celery, cherries, imported grapes, nectarines, peaches, pears, potatoes, red raspberries, spinach, and strawberries. Experts also recommend buying organic beef, poultry, eggs, dairy products, and baby food. Fruits and vegetables that carry little pesticide residue whether grown conventionally or organically include asparagus, avocados, bananas, broccoli, cauliflower, corn, kiwi, mangoes, onions, papaya, pineapples, and peas. All foods are subject to strict pesticide limits; the debate about the health effects of small amounts of residue is ongoing.

Whether organic foods are better for your health cannot be said for certain, but organic farming is better for the environment. It helps maintain biodiversity of crops and replenish the Earth's resources. It is less likely to degrade soil, contaminate water, or expose farm workers to toxic chemicals. As multinational food companies get into the organic food business, however, consumers who want to support environmentally friendly farming methods should look for foods that are not only organic but also locally grown.

Guidelines for Fish Consumption A specific area of concern has been possible mercury contamination in fish. Overall, fish and shellfish are healthy sources of protein, omega-3 fats, and other nutrients, and experts continue to encourage consumption of both wild-caught and farmed fish. Prudent choices can minimize the risk of any possible negative health effects. High mercury concentrations are most likely to be found in predator fish—large fish that eat smaller fish. Mercury can cause brain damage to fetuses and young children. According to FDA and Environmental Protection Agency (EPA) guidelines, women who are or who may become pregnant and nursing mothers should follow these guidelines to minimize their exposure to mercury:

- Do not eat shark, swordfish, king mackerel, or tilefish.
- Eat 8–12 ounces a week of a variety of fish and shellfish that are lower in mercury, such as shrimp, canned light tuna, salmon, pollock, and catfish. Limit consumption of albacore tuna to 6 ounces per week.

- Check advisories about the safety of recreationally caught fish from local lakes, rivers, and coastal areas. If no information is available, limit consumption to 6 ounces per week.

The same guidelines apply to children, although they should consume smaller servings.

A PERSONAL PLAN: APPLYING NUTRITIONAL PRINCIPLES

Based on your particular nutrition and health status, there probably is an ideal diet for you, but no single type of diet provides optimal health for everyone. Many cultural dietary patterns can meet people's nutritional requirements (see the box "Ethnic Foods"). Customize your food plan based on your age, gender, weight, activity level, medical risk factors, and personal tastes.

Assessing and Changing Your Diet

The first step in planning a healthy diet is to examine what you currently eat. Labs 8.1 and 8.2 help you analyze your current diet and compare it with optimal dietary goals. (This analysis can be completed using a nutritional analysis software program or one of several websites.)

To put your plan into action, use the behavioral self-management techniques and tips described in Chapter 1. If you identify several changes you want to make, focus on one at a time. You might start, for example, by substituting water for sugar-sweetened beverages. When you become used to that, you can try substituting whole-wheat bread for white bread. The information on eating behavior in Lab 8.1 will help you identify and change unhealthy patterns of eating.

Staying Committed to a Healthy Diet

Beyond knowledge and information, you also need support in difficult situations. Keeping to your plan is easiest when you choose and prepare your own food at home. Advance planning is the key: mapping out meals and shopping appropriately, cooking in advance when possible, and preparing enough food for leftovers. A tight budget does not necessarily make it difficult to eat healthy meals. It makes good health sense and good budget sense to use only small amounts of meat and to have a few meatless meals each week.

In restaurants, sticking to food plan goals becomes somewhat more difficult. Portion sizes in restaurants tend to be larger than MyPlate serving size equivalents, but by remaining focused on your goals, you can eat only part of your meal and take the rest home for a meal later in the week. Don't hesitate to ask questions when you're eating in a restaurant. Most restaurant personnel are glad to explain how menu selections are prepared and to make small adjustments, such as serving salad dressings and sauces on the side so they can be avoided or used sparingly.

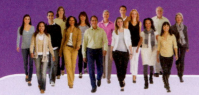

DIVERSITY MATTERS
Ethnic Foods

Every diet has advantages and disadvantages, and within each cuisine, some foods are more healthful choices. As the table below shows, the dietary guidelines described in this chapter can be applied to any ethnic cuisine.

	Choose More Often	Choose Less Often
Chinese	Dishes that are steamed, poached (jum), boiled (chu), roasted (kow), barbecued (shu), or lightly stir-fried Hoisin sauce, oyster sauce, wine sauce, plum sauce, velvet sauce, or hot mustard Fresh fish and seafood, skinless chicken, tofu Mixed vegetables, Chinese greens Steamed rice, steamed spring rolls, soft noodles	Fried wontons or egg rolls Crab rangoon Crispy (Peking) duck or chicken Sweet-and-sour dishes made with breaded and deep-fried meat, poultry, or fish Fried or crispy noodles Fried rice
French	Dishes prepared au vapeur (steamed), en brochette (skewered and broiled), or grillé (grilled) Fresh fish, shrimp, scallops, mussels, or skinless chicken, without sauces Clear soups	Dishes prepared á la créme (in cream sauce), au gratin or gratinée (baked with cream and cheese), or en croûte (in pastry crust) Drawn butter, hollandaise sauce, and remoulade (mayonnaise-based sauce)
Greek	Dishes that are stewed, broiled, or grilled, including shish kabobs (souvlaki) Dolmas (grape leaves) stuffed with rice Tzatziki (yogurt, cucumbers, and garlic) Tabouli (bulgur-based salad) Pita bread, especially whole wheat	Moussaka, saganaki (fried cheese) Vegetable pies such as spanakopita and tyropita Baba ghanoush (eggplant and olive oil) Deep-fried falafel (chickpea patties) Gyros stuffed with ground meat Baklava
Indian	Dishes prepared masala (curry), tandoori (roasted in a clay oven), or tikke (pan roasted); kabobs Raita (yogurt and cucumber salad) and other yogurt-based dishes and sauces Dal (lentils), pullao or pilau (basmati rice) Chapati (baked bread)	Ghee (clarified butter) Korma (meat in cream sauce) Samosas, pakoras (fried dishes) Molee and other coconut milk-based dishes Poori, bhatura, or paratha (fried breads)
Italian	Pasta primavera or pasta, polenta, risotto, or gnocchi with marinara, red or white wine, white or red clam, or light mushroom sauce Dishes that are grilled or prepared cacciatore (tomato-based sauce), marsala (broth and wine sauce), or piccata (lemon sauce) Cioppino (seafood stew) Vegetable soup, minestrone or fagioli (beans)	Antipasto (cheese, smoked meats) Dishes that are prepared alfredo, frito (fried), crema (creamed), alla panna (with cream), or carbonara Veal scaloppini Chicken, veal, or eggplant parmigiana Italian sausage, salami, and prosciutto Buttered garlic bread Cannoli
Japanese	Dishes prepared nabemono (boiled), shabu-shabu (in boiling broth), mushimono (steamed), nimono (simmered), yaki (broiled), or yakimono (grilled) Sushi or domburi (mixed rice dish) Steamed rice or soba (buckwheat), udon (wheat), or rice noodles	Tempura (battered and fried) Agemono (deep fried) Katsu (fried pork cutlet) Sukiyaki Fried tofu
Mexican	Soft corn or wheat tortillas Burritos, fajitas, enchiladas, soft tacos, and tamales filled with beans, vegetables, or lean meats Refried beans, nonfat or low-fat; rice and beans Ceviche (fish marinated in lime juice) Gazpacho, menudo, or black bean soup Fruit or flan for dessert	Crispy, fried tortillas Dishes that are fried, such as chile rellenos, chimichangas, flautas, and tostadas Nachos and cheese, chili con queso, and other dishes made with cheese or cheese sauce Refried beans made with lard Fried ice cream
Thai	Dishes that are barbecued, sautéed, broiled, boiled, steamed, braised, or marinated Sáte (skewered and grilled meats) Fish sauce, basil sauce, chili or hot sauces Bean thread noodles, Thai salad	Coconut milk soup Peanut sauce or dishes topped with nuts Mee-krob (crispy noodles) Red, green, and yellow curries, which typically contain coconut milk

Strategies like these are helpful, but small changes cannot change a fundamentally high-fat, high-calorie meal into a moderate, healthful one. Often, the best advice is to bypass a large steak with potatoes au gratin for a flavorful but low-fat entree. Many of the selections offered in ethnic restaurants are healthy choices (refer to the "Ethnic Foods" box for suggestions).

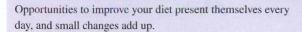

TIPS FOR TODAY AND THE FUTURE

Opportunities to improve your diet present themselves every day, and small changes add up.

RIGHT NOW YOU CAN

- Substitute a healthy snack for an unhealthy one.
- Drink a glass of water and put a bottle of water in your backpack for tomorrow.
- Plan to make healthy selections when you eat out, such as steamed vegetables instead of french fries or salmon instead of steak.

IN THE FUTURE YOU CAN

- Visit the MyPlate website at http://www.choosemyplate.gov and use the online tools to create a personalized nutrition plan and begin tracking your eating habits.
- Learn to cook healthier meals. There are hundreds of free websites and low-cost cookbooks that provide recipes for healthy dishes.

SUMMARY

- The six classes of nutrients are proteins, fats, carbohydrates, vitamins, minerals, and water.

- The nutrients essential to humans are released into the body through digestion. Nutrients in foods provide energy, measured in kilocalories (commonly called calories), build and maintain body tissues, and regulate body functions.

- Protein, an important component of body tissue, is composed of amino acids; nine are essential to good health. Foods from animal sources provide complete proteins. Plants provide incomplete proteins.

- Fats, a major source of energy, also insulate the body and cushion the organs. Just 3–4 teaspoons of vegetable oil per day supply the essential fats. Unsaturated fats should be favored over saturated fats. Trans fats should be avoided.

- Carbohydrates provide energy to the brain, nervous system, and blood and to muscles during high-intensity exercise. Naturally occurring simple carbohydrates and unrefined complex carbohydrates should be favored over added sugars and refined carbohydrates.

- Fiber includes plant substances that are impossible for the human body to digest. It helps reduce cholesterol levels and promotes the passage of wastes through the intestines.

- The 13 essential vitamins are organic substances that promote specific chemical and cell processes and act as antioxidants. The 17 known essential minerals are inorganic substances that regulate body functions, aid in growth and tissue maintenance, and help in the release of energy from food. Deficiencies in vitamins and minerals can cause severe symptoms over time, but excess doses are also dangerous.

- Water aids in digestion and food absorption, allows chemical reactions to take place, serves as a lubricant or cushion, and helps regulate body temperature.

- Foods contain other substances, such as phytochemicals, that may not be essential nutrients but that may protect against chronic diseases.

- The Dietary Reference Intakes, Dietary Guidelines for Americans, and MyPlate food guidance system provide standards and recommendations for getting all essential nutrients from a varied, balanced diet and for eating in ways that protect against chronic disease.

- The Dietary Guidelines for Americans advise us to reduce consumption of sodium, solid fats, added sugars, and refined grains; increase consumption of fruits, vegetables, and whole grains; and follow a healthy eating pattern.

- Choosing the right amount of foods from each group in MyPlate every day helps ensure the appropriate amounts of calories and necessary nutrients.

- A vegan diet requires special planning but can meet all human nutritional needs.

- Different population groups, such as college students and athletes, face special dietary challenges and should plan their diets to meet their particular needs.

- Consumers can get help applying nutritional principles by reading the standardized labels that appear on all packaged foods and on dietary supplements.

- Although nutritional basics are well established, no single diet provides wellness for everyone. Individuals should focus on their particular needs and adapt general dietary principles to meet them.

FOR FURTHER EXPLORATION

Academy of Nutrition and Dietetics. Provides a wide variety of educational materials on nutrition.
http://www.eatright.org

American Heart Association: Delicious Decisions. Provides basic information about nutrition, tips for shopping and eating out, and heart-healthy recipes.
http://www.heart.org/HEARTORG/GettingHealthy/NutritionCenter/Recipes/Delicious-Decisions-Cookbooks-and-Recipes-from-American-Heart-Association_UCM_452733_SubHomePage.jsp

COMMON QUESTIONS ANSWERED

Q **MyPlate recommends such large amounts of vegetables and fruit. How can I possibly eat that many servings without gaining weight?**

A First, consider your typical portion sizes; you may be closer to meeting the recommendations than you think. Many people consume large servings of foods and underestimate the size of their portions. For example, a large banana may contain the equivalent of a cup of fruit. Likewise, a small salad may easily contain one cup of leafy greens and count as one-half cup of vegetables. Use a measuring cup or a food scale for a few days to train your eye to accurately estimate food portion sizes. The http://www.ChooseMyPlate.gov website includes charts of portion-size equivalents for each food group.

If you need to increase your overall intake of fruits and vegetables, look for healthy substitutions. If you are like most Americans, you are consuming more than the recommended number of calories from added sugars and solid fats; trim some of these calories to make room for additional servings of fruits and vegetables. Your beverage choices may be a good place to start. Do you routinely consume regular sodas, sweetened energy or fruit drinks, or whole milk? One regular 12-ounce soda contains the equivalent of about 150 calories of added sugars; an 8-ounce glass of whole milk provides about 75 calories as discretionary fats. Substituting water or low-fat milk would free up calories for additional servings of fruits and vegetables. A half-cup of carrots, tomatoes, apples, or melon has only about 25 calories; you could consume six cups of these foods for the calories in one can of regular soda. Substituting lower-fat condiments for full-fat butter, mayonnaise, and salad dressing is another good way to trim calories to make room for additional servings of nutrient-rich fruits and vegetables.

Also consider your portion sizes and/or the frequency with which you consume foods high in discretionary calories: You may not need to eliminate a favorite food—instead, just cut back. For example, cut your consumption of fast-food fries from four times a week to once a week, or reduce the size of your ice cream dessert from a cup to one-half cup. Treats should be consumed infrequently and in small amounts.

For additional help on improving food choices to meet dietary recommendations, visit http://www.ChooseMyPlate.gov and the family-friendly chart of "We Can! Go, Slow, and Whoa" foods at the site for the National Heart, Lung, and Blood Institute (http://www.nhlbi.nih.gov/health/public/heart/obesity/wecan/downloads/gswtips.pdf).

Q **What exactly are genetically modified foods? Are they safe? How can I recognize them on the shelf, and how can I know when I'm eating them?**

A Genetic engineering involves altering the characteristics of a plant, animal, or microorganism by adding, rearranging, or replacing genes in its DNA; the result is a genetically modified (GM) organism. New DNA may come from related species of organisms or from entirely different types of organisms. Many GM crops are already grown in the United States: About 94% of the current U.S. soybean crop and more than 79% of the cotton crop has been genetically modified. Products made with GM organisms include juice, soda, nuts, tuna, frozen pizza, spaghetti sauce, canola oil, chips, salad dressing, and soup.

The potential benefits of GM foods cited by supporters include improved yields overall and in difficult growing conditions, increased disease resistance, improved nutritional content, lower prices, and less use of pesticides. Critics of biotechnology argue that unexpected effects may occur: Gene manipulation could elevate levels of naturally occurring toxins or

FDA: Food. Offers information and interactive tools about topics such as food labeling, food additives, dietary supplements, and foodborne illness.
http://www.fda.gov/food/default.htm

Food Safety Hotlines. Provide information on the safe purchase, handling, cooking, and storage of food.
1-888-723-3366

Forks over Knives. Shares articles by doctors from Cleveland Clinic and Cornell on plant-based diets; also includes recipe ideas.
http://www.forksoverknives.com

Fruits and Veggies—More Matters. Hosted by the Produce for Better Health Foundation; promotes the consumption of fruits and vegetables every day.
http://www.fruitsandveggiesmorematters.org/

Gateways to Government Nutrition Information. Provides access to government resources relating to food safety, including consumer advice and information on specific pathogens.

http://www.foodsafety.gov
http://www.nutrition.gov

Harvard School of Public Health: The Nutrition Source. Provides knowledge for healthy eating, including advice on interpreting news on nutrition; and suggestions for building a healthy diet.
http://www.hsph.harvard.edu/nutritionsource

International Food Information Council. Food Insight. Provides information on food safety and nutrition for consumers, journalists, and educators.
http://www.foodinsight.org/

MedlinePlus: Nutrition. Provides links to information from government agencies and major medical associations on a variety of nutrition topics.
http://www.nlm.nih.gov/medlineplus/nutrition.html

MyPlate. Provides personalized dietary plans and interactive food and activity tracking tools.
http://www.choosemyplate.gov

allergens, permanently change the gene pool and reduce biodiversity, and produce pesticide-resistant insects through the transfer of genes. In 2000, a form of GM corn approved for use only in animal feed was found to have commingled with other varieties of corn and to have been used in human foods; this mistake sparked fears of allergic reactions and led to recalls. Opposition to GM foods is particularly strong in Europe; in many developing nations that face food shortages, responses to GM crops have tended to be more positive.

In April 2000, the National Academy of Sciences released a report stating that there is no proof that GM food on the market is unsafe but that changes are needed to better coordinate regulation of GM foods and to assess potential problems.

At the time this text was written, the National Academy report was scheduled to be updated in 2016.

Labeling has been another major concern. Surveys indicate that the majority of Americans want to know if their foods contain GM organisms. However, under current rules, the FDA requires special labeling only when a food's composition is changed significantly or when a known allergen is introduced. For example, soybeans that contain a gene from a peanut would have to be labeled because peanuts are a common allergen. The only foods guaranteed not to contain GM ingredients are those certified as organic.

Q How can I tell if I'm allergic to a food?

A A true food allergy is a reaction of the body's immune system to a food or food ingredient, usually a protein. This immune reaction can occur within minutes of ingesting the food, resulting in symptoms such as hives, diarrhea, difficulty breathing, or swelling of the lips or tongue. The most severe response is a systemic reaction called anaphylaxis, which involves a potentially life-threatening drop in blood pressure. Food allergies affect only about 2% of the adult population and approximately 5% of infants and young children. People with food allergies, especially children, are more likely to have asthma or other allergic conditions.

Just eight foods account for more than 90% of the food allergies in the United States: cow's milk, eggs, peanuts, tree nuts (walnuts, cashews, and so on), soy, wheat, fish, and shellfish. Food manufacturers are now required to state the presence of these eight allergens in plain language in the list of ingredients on food labels.

Many people who believe they have food allergies may actually suffer from a food intolerance, a much more common source of adverse food reactions that typically involves problems with metabolism rather than with the immune system. The body may not be able to adequately digest a food or the body may react to a particular food compound. Food intolerances have been attributed to lactose (milk sugar), gluten (a protein in some grains), tartrazine (yellow food coloring), sulfite (a food additive), MSG, and the sweetener aspartame. Although symptoms of a food intolerance may be similar to those of a food allergy, they are typically more localized and not life-threatening. Many people with food intolerance can safely and comfortably consume small amounts of the food that affects them.

If you suspect you have a food allergy or intolerance, a good first step is to keep a food diary. Note everything you eat or drink, any symptoms you develop, and how long after eating the symptoms appear. Then make an appointment with your physician to go over your diary and determine if any additional tests are needed. People at risk for severe allergic reactions must diligently avoid trigger foods and carry medications to treat anaphylaxis.

SOURCE FOR REVISED DATA: Tables at http://www.ers.usda.gov/data-products/adoption-of-genetically-engineered-crops-in-the-us.aspx

---

National Academies' Food and Nutrition Board. Provides information about the Dietary Reference Intakes and related guidelines.
   http://www.iom.edu/About-IOM/Leadership-Staff/Boards/Food-and-Nutrition-Board.aspx

National Institutes of Health: Osteoporosis and Related Bone Diseases' National Resource Center. Provides information about osteoporosis prevention and treatment; includes a special section on men and osteoporosis.
   http://www.niams.nih.gov/Health_Info/Bone/

National Osteoporosis Foundation. Provides information on the causes, prevention, detection, and treatment of osteoporosis.
   http://www.nof.org

USDA Center for Nutrition Policy and Promotion. Includes information on the Dietary Guidelines and MyPlate.
   http://www.cnpp.usda.gov

USDA Food and Nutrition Information Center. Provides a variety of materials relating to the Dietary Guidelines, food labels, MyPlate, and many other topics.
   http://www.nal.usda.gov/fnic

USDA Hotline. Use this hotline for questions about meat and poultry.
   800-535-4555

Vegetarian Resource Group. Provides information and links for vegetarians and people interested in learning more about vegetarian diets.
   http://www.vrg.org

USDA Nutrient Data Laboratory Provides nutrient breakdowns of individual food items.
   http://www.ars.usda.gov/ba/bhnrc/ndl

See also the resources listed in Chapters 9, 11, and 12.

Adebamowo, S. N., et al. 2015. Association between intakes of magnesium, potassium, and calcium and risk of stroke: 2 cohorts of US women and updated meta-analyses. *American Journal of Clinical Nutrition* 101(6): 1269–1277.

American Diabetes Association. 2013. *Glycemic Index and Diabetes.* (http://www.diabetes.org/food-and-fitness/food/planning-meals/glycemic-index-and-diabetes.html?keymatch=glycemic-index; retrieved April 16, 2015).

American Dietetic Association. 2009. Position of the American Dietetic Association: functional foods. *Journal of the American Dietetic Association* 109(4): 735–746.

American Heart Association. 2010. *Fish and Omega-3 Fatty Acids.* (http://www.heart.org/HEARTORG/GettingHealthy/NutritionCenter/HealthyDietGoals/Fish-and-Omega-3-Fatty-Acids_UCM_303248_Article.jsp; retrieved April 20, 2015).

American Heart Association. 2010. *Trans Fats.* (http://www.heart.org/HEARTORG/GettingHealthy/FatsAndOils/Fats101/Trans-Fats_UCM_301120_Article.jsp; retrieved April 22, 2015).

American Heart Association. 2014. *Science Advisory: Omega-6 Fatty Acids.* (http://www.heart.org/HEARTORG/GettingHealthy/FatsAndOils/Fats101/Omega-6-Fatty-Acids---Science-Advisory_UCM_306808_Article.jsp, April 20, 2015).

American Heart Association. 2015. *Diet and Lifestyle Recommendations.* (http://www.heart.org/HEARTORG/GettingHealthy/Diet-and-Lifestyle-Recommendations_UCM_305855_Article.jsp, April 20, 2015).

Bernstein, M., Munoz, N. August 2012. Position of the Academy of Nutrition and Dietetics: food and nutrition for older adults: promoting health and wellness. *Journal of the Academy of Nutrition and Dietetics* 112(8): 1255–1277. doi: 10.1016/j.jand.2012.06.015.

Byrd-Bredbenner, C., et al. 2012. *Wardlaw's Perspectives in Nutrition,* 9th ed. New York: McGraw-Hill Education.

Carlsen, M. H., et al. January 2010. The total antioxidant content of more than 3100 foods, beverages, spices, herbs and supplements used worldwide. *Nutrition Journal* 9:3. doi: 10.1186/1475-2891-9-3.

Centers for Disease Control and Prevention. 2014. *Estimates of Foodborne Illness in the United States.* (http://www.cdc.gov/foodborneburden/index.html; retrieved April 20, 2015).

Centers for Disease Control and Prevention. 2015. *Food Safety.* (http://www.cdc.gov/foodsafety/; April 20).

Centers for Disease Control and Prevention. 2014. *Incidence and Trends of Foodborne Illness, 2013.* (http://www.cdc.gov/features/dsfoodnet/, April 20, 2015).

Centers for Disease Control and Prevention. 2015. *Listeria (Listeriosis).* (http://www.cdc.gov/listeria/, April 20, 2015).

Centers for Disease Control and Prevention. 2015. *Salt.* (http://www.cdc.gov/salt/, April 20, 2015).

Chowdhury, R., et al. 2014. Association of dietary, circulating, and supplement fatty acids with coronary risk: A systematic review and metaanalysis. *Annals of Internal Medicine* 160(6): 398–406.

Coleman-Jensen, A., et al. 2012. *Household Food Security in the United States in 2011. Economic Research Report No. (ERR-141), September.* (http://www.ers.usda.gov/publications/err-economic-research-report/err141.aspx, April 20, 2015).

Council for Responsible Nutrition. 2009. *Dietary Supplements: Safe, Regulated and Beneficial.* (http://www.crnusa.org/pdfs/CRN_FACT_DSSafeRegulatedBeneficial_09.pdf, April 20, 2015).

Delgado-Lista, J., et. al. June 2012. Long chain omega-3 fatty acids and cardiovascular disease: a systematic review. *British Journal of Nutrition* 107(Suppl 2): S201–13. doi: 10.1017/S0007114512001596.

Duyff, R. L. 2012. *ADA Complete Food and Nutrition Guide,* 4th ed. Hoboken, N.J.: Wiley.

Eckel R. H., et al. 2013. AHA/ACC Guideline on Lifestyle Management to Reduce Cardiovascular Risk: A Report of the American College of Cardiology/American Heart Association Task Force on Practice Guidelines. *Journal of the American College of Cardiology* 63 (25_PA).

El Khoury, D. et al. 2012. Beta glucan: health benefits in obesity and metabolic syndrome. *Journal of Nutrition and Metabolism,* Article ID 851362. doi:10.1155/2012/851362.

Estruch R., et al. April 2013. Primary prevention of cardiovascular disease with a Mediterranean diet. *New England Journal of Medicine* 368(14): 1279–90. doi: 10.1056/NEJMoa1200303. Epub February 25, 2013.

Fitch C., Keim, K. S.; Academy of Nutrition and Dietetics. May 2012. *Position of the Academy of Nutrition and Dietetics: use of nutritive and nonnutritive sweeteners. Journal of the Academy of Nutrition and Dietetics* 112(5): 739–758. doi: 10.1016/j.jand.2012.03.009. Epub April 25, 2012.

Food and Nutrition Board, Institute of Medicine. 2005. *Dietary Reference Intakes for Energy, Carbohydrate, Fiber, Fat, Fatty Acids, Cholesterol, Protein, and Amino Acids.* Washington, D.C.: National Academy Press.

Food and Nutrition Board, Institute of Medicine. 2005. *Dietary Reference Intakes for Water, Potassium, Sodium, Chloride, and Sulfate.* Washington, D.C.: National Academy Press.

Giacosa A., et al. January 2013. Cancer prevention in Europe: the Mediterranean diet as a protective choice. *European Journal of Cancer Prevention* 22(1): 90–5. doi: 10.1097/CEJ.0b013e328354d2d7.

Grisenbeck, J. S., et al. 2010. Maternal characteristics associated with the dietary intake of nitrates, nitrites, and nitrosamines in women of childbearing age: a cross-sectional study. *Environmental Health* 9(1): 10.

Han, E., and Powell, L. M. January 2013. Consumption patterns of sugar-sweetened beverages in the United States. *Journal of the Academy of Nutrition and Dietetics* 113(1): 43–53. doi: 10.1016/j.jand.2012.09.016.

Hasler, C. M., et al. 2009. Position of the American Dietetic Association: functional foods. *Journal of the American Dietetic Association* 109(4): 735–736.

Hooper, L., et al. 2015. Reduction in saturated fat intake for cardiovascular disease. *Cochrane Database of Systematic Reviews* 6:CD011737.

Insel, P., et al. 2014. *Nutrition,* 5th ed. Burlington, Mass.: Jones & Bartlett.

Jalonick, M. C. 2015. Major shift in new federal dietary guidelines proposed. *Huffpost* February 19, 2015. (http://www.huffingtonpost.com/2015/02/19/federal-dietary-guidelines_n_6716130.html).

Katz, D. L., and S. Meller. 2014. Can we say what diet is best for health? *Annual Review of Public Health* 35: 83–103.

Kiage, J. N., et al. 2013. Trans fat intake and all-cause mortality in the Reasons for Geographical and Racial Differences in Stroke (REGARDS) cohort. *American Journal of Clinical Nutrition* 97: 1121–1128.

Liu, R., et al. 2012. Caffeine intake, smoking, and risk of Parkinson disease in men and women. *American Journal of Epidemiology* 175(11): 1200–1207.

Maki, K. C., et al. 2010. Whole-grain ready-to-eat oat cereal, as part of a dietary program for weight loss, reduces low-density lipoprotein cholesterol in adults with overweight and obesity more than a dietary program including low-fiber control foods. *Journal of the American Dietetic Association* 110(2): 205–214.

Mayo Clinic. 2015. *Pyramid or plate? Explore These Healthy Diet Options Updated June 18, 2011.* (http://www.mayoclinic.com/health/healthy-diet/NU00190, April 20, 2015).

Miller, P. E., and Snyder, D. C. October 2012. Phytochemicals and cancer risk: a review of the epidemiological evidence. *Nutrition in Clinical Practice* 27(5): 599–612. doi: 10.1177/0884533612456043. Epub August 9, 2012.

Nestle, M. 2007. *What to Eat.* New York: North Point Press.

Okarter N., and Liu, R. H. March 2010. Health benefits of whole grain phytochemicals. *Critical Reviews in Food and Science Nutrition* 50(3): 193–208. doi: 10.1080/10408390802248734.

Orlich, M. J., et al. 2015. Vegetarian dietary patterns and the risk of colorectal cancers. *JAMA Internal Medicine* 175(5): 767–776.

Pollan, Michael. 2009. *In Defense of Food.* New York: Penguin.

Remig, V., et al. April 2010. Trans fats in America: a review of their use, consumption, health implications, and regulation. *Journal of the American Dietetic Assocation* 110(4): 585–92. doi: 10.1016/j.jada.2009.12.024.

Ross, S. M. 2015. Cardiovascular disease mortality: The deleterious effects of excess dietary sugar intake. *Holistic Nursing Practice* 29(1): 53–57.

Satya, S. J., et al. 2011. Putting the whole grain puzzle together: Health benefits associated with whole grains—Summary of American Society for Nutrition 2010 Satellite Symposium. *Journal of Nutrition.* doi: 10.3945/jn.110.132944.

Siri-Tarino, P. W., et al. 2010. Meta-analysis of prospective cohort studies evaluating the association of saturated fat with cardiovascular disease. *American Journal of Clinical Nutrition* 91(3): 535–546.

Sirsikar, S., Sirsikar, A. 2015. Prevention and management of postmenopausal osteoporosis. *International Journal of Innovative and Applied Research* 3(6):15–26.

Slavin, J. L., and Lloyd, B. July 2012. Health benefits of fruits and vegetables. *Advances in Nutrition* 3(4):506–516. doi: 10.3945/an.112.002154.

Sofi, F., et al. November 2010. Accruing evidence on benefits of adherence to the Mediterranean diet on health: an updated systematic review and meta-analysis.

American Journal of Clinical Nutrition 92(5): 1189–1196. doi: 10.3945/ajcn.2010.29673. Epub September 1, 2010.

Trump, D. L., et al. 2010. Vitamin D: Considerations in the continued development as an agent for cancer prevention and therapy. *Cancer Journal* 16(1): 1–9.

U. S. Department of Agriculture. 2015. Scientific Report of the 2015 Dietary Guidelines Advisory Committee. Available from: http://www.health.gov/dietaryguidelines/2015-scientific-report.

U.S. Department of Agriculture 2015. *Biotechnology Frequently Asked Questions (FAQs).* (http://www.usda.gov/wps/portal/usda/usdahome?contentid=Biotechnology FAQs.xml&navid=AGRICULTURE, April 20, 2015).

U.S. Department of Agriculture and U.S. Department of Health and Human Services. Dietary Guidelines for Americans, 2010, 7th ed. Washington, DC: U.S. Government Printing Office, December 2010.

U.S. Food and Drug Administration. 2014. *Food Allergies: What You Need to Know* (http://www.fda.gov/Food/IngredientsPackagingLabeling/Food Allergens/ucm079311.htm, April 20, 2015).

U.S. Food and Drug Administration. 2015. Calorie labeling on restaurant menus and vending machines: what you need to know. http://www.fda.gov/Food/IngredientsPackagingLabeling/LabelingNutrition/ucm436722.htm.

U.S. Food and Drug Administration. 2015. FDA cuts trans fats in processed foods. http://www.fda.gov/ForConsumers/ConsumerUpdates/ucm372915.htm.

Varraso, R., et al. April 2010. Prospective study of dietary fiber and risk of chronic obstructive pulmonary disease among U.S. women and men. *American Journal of Epidemiology* 171(7): 776–784. (http://www.ncbi.nlm.nih.gov/pmc/articles/PMC2877480/).

Wang, X., et al. 2014. Fruit and vegetable consumption and mortality from all causes, cardiovascular disease, and cancer: systematic review and dose-response meta-analysis of prospective cohort studies. *BMJ* 349:g4490.

Willett, W. C. July 2012. Dietary fats and coronary heart disease. *Journal of Internal Medicine* 272(1): 13–24. (http://www.ncbi.nlm.nih.gov/pubmed/22583051, April 20, 2015). doi: 10.1111/j.1365-2796.2012.02553.x.

NUTRITION RESOURCES

Healthy US-Style Food Patterns

Calorie level of pattern	1600	1800	2000	2200	2400	2600	2800	3000
Food Group	**Daily amount** of food from each group (vegetable and protein foods subgroup amounts are per week)							
Fruits	1.5 c	1.5 c	2 c	2 c	2 c	2 c	2.5 c	2.5 c
Vegetables	2 c	2.5 c	2.5 c	3 c	3 c	3.5 c	3.5 c	4 c
Dark green veg	1.5 c/wk	1.5 c/wk	1.5 c/wk	2 c/wk	2 c/wk	2.5 c/wk	2.5 c/wk	2.5 c/wk
Red/Orange veg	4 c/wk	5.5 c/wk	5.5 c/wk	6 c/wk	6 c/wk	7 c/wk	7 c/wk	7.5 c/wk
Beans and peas	1 c/wk	1.5 c/wk	1.5 c/wk	2 c/wk	2 c/wk	2.5 c/wk	2.5 c/wk	3 c/wk
Starchy veg	4 c/wk	5 c/wk	5 c/wk	6 c/wk	6 c/wk	7 c/wk	7 c/wk	8 c/wk
Other veg	3.5 c/wk	4 c/wk	4 c/wk	5 c/wk	5 c/wk	5.5 c/wk	5.5 c/wk	7 c/wk
Grains	5 oz eq	6 oz eq	6 oz eq	7 oz eq	8 oz eq	9 oz eq	10 oz eq	10 oz eq
Whole grains	3 oz eq	3 oz eq	3 oz eq	3.5 oz eq	4 oz eq	4.5 oz eq	5 oz eq	5 oz eq
Other grains	2 oz eq	3 oz eq	3 oz eq	3.5 oz eq	4 oz eq	4.5 oz eq	5 oz eq	5 oz eq
Protein foods	5 oz eq	5 oz eq	5.5 oz eq	6 oz eq	6.5 oz eq	6.5 oz eq	7 oz eq	7 oz eq
Meat poultry, eggs	23 oz eq/wk	23 oz eq/wk	26 oz eq/wk	28 oz eq/wk	31 oz eq/wk	31 oz eq/wk	33 oz eq/wk	33 oz eq/wk
Seafood	8 oz eq/wk	8 oz eq/wk	8 oz eq/wk	9 oz eq/wk	10 oz eq/wk	10 oz eq/wk	10 oz eq/wk	10 oz eq/wk
Nuts, seeds, soy	4 oz eq/wk	4 oz eq/wk	5 oz eq/wk	5 oz eq/wk	5 oz eq/wk	5 oz eq/wk	6 oz eq/wk	6 oz eq/wk
Dairy	3 c	3 c	3 c	3 c	3 c	3 c	3 c	3 c
Oils	22 g	24 g	27 g	29 g	31 g	34 g	36 g	44 g
Limits for solid fats and added sugars								
Solid fats	8 g	11 g	18 g	18 g	23 g	25 g	26 g	31 g
Added sugars	14 g	19 g	30 g	32 g	39 g	43 g	45 g	53 g

Food group amounts shown in cup (c) or ounce equivalents (oz eq). Oils, solid fats, and added sugars are shown in grams (g).
Quantity equivalents for each food group are:
- Grains, 1 ounce equivalent is: ½ cup cooked rice, pasta, or cooked cereal; 1 ounce dry pasta or rice; 1 slice bread; 1 cup ready-to-eat cereal flakes.
- Fruits and vegetables, 1 cup equivalent is: 1 cup raw or cooked fruit or vegetable, 1 cup fruit or vegetable juice, 2 cups leafy salad greens.
- Protein Foods, 1 ounce equivalent is: 1 ounce lean meat, poultry, or seafood; 1 egg; ¼ cup cooked beans or tofu; 1 Tbsp peanut butter; ½ ounce nuts/seeds.
- Dairy, 1 cup equivalent is: 1 cup milk or yogurt, 1½ ounces natural cheese such as cheddar cheese or 2 ounces of processed cheese.

FIGURE 1 Healthy US-Style Food Patterns

SOURCE: U.S. Department of Health and Human Services and U.S. Department of Agriculture. 2015. Scientific Report of the 2015 Dietary Guidelines Advisory Committee, Appendix E-3, Table E3.1.A1. Available from: http://www.health.gov/dietaryguidelines/2015-scientific-report/.

Healthy Vegetarian Patterns

Calorie level of pattern	1600	1800	2000	2200	2400	2600	2800	3000
Food Group	**Daily amount[a]** of food from each group (vegetable and protein foods subgroup amounts are per week)							
Fruits	1.5 c	1.5 c	2 c	2 c	2 c	2 c	2.5 c	2.5 c
Vegetables	2 c	2.5 c	2.5 c	3 c	3 c	3.5 c	3.5 c	4 c
Dark green veg	1.5 c/wk	1.5 c/wk	1.5 c/wk	2 c/wk	2 c/wk	2.5 c/wk	2.5 c/wk	2.5 c/wk
Red/Orange veg	4 c/wk	5.5 c/wk	5.5 c/wk	6 c/wk	6 c/wk	7 c/wk	7 c/wk	7.5 c/wk
Beans and peas	1 c/wk	1.5 c/wk	1.5 c/wk	2 c/wk	2 c/wk	2.5 c/wk	2.5 c/wk	3 c/wk
Starchy veg	4 c/wk	5 c/wk	5 c/wk	6 c/wk	6 c/wk	7 c/wk	7 c/wk	8 c/wk
Other veg	3.5 c/wk	4 c/wk	4 c/wk	5 c/wk	5 c/wk	5.5 c/wk	5.5 c/wk	7 c/wk
Grains	5.5 oz eq	6.5 oz eq	6.5 oz eq	7.5 oz eq	8.5 oz eq	9.5 oz eq	10.5 oz eq	10.5 oz eq
Whole grains	3.5 oz eq	3.5 oz eq	3.5 oz eq	4 oz eq	4.5 oz eq	5 oz eq	5.5 oz eq	5.5 oz eq
Other grains	2 oz eq	3 oz eq	3 oz eq	3.5 oz eq	4 oz eq	4.5 oz eq	5 oz eq	5 oz eq
Protein foods	2.5 oz eq	3 oz eq	3.5 oz eq	4 oz eq	4 oz eq	5 oz eq	5 oz eq	5.5 oz eq
Beans and peas[b]	4 oz eq/wk	6 oz eq/wk	6 oz eq/wk	8 oz eq/wk	8 oz eq/wk	10 oz eq/wk	10 oz eq/wk	12 oz eq/wk
Eggs	3 oz eq/wk	3 oz eq/wk	3 oz eq/wk	3 oz eq/wk	3 oz eq/wk	3 oz eq/wk	4 oz eq/wk	4 oz eq/wk
Nuts and seeds	5 oz eq/wk	6 oz eq/wk	7 oz eq/wk	8 oz eq/wk	9 oz eq/wk	10 oz eq/wk	11 oz eq/wk	12 oz eq/wk
Tofu/processed soy	5 oz eq/wk	6 oz eq/wk	7 oz eq/wk	8 oz eq/wk	9 oz eq/wk	10 oz eq/wk	11 oz eq/wk	12 oz eq/wk
Dairy	3 c	3 c	3 c	3 c	3 c	3 c	3 c	3 c
Oils	22 g	24 g	27 g	29 g	31 g	34 g	36 g	44 g
Limits for solid fats and added sugars								
Solid fats	12 g	12 g	19 g	19 g	23 g	23 g	23 g	27 g
Added sugars	21 g	20 g	32 g	32 g	39 g	40 g	40 g	46 g

[a]Food group amounts shown in cup (c) or ounce equivalents (oz eq). Oils, solid fats, and added sugars are shown in grams (g).
Quantity equivalents for each food group are:
- Grains, 1 ounce equivalent is: ½ cup cooked rice, pasta, or cooked cereal; 1 ounce dry pasta or rice; 1 slice bread; 1 cup ready-to-eat cereal flakes.
- Fruits and vegetables, 1 cup equivalent is: 1 cup raw or cooked fruit or vegetable, 1 cup fruit or vegetable juice, 2 cups leafy salad greens.
- Protein Foods, 1 ounce equivalent is: 1 ounce lean meat, poultry, or seafood; 1 egg; ¼ cup cooked beans or tofu; 1 tbsp peanut butter; ½ ounce nuts/seeds.
- Dairy, 1 cup equivalent is: 1 cup milk or yogurt, 1½ ounces natural cheese (e.g. cheddar cheese) or 2 ounces of processed cheese.

[b]About half of total beans and peas are shown as vegetables, in cup eqs, and half as protein foods, in ounce eqs. Total beans and peas in cup eq is amount in vegetables plus the amount in protein foods/4:

	1600	1800	2000	2200	2400	2600	2800	3000
Total beans/peas	2 c eq/wk	3 c eq/wk	3 c eq/wk	4 c eq/wk	4 c eq/wk	5 c eq/wk	5 c eq/wk	6 c eq/wk

FIGURE 2 Healthy Vegetarian Patterns

SOURCE: U.S. Department of Health and Human Services and U.S. Department of Agriculture. 2015. Scientific Report of the 2015 Dietary Guidelines Advisory Committee, Appendix E-3, Table A1. Available from: http://www.health.gov/dietaryguidelines/2015-scientific-report/.

Healthy Mediterranean-Style Patterns

Calorie level of pattern	1600	1800	2000	2200	2400	2600	2800	3000
Food Group	**Daily amount** of food from each group (vegetable and protein foods subgroup amounts are per week)							
Fruits	1.5 c	2 c	2.5 c	2.5 c	2.5 c	2.5 c	3 c	3 c
Vegetables	2 c	2.5 c	2.5 c	3 c	3 c	3.5 c	3.5 c	4 c
Dark green veg	1.5 c/wk	1.5 c/wk	1.5 c/wk	2 c/wk	2 c/wk	2.5 c/wk	2.5 c/wk	2.5 c/wk
Red/Orange veg	4 c/wk	5.5 c/wk	5.5 c/wk	6 c/wk	6 c/wk	7 c/wk	7 c/wk	7.5 c/wk
Beans and peas	1 c/wk	1.5 c/wk	1.5 c/wk	2 c/wk	2 c/wk	2.5 c/wk	2.5 c/wk	3 c/wk
Starchy veg	4 c/wk	5 c/wk	5 c/wk	6 c/wk	6 c/wk	7 c/wk	7 c/wk	8 c/wk
Other veg	3.5 c/wk	4 c/wk	4 c/wk	5 c/wk	5 c/wk	5.5 c/wk	5.5 c/wk	7 c/wk
Grains	5 oz eq	6 oz eq	6 oz eq	7 oz eq	8 oz eq	9 oz eq	10 oz eq	10 oz eq
Whole grains	3 oz eq	3 oz eq	3 oz eq	3.5 oz eq	4 oz eq	4.5 oz eq	5 oz eq	5 oz eq
Other grains	2 oz eq	3 oz eq	3 oz eq	3.5 oz eq	4 oz eq	4.5 oz eq	5 oz eq	5 oz eq
Protein foods	5.5 oz eq	6 oz eq	6.5 oz eq	7 oz eq	7.5 oz eq	7.5 oz eq	8 oz eq	8 oz eq
Meat, poultry, eggs	23 oz eq/wk	23 oz eq/wk	26 oz eq/wk	28 oz eq/wk	31 oz eq/wk	31 oz eq/wk	33 oz eq/wk	33 oz eq/wk
Seafood	11 oz eq/wk	15 oz eq/wk	15 oz eq/wk	16 oz eq/wk	16 oz eq/wk	17 oz eq/wk	17 oz eq/wk	17 oz eq/wk
Nut seeds, soy	4 oz eq/wk	4 oz eq/wk	5 oz eq/wk	5 oz eq/wk	5 oz eq/wk	5 oz eq/wk	6 oz eq/wk	6 oz eq/wk
Dairy	2 c	2 c	2 c	2 c	2 c	2.5 c	2.5 c	2.5 c
Oils	22 g	24 g	27 g	29 g	31 g	34 g	36 g	44 g
Limits for solid fats and added sugars								
Solid fats	12 g	11g	17 g	18 g	20 g	22 g	23 g	28 g
Added sugars	21 g	18 g	29 g	31 g	34 g	37 g	40 g	48 g

Food group amounts shown in cup (c) or ounce equivalents (oz eq). Oils, solid fats, and added sugars are shown in grams (g).
Quantity equivalents for each food group are:
- Grains, 1 ounce equivalent is: ½ cup cooked rice, pasta, or cooked cereal; 1 ounce dry pasta or rice; 1 slice bread; 1 cup ready-to-eat cereal flakes.
- Fruits and vegetables, 1 cup equivalent is: 1 cup raw or cooked fruit or vegetable, 1 cup fruit or vegetable juice, 2 cups leafy salad greens.
- Protein Foods, 1 ounce equivalent is: 1 ounce lean meat, poultry, or seafood; 1 egg; ¼ cup cooked beans or tofu; 1 Tbsp peanut butter; ½ ounce nuts/seeds.
- Dairy, 1 cup equivalent is: 1 cup milk or yogurt, 1½ ounces natural cheese such as cheddar cheese or 2 ounces of processed cheese.

FIGURE 3   Healthy Mediterranean-Style Patterns

SOURCE: U.S. Department of Health and Human Services and U.S. Department of Agriculture. 2015. Scientific Report of the 2015 Dietary Guidelines Advisory Committee, Appendix E-3, Table A2. Available from: http://www.health.gov/dietaryguidelines/2015-scientific-report/.

Number of servings per day (or per week, as noted)

Food groups	1600 calories	2000 calories	2600 calories	3100 calories	Serving sizes and notes
Grains	6	6–8	10–11	12–13	1 slice bread, 1 oz dry cereal, 1/2 cup cooked rice, pasta, or cereal; choose whole grains
Vegetables	3–4	4–5	5–6	6	1 cup raw leafy vegetables, 1/2 cup cooked vegetables, 1/2 cup vegetable juice
Fruits	4	4–5	5–6	6	1/2 cup fruit juice, 1 medium fruit, 1/4 cup dried fruit, 1/2 cup fresh, frozen, or canned fruit
Low-fat or fat-free dairy foods	2–3	2–3	3	3–4	1 cup milk; 1 cup yogurt, 1 1/2 oz cheese; choose fat-free or low-fat types
Meat, poultry, fish	3–6	6 or less	6	6–9	1 oz cooked meats, poultry, or fish: select only lean; trim away visible fats; broil, roast, or boil instead of frying; remove skin from poultry
Nuts, seeds, legumes	3 servings per week	4–5 servings per week	1	1	1/3 cup or 1 1/2 oz nuts, 2 Tbsp or 1/2 oz seeds, 1/2 cup cooked dry beans/peas, 2 Tbsp peanut butter
Fats and oils	2	2–3	3	4	1 tsp soft margarine, 1 Tbsp low-fat mayonnaise, 2 Tbsp light salad dressing, 1 tsp vegetable oil; DASH has 27% of calories as fat (low in saturated fat)
Sweets	0	5 servings/ week or less	2	2	1 Tbsp sugar, 1 Tbsp jelly or jam, 1/2 cup sorbet, 1 cup lemonade; sweets should be low in fat

FIGURE 4   The DASH Eating Plan.

SOURCE: National Institutes of Health, National Heart, Lung, and Blood Institute. 2006. *Your Guide to Lowering Your Blood Pressure with DASH: How Do I Make the Dash?* NIH Publication No. 06-4082 (http://www.nhlbi.nih.gov/health/public/heart/hbp/dash/new_dash.pdf, April 20, 2015).

Name _____ Section _____ Date _____

LAB 8.1   Your Daily Diet versus MyPlate

Make three photocopies of the worksheet in this lab and use them to keep track of everything you eat for three consecutive days. Break down each food item into its component parts, and list them separately in the column labeled "Food." Then enter the portion size you consumed in the correct food-group column. For example, a turkey sandwich might be listed as follows: whole-wheat bread, 2 oz-equiv of whole grains; turkey, 2 oz-equiv of meat/beans; tomato, ⅓ cup other vegetables; romaine lettuce, ¼ cup dark green vegetables; 1 tablespoon mayonnaise dressing, 1 teaspoon oils. It can be challenging to track values for added sugars and oils and fats, but use food labels to be as accurate as you can. Additional guidelines for counting discretionary calories can be found at http://www.ChooseMyPlate.gov.

For vegetables, enter your portion sizes in both the "Total" column and the column corresponding to the correct subgroup; for example, the spinach in a spinach salad would be entered under "Dark Green" and carrots would be entered under "Orange." For the purpose of this three-day activity, you will compare only your total vegetable consumption against MyPlate guidelines; as described in the chapter, vegetable subgroup recommendations are based on weekly consumption. However, it is important to note which vegetable subgroups are represented in your diet; over a three-day period, you should consume several servings from each of the subgroups.

Date: _____

Food	Grains (oz-eq)		Vegetable (cups)						Fruits (cups)	Milk (cups)	Meat/ Beans (oz-eq)	Oils (tsp)	Discretionary Calories	
	Whole	Other	Total	Dark Green	Orange	Legume	Starchy	Other					Solid Fats (g)	Added Sugars (g/tsp)
Daily Total														

LABORATORY ACTIVITIES

Next, average your daily intake totals for the three days and enter them in the chart below. For example, if your three daily totals for the fruit group were 1 cup, 1½ cups, and 2 cups, your average daily intake would be 1½ cups. Fill in the recommended intake totals that apply to you from ChooseMyPlate.gov or your chosen dietary pattern from the Nutrition Resources section.

MyPlate Food Group	Recommended Daily Amounts or Limits	Your Actual Average Daily Intake
Grains (total)	oz-eq	oz-eq
Whole grains	oz-eq	oz-eq
Other grains	oz-eq	oz-eq
Vegetables (total)	cups	cups
Fruits	cups	cups
Milk	cups	cups
Meat and beans	oz-eq	oz-eq
Oils	tsp	tsp
Solid fats	g	g
Added sugars	g/tsp	g/tsp

Using Your Results

How did you score? How close is your diet to that recommended by MyPlate? Are you surprised by the amount of food you are consuming from each food group or from added sugars and solid fats?

What should you do next? If the results of the assessment indicate that you could boost your level of wellness by improving your diet, set realistic goals for change. Do you need to increase or decrease your consumption of any food groups? List any areas of concern below, along with a goal for change and strategies for achieving the goal you've set. If you see that you are falling short in one food group, such as fruits or vegetables but have many foods that are rich in discretionary calories from solid fats and added sugars, try decreasing those items in favor of an apple, a bunch of grapes, or some baby carrots. Think carefully about the reasons behind your food choices. For example, if you eat doughnuts for breakfast every morning because you feel rushed, make a list of ways to save time to allow for a healthier breakfast.

Problem: _____

Goal: _____

Strategies for change: _____

_____

_____

Problem: _____

Goal: _____

Strategies for change: _____

_____

_____

Problem: _____

Goal: _____

Strategies for change: _____

_____

_____

Enter the results of this lab in the Preprogram Assessment column in Appendix C. If you've set goals and identified strategies for change, begin putting your plan into action. After several weeks of your program, complete this lab again and enter the results in the Postprogram Assessment column of Appendix C. How do the results compare?

Name _____ **Section** _____ **Date** _____

LAB 8.2 Dietary Analysis

You can complete this activity using either a nutrition analysis software program or information about the nutrient content of foods available online; see the For Further Exploration section and page A–1 for recommended websites. (This lab asks you to analyze one day's diet. For a more complete and accurate assessment of your diet, analyze the results from several different days, including a weekday and a weekend day.)

DATE _____   DAY: M Tu W Th F Sa Su

Food	Amount	Calories	Protein (g)	Carbohydrate (g)	Dietary fiber (g)	Fat, total (g)	Saturated fat (g)	Sodium (mg)	Vitamin A (RE)	Vitamin C (mg)	Calcium (mg)	Iron (mg)
Recommended totals*			10–35%	45–65%	25–38 g	20–35%	<10%	≤2300 mg	RE	mg	mg	mg
Actual totals**		cal	g / %	g / %	g	g / %	g / %	mg	RE	mg	mg	mg

*Fill in the appropriate DRI values for vitamin A, vitamin C, calcium, and iron from Tables 8.6 and 8.7 or by visiting the Interactive DRI website: **http://fnic.nal.usda.gov/fnic/interactiveDRI**.

**Total the values in each column. Protein and carbohydrate provide 4 calories per gram; fat provides 9 calories per gram. For example, if your day's total energy intake was 2,000 calories, including 270 grams of carbohydrate, you would calculate your percentage of total calories from carbohydrate as follows: (270 g X 4 cal/g) ÷ 2,000 = 54%. Percentages may not total 100% due to rounding.

Using Your Results

How did you score? How close is your diet to that recommended in this chapter? Are you surprised by any of the results of this assessment?

What should you do next? Enter the results of this lab in the Preprogram Assessment column in Appendix C. If your daily diet meets all the recommended intakes, congratulations—and keep up the good work. If the results of the assessment pinpoint areas of concern, then work with your food record on the previous page to determine what changes you could make to meet all the guidelines. Make changes, additions, and deletions until it conforms to all or most of the guidelines. Or, if you prefer, start from scratch to create a day's diet that meets the guidelines. Use the chart below to experiment and record your final, healthy sample diet for one day. Then put what you learned from this exercise into practice in your daily life. After several weeks of your program, complete this lab again and enter the results in the Postprogram Assessment column of Appendix C. How do the results compare?

DATE _____   DAY: **M**   **Tu**   **W**   **Th**   **F**   **Sa**   **Su**

Food	Amount	Calories	Protein (g)	Carbohydrate (g)	Dietary fiber (g)	Fat, total (g)	Saturated fat (g)	Sodium (mg)	Vitamin A (RE)	Vitamin C (mg)	Calcium (mg)	Iron (mg)
Recommended totals*			10–35%	45–65%	25–38 g	20–35%	<10%	≤2300 mg	RE	mg	mg	mg
Actual totals**		cal	g / %	g / % g	g / %	g / %	mg	RE	mg	mg	mg

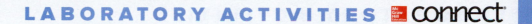

Name _____ Section _____ Date _____

LAB 8.3 Informed Food Choices

Part I Using Food Labels

Choose three food items to evaluate. You might want to select three similar items, such as regular, low-fat, and nonfat salad dressing, or three very different items. Record the information from their food labels in the table below.

Food Items			
Serving size			
Total calories	cal	cal	cal
Total fat—grams	g	g	g
—% Daily Value	%	%	%
Saturated fat—grams	g	g	g
—% Daily Value	%	%	%
Trans fat—grams	g	g	g
Sodium—milligrams	mg	mg	mg
—% Daily Value	%	%	%
Carbohydrates (total)—gram	g	g	g
—% Daily Value	%	%	%
Dietary fiber—grams	g	g	g
—% Daily Value	%	%	%
Sugars—grams	g	g	g
Protein—grams	g	g	g
Vitamin A—% Daily Value	%	%	%
Vitamin C—% Daily Value	%	%	%
Calcium—% Daily Value	%	%	%
Iron—% Daily Value	%	%	%

How do the items you chose compare? You can do a quick nutrient check by totaling the Daily Value percentages for nutrients you should limit (saturated fat, sugars, sodium) and the nutrients you should favor (dietary fiber, vitamin A, vitamin C, calcium, iron) for each food. Which food has the largest percent Daily Value sum for nutrients to limit? For nutrients to favor?

Food Items			
Calories	cal	cal	cal
% Daily Value total for nutrients to limit (saturated fat, sugars, sodium)	%	%	%
% Daily Value total for nutrients to favor (fiber, vitamin A, vitamin C, calcium, iron)	%	%	%

LABORATORY ACTIVITIES

Part II Evaluating Fast Food

Use the nutritional information available from fast-food restaurants to complete the chart on this page for the last fast-food meal you ate. Add up your totals for the meal. Compare the values for fat, protein, carbohydrate, and sodium content for each food item and for the meal as a whole with the levels suggested by the Dietary Guidelines for Americans. Calculate the percent of total calories derived from fat, saturated fat, protein, and carbohydrate using the formulas given.

To get fast-food nutritional information, ask for a nutrition information brochure when you visit the restaurant, or visit restaurant websites: Arby's (http://www.arbysrestaurant.com), Burger King (http://www.burgerking.com), Domino's Pizza (http://www.dominos.com), Jack in the Box (http://www.jackinthebox.com), KFC (http://www.kfc.com), McDonald's (http://www.mcdonalds.com), Subway (http://www.subway.com), Taco Bell (http://www.tacobell.com), Wendy's (http://www.wendys.com).

If you haven't recently been to a fast-food restaurant, fill in the chart for any sample meal you might eat.

FOOD ITEMS

	Dietary Guidelines							Total**
Serving size (g)		g	g	g	g	g	g	g
Calories		cal	cal	cal	cal	cal	cal	cal
Total fat—grams		g	g	g	g	g	g	g
—% calories*	20–35%	%	%	%	%	%	%	%
Saturated fat—grams		g	g	g	g	g	g	g
—% calories*	<10%	%	%	%	%	%	%	%
Protein—grams		g	g	g	g	g	g	g
—% calories*	10–35%	%	%	%	%	%	%	%
Carbohydrate—grams		g	g	g	g	g	g	g
—% calories*	45–65%	%	%	%	%	%	%	%
Sodium†	800 mg	mg	mg	mg	mg	mg	mg	mg

*To calculate the percent of total calories from each food energy source (fat, carbohydrate, protein), use the following formula:

$$\frac{(\text{number of grams of energy source}) \times (\text{number of calories per gram of energy source})}{(\text{total calories in serving of food item})}$$

(*Note:* Fat and saturated fat provide 9 calories per gram; protein and carbohydrate provide 4 calories per gram.) For example, the percent of total calories from protein in a 150-calorie dish containing 10 grams of protein is

$$\frac{(10 \text{ grams of protein}) \times (4 \text{ calories per gram})}{(150 \text{ calories})} = \frac{40}{150} = 0.27, \text{ or } 27\% \text{ of total calories from protein}$$

**For the Total column, add up the total grams of fat, carbohydrate, and protein contained in your sample meal and calculate the percentages based on the total calories in the meal. (Percentages may not total 100% due to rounding.) For cholesterol and sodium values, add up the total number of milligrams.
†Recommended daily limit of sodium is divided by 3 here to give an approximate recommended limit for a single meal.

SOURCE: Insel, P. M., and W. T. Roth. 2016. Wellness Worksheet 66. *Core Concepts in Health,* 14th ed. Copyright © 2016 The McGraw-Hill Companies, Inc. Reprinted with permission.

APPENDIXES

NUTRITIONAL CONTENT OF COMMON FOODS

If you are developing a behavior change plan to improve your diet, or if you simply want to choose healthier foods, you may want to know more about the nutritional content of common food items.

You can track your daily food intake, calculate your nutrient intake from foods, and compare your intake with the U.S. Department of Agriculture's recommendations for your age, sex, height, and weight at the MyPlate website (**www.choosemyplate.gov**).

You can also look up the nutrient content of the foods you eat in the USDA Agricultural Research Service National Nutrient Database, which lists foods both by description and by nutrient content (**www.ars.usda.gov/Services/docs.htm?docid=17477**). For example, under "protein," you can find out how much protein there is in a chicken pot pie or what foods have the most protein per serving. Although cumbersome, the database is comprehensive.

Nutritional Content of Popular Items from Fast-Food Restaurants

Although most foods served at fast-food restaurants are high in calories, fat, saturated fat, cholesterol, sodium, and sugar, some items are healthier than others. If you eat at fast-food restaurants, knowing the nutritional content of various items can help you make better choices. Fast-food restaurants provide nutritional information both online and in print brochures available at most restaurant locations. To learn more about the items you order, visit the restaurants' websites:

Arby's:	http://arbys.com/	Pizza Hut:	http://www.pizzahut.com
Burger King:	http://www.bk.com/	Starbucks:	http://www.starbucks.com
Chiptole:	http://www.chipotle.com	Subway:	http://www.subway.com
Domino's Pizza:	www.dominos.com		/subwayroot/default.aspx
Hardees:	www.hardees.com	Taco Bell:	www.tacobell.com
KFC:	www.kfc.com	Wendy's:	www.wendys.com
McDonald's:	www.mcdonalds.com	White Castle:	www.whitecastle.com
Papa John's Pizza:	http://www.papajohns		
	.com/index.html		

INJURY PREVENTION AND PERSONAL SAFETY

Unintentional injuries are the leading cause of death in the United States for people under age 45. The greatest number of disabling injuries occur in the home; falls are the leading cause of nonfatal, unintentional injuries that are treated in hospital emergency departments. In all these arenas, the action you take can mean the difference between injury or death and no injury at all.

Injuries are generally classified into four categories, based on where they occur: motor vehicle injuries, home injuries, leisure injuries, and work injuries.

MOTOR VEHICLE INJURIES

According to the National Safety Council (NSC), nearly 35,000 Americans were killed and nearly 3.7 million were injured in motor vehicle crashes in 2011. Those most affected by motor vehicle crashes are people 15–24 years of age. It is more likely that your death will be caused by a motor vehicle crash than by any other type of unintentional or intentional injury. Motor vehicle injuries also result in the majority of cases of paralysis due to spinal injuries, and they are the leading cause of severe brain injury in the United States.

Factors in Motor Vehicle Injuries

Driving Habits Nearly two-thirds of motor vehicle injuries are caused by bad driving, especially speeding. As speed increases, momentum and force of impact increase and the time available for the driver to react decreases. Speed limits are posted to establish the safest *maximum* speed limit for a given area under *ideal* conditions. Aggressive driving—characterized by speeding, frequent and abrupt lane changes, tailgating, and passing on the shoulder—also increases the risk of crashes.

Distracted driving contributes to 25 to 50% of all crashes. Anything that distracts a driver—sleepiness, bad mood, children or pets in the car, use of a cell phone—can increase the risk of a crash. Sleepiness reduces reaction time, coordination, and speed of information processing and can be as dangerous as drug and alcohol use. Even mild sleep deprivation causes a deterioration in driving ability comparable to that caused by a 0.05% blood alcohol concentration.

Cell phone users respond to hazards about 20% slower than undistracted drivers and are about twice as likely to rear-end a braking car in front of them. According to 2011 statistics from the AAA Foundation for Traffic Safety, drivers who use cell phones are nearly four times as likely to be involved in a crash as drivers who don't. Hands-free devices do not help significantly; the mental distraction of talking is the factor in crashes rather than holding a phone. Newer research shows that text-messaging (texting) on a cell phone while driving is even more dangerous than talking. Estimates provided by the NSC attribute 1.3 million traffic crashes (about 24% of all crashes) to the use of cell phones and text messaging. Many cities and states have outlawed the use of cell phones while driving.

Safety Belts and Air Bags A person who doesn't wear a safety belt is twice as likely to be injured in a crash as a person who does wear one. Safety belts not only prevent occupants from being thrown from the car at the time of the crash but also provide protection from the "second collision," which occurs when the occupant of the car hits something inside the car, such as the steering column or windshield. The safety belt also spreads the stopping force of a collision over the body.

Since 1998, all new cars have been equipped with dual air bags—one for the driver and one for the front passenger seat. Air bags provide supplemental protection in a collision but are most useful in head-on collisions. (Many newer vehicles feature side air bags to offer protection in a side-impact crash.) They also deflate immediately after inflating and so do not provide protection in collisions involving multiple impacts. To ensure that air bags work as intended, follow these guidelines:

- Place infants in rear-facing infant seats in the backseat.
- Transport children age 12 and under in the backseat.
- Always use safety belts or appropriate safety seats.
- Keep at least 10 inches between the air bag cover and the breastbone of the driver or passenger.

If you cannot comply with these guidelines, you can apply to the National Highway Traffic Safety Administration for permission to install an on-off switch that temporarily disables the air bag.

Alcohol and Other Drugs Alcohol is involved in about 3 out of 10 fatal crashes. Alcohol-impaired driving, defined by blood alcohol concentration (BAC), is illegal. The legal BAC limit is 0.08% in all states, but driving ability is impaired at much lower BACs. All psychoactive drugs have the potential to impair driving ability.

Preventing Motor Vehicle Injuries

About 75% of all motor vehicle collisions occur within 25 miles of home and at speeds lower than 40 mph. These crashes often occur because the driver believes safety measures are not necessary for short trips. Clearly, the statistics prove otherwise.

To prevent motor vehicle injuries:

- Obey the speed limit. If you have to speed to get to your destination on time, you're not allowing enough time.
- Always wear a safety belt and ask passengers to do the same. Strap infants and toddlers into government-approved car seats in the back seat. Children who have outgrown child safety seats but who are still too small for adult safety belts alone (usually age 4–8) should be secured using booster seats. All children under 12 should ride in the backseat.

- Never drive under the influence of alcohol or other drugs or with a driver who is.
- Do not drive when you are sleepy or have been awake for 18 or more hours.
- Avoid using your cell phone while driving—your primary obligation is to pay attention to the road. If you do make calls, follow laws set by your city or state. Place calls when you are at a stop, and keep them short. Pull over if the conversation is stressful or emotional.
- Never text while driving.
- Keep your car in good working order. Regularly inspect tires, oil and fluid levels, windshield wipers, spare tire, and so on.
- Always allow enough following distance. Follow the "3-second rule": When the vehicle ahead passes a reference point, count out 3 seconds. If you pass the reference point before you finish counting, drop back and allow more following distance.
- Always increase following distance and slow down if weather or road conditions are poor.
- Choose major highways rather than rural roads. Highways are much safer because of better visibility, wider lanes, fewer surprises, and other factors.
- Always signal before turning or changing lanes.
- Stop completely at stop signs. Follow all traffic laws.
- Take special care at intersections. Always look left, right, and then left again. Make sure you have plenty of time to complete your maneuver in the intersection.
- Don't pass on two-lane roads unless you are in a designated passing area and have a clear view ahead.

Motorcycles and Scooters

About 1 out of every 7 traffic fatalities among people age 15–34 involves someone riding a motorcycle. Injuries from motorcycle collisions are generally more severe than those involving automobiles because motorcycles provide little, if any, protection. Scooter riders face additional challenges. Motorized scooters usually have a maximum speed of 30–35 mph and have less power for maneuverability.

To prevent motorcycle and scooter injuries:

- Make yourself easier to see by wearing light-colored clothing, driving with your headlights on, and correctly positioning yourself in traffic.
- Develop the necessary skills. Lack of skill, especially when evasive action is needed to avoid a collision, is a major factor in motorcycle and moped injuries. Skidding from improper braking is the most common cause of loss of control.
- Wear a close-fitting helmet, one marked with the symbol DOT (for Department of Transportation).
- Protect your eyes with goggles, a face shield, or a windshield.
- Drive defensively and never assume that other drivers see you.

Pedestrians and Bicycles

Injuries to pedestrians and bicyclists are considered motor vehicle–related because they usually involve motor vehicles. About 1 in 7 motor vehicle deaths involves pedestrians, and more than 160,000 pedestrians are injured each year.

To prevent injuries when walking or jogging:

- Walk or jog in daylight.
- Make yourself easier to see by wearing light-colored, reflective clothing.
- Face traffic when walking or jogging along a roadway, and follow traffic laws.
- Avoid busy roads or roads with poor visibility.
- Cross only at marked crosswalks and intersections.
- Don't use headphones while walking or jogging.
- Don't hitchhike. Hitchhiking places you in a potentially dangerous situation.

Bicycle injuries result primarily from not knowing or understanding the rules of the road, failing to follow traffic laws, and not having sufficient skill or experience to handle traffic conditions. Bicycles are considered vehicles; bicycle riders must obey all traffic laws that apply to automobile drivers, including stopping at traffic lights and stop signs.

To prevent injuries when riding a bike:

- Wear safety equipment, including a helmet, eye protection, gloves, and proper footwear. Secure the bottom of your pant legs with clips and secure your shoelaces so they don't get tangled in the chain.
- Make yourself easier to see by wearing light-colored, reflective clothing. Equip your bike with reflectors and use lights, especially at night or when riding in wooded or other dark areas.
- Ride with the flow of traffic, not against it, and follow traffic laws. Use bike paths when they are available.
- Ride defensively; never assume that drivers can see you. Be especially careful when turning or crossing at corners and intersections. Watch for cars turning right.
- Stop at all traffic lights and stop signs. Know and use hand signals.
- Continue pedaling at all times when moving (don't coast) to help keep the bike stable and to maintain your balance.
- Properly maintain your bike.

Aggressive Driving

Aggressive driving, known as *road rage*, has increased more than 50% since 1990. Aggressive drivers increase the risk of crashes for themselves and others. They further increase the risk of injuries if they stop their vehicles and confront each other. Even if you are successful at controlling your own aggressive driving impulses, you may still encounter an aggressive driver.

To avoid being the victim of an aggressive driver:

- Always keep distance between your car and others. If you are behind a very slow driver and can't pass, slow down to increase distance in case that driver does something unexpected. If you are being tailgated, do not increase your speed; instead, let the other driver pass you. If you are in the left lane when being tailgated, signal and pull over to let the other driver go by, even if you are traveling at the speed limit. When you are merging, make sure you have plenty of room. If you are cut off by a merging driver, slow down to make room.
- Be courteous, even if the other driver is not. Use your horn rarely, if ever. Avoid making gestures of irritation, even shaking

your head. When parking, let the other driver have the space that both of you found.

- Refuse to join in a fight. Avoid eye contact with an angry driver. If someone makes a rude gesture, ignore it. If you think another car is following you and you have a cell phone, call the police. Otherwise, drive to a public place and honk your horn to get someone's attention.
- If you make a mistake while driving, apologize. Raise or wave your hand or touch or knock your head with the palm of your hand to indicate "What was I thinking?" You can also mouth the words "I'm sorry."

HOME INJURIES

Contrary to popular belief, home is one of the most dangerous places to be. The most common fatal home injuries are caused by falls, poisoning, fires, suffocation and choking, and incidents involving firearms.

Falls

About 90% of fatal falls involve people age 45 and older, but falls are a significant cause of unintentional death for people under age 25. Most deaths occurring from falls involve falling on stairs or steps or from one level to another. Falls also occur on the same level, from tripping, slipping, or stumbling. Alcohol is a contributing factor in many falls.

To prevent injuries from falls:

- Install handrails and nonslip surfaces in the shower and bathtub. Place skidproof backing on rugs and carpets.
- Keep floors, stairs, and outside areas clear of objects or conditions that could cause slipping or tripping, such as heavy wax coating, electrical cords, and toys.
- Put a light switch by the door of every room so no one has to walk across a room to turn on a light. Use night lights in bedrooms, halls, stairways, and bathrooms.
- Outside the house, clear dangerous surfaces created by ice, snow, fallen leaves, or rough ground.
- Install handrails on stairs. Keep stairs well lit and clear of objects.
- When climbing a ladder, use both hands. Never stand higher than the third step from the top. When using a stepladder, make sure the spreader brace is in the locked position. With straight ladders, set the base out 1 foot for every 4 feet of height. Don't stand on chairs to reach things.
- If there are small children in the home, place gates at the top and bottom of stairs. Never leave a baby unattended.

Poisoning

More than 2.5 million poisonings and more than 35,000 poison-related deaths occur every year in the United States.

To prevent poisoning:

- Store all medicines out of the reach of children. Use medicines only as directed on the label or by a physician.
- Use cleaners, pesticides, and other dangerous substances only in areas with proper ventilation. Store them out of the reach of children.

- Never operate a vehicle in an enclosed space. Have your furnace inspected yearly. Use caution with any substance that produces potentially toxic fumes, such as kerosene. If appropriate, install carbon monoxide detectors.
- Keep poisonous plants out of the reach of children. These include azalea, oleander, rhododendron, wild mushrooms, daffodil and hyacinth bulbs, mistletoe berries, apple seeds, morning glory seeds, wisteria seeds, and the leaves and stems of potato, rhubarb, and tomato plants.

To be prepared in case of poisoning:

- Keep the number of the nearest Poison Control Center (or emergency room) in an accessible location. A call to the national poison control hotline (800-222-1222) will be routed to a local center.

Emergency first aid for poisonings:

1. Remove the poison from contact with eyes, skin, or mouth, or remove the victim from contact with poisonous fumes or gases.
2. Call the Poison Control Center immediately for instructions. Have the container with you.
3. Do not follow emergency instructions on labels. Some may be out-of-date and carry incorrect treatment information.
4. If you are instructed to go to an emergency room, take the poisonous substance or its container with you.

Guidelines for specific types of poisons:

- *Swallowed poisons.* Call the Poison Control Center or a physician for advice. Do not induce vomiting.
- *Poisons on the skin.* Remove any affected clothing. Flood affected parts of the skin with warm water, wash with soap and water, and rinse. Then call for advice.
- *Poisons in the eye.* For children, flood the eye with lukewarm water poured from a pitcher held 3–4 inches above the eye for 15 minutes; alternatively, irrigate the eye under a faucet. For adults, get in the shower and flood the eye with a gentle stream of lukewarm water for 15 minutes. Then call for advice.
- *Inhaled poisons.* Immediately carry or drag the person to fresh air and, if necessary, give rescue breaths (Figure A.1). If the victim is not breathing easily, call 9-1-1 for help. Ventilate the area. Then call the Poison Control Center for advice.

Fires

Each year, about 85% of fire deaths and 65% of fire injuries occur in the home. Careless smoking is the leading cause of home fire deaths. Cooking is the leading cause of home fire injuries.

To prevent fires:

- Dispose of all cigarettes in ashtrays. Never smoke in bed.
- Do not overload electrical outlets. Do not place extension cords under rugs or where people walk. Replace worn or frayed extension cords.
- Place a wire screen in front of fireplaces and woodstoves. Remove ashes carefully and store them in airtight metal containers, not paper bags.
- Properly maintain electrical appliances, kerosene heaters, and furnaces. Clean flues and chimneys annually.

EMERGENCY CARE FOR CHOKING

- If the victim is coughing, encourage the coughing to clear the object from the airway.
- If the victim is not coughing, follow the steps in "Choking Care for Responsive Adult or Child."

Choking Care for Responsive Adult or Child

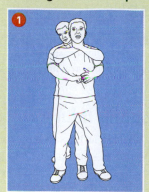

1 Stand behind an adult victim with one leg forward between the victim's legs. (With a child, kneel behind the victim.) Keep your head slightly to one side. Reach around the abdomen with both arms. Make a fist with one hand and place the thumb side of the fist against the abdomen just above the navel.

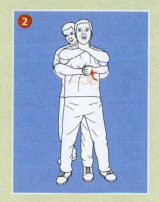

2 Grasp your fist with your other hand and thrust inward and upward into the victim's abdomen with quick jerks. Continue abdominal thrusts until the victim expels the object or becomes unresponsive. If the victim becomes unresponsive while you are administering abdominal thrusts, lower the victim to the floor onto his or her back, and follow the steps in "Choking Care for Unresponsive Adult or Child."

Choking Care for Unresponsive Adult or Child: CPR

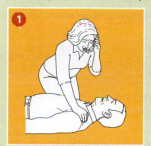

1 Call 911 and begin CPR.

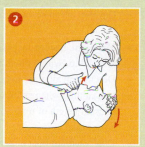

2 Open the airway to see if the victim is breathing. Use the "head tilt–chin lift" maneuver to open the airway: Push down on the forehead and lift the chin.

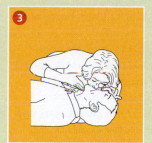

3 If the victim is not breathing, give two rescue breaths, each lasting 1 second. Pinch the victim's nose shut and blow a normal breath into the victim's mouth. If the first breath does not go in (the chest does not rise), reposition the head to open the airway and try again. Each time you give a rescue breath, look for an object in the victim's mouth and remove it if present.

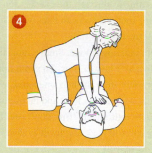

4 If the obstruction remains, begin chest compressions. Place the heel of one hand in the center of the chest between the nipples and the other hand on top of the first. Position your shoulders over your hands and lock your elbows. Give 30 chest compressions at a rate of 100 per minute. The chest should go down by 1½ to 2 inches. Then give two breaths, looking in the mouth for an expelled object. Continue chest compressions until help arrives. **Remember: Push hard and push fast at a rate of 100 compressions per minute.**

EMERGENCY CARE FOR CARDIAC ARREST

For cardiac arrest, the American Heart Association's revised (2005) Emergency Cardiac Care guidelines are as follows:

1 Call 911.

2 Start CPR (100 compressions per minute, stopping every 30 to 60 seconds to give two rescue breaths).

3 If an automated external defibrillator (AED) is available, or when one arrives, give one shock to restart the victim's heart.

4 Go back to CPR immediately after the shock.

Hands-Only CPR

In 2008, the American Heart Association reported that hands-only (compression-only) CPR can be as effective as conventional CPR. There are only two steps:

1 Call 911.

2 Push hard and fast in the center of the chest.

Don't wait for an emergency to learn how to use an AED or perform CPR.
To find a course in your area, contact the American Heart Association (800 242-8721) or the American Red Cross (202 303-4498).

FIGURE A.1 Emergency care for choking and for cardiac arrest.

SOURCES: Adapted from American Heart Association. 2008. Hands-only (compression-only) cardiopulmonary resuscitation: A call to action for bystander response to adults who experience out-of-hospital sudden cardiac arrest. *Circulation* 117: 2162–2167; National Safety Council. 2007. *First Aid: Taking Action.* New York: McGraw-Hill; American Heart Association. 2005. Adult basic life support. *Circulation* 112: 19–34; New CPR guidelines: Simplicity to the rescue. 2006. *Harvard Health Letter,* March, Streamlined CPR guidelines a life-saving move. 2006. *Harvard Heart Letter,* February.

- Keep portable heaters at least three feet away from curtains, bedding, towels, or anything that might catch fire. Never leave operating heaters unattended.

To be prepared for a fire:

- Plan at least two escape routes out of each room. Designate a location outside the home as a meeting place. Stage a home fire drill.
- Install a smoke detection device on every level of your home. Clean the detectors and test batteries once a month, and replace the batteries at least once a year.
- Keep a fire extinguisher in your home and know how to use it.

To prevent injuries from fire:

- Get out as quickly as possible and go to the designated meeting place. Don't stop for a keepsake or a pet. Never hide in a closet or under a bed. Once outside, count heads to see if everyone is out. If you think someone is still inside the burning building, tell the firefighters. Never go back inside a burning building.
- If you're trapped in a room, feel the door. If it is hot or if smoke is coming in through the cracks, don't open it; use the alternative escape route. If you can't get out of a room, go to the window and shout or wave for help.
- Avoid inhaling smoke. Smoke inhalation is the largest cause of death and injury in fires. To avoid inhaling smoke, crawl along the floor away from the heat and smoke. Cover your mouth and nose, ideally with a wet cloth, and take short, shallow breaths.
- If your clothes catch fire, don't run. Drop to the ground, cover your face, and roll back and forth to smother the flames. Remember: Stop-drop-roll.

Suffocation and Choking

Suffocation and choking account for over 6,000 deaths annually in the United States. Children can suffocate if they put small items in their mouths, get tangled in their crib bedding, or get trapped in airtight appliances like old refrigerators. Keep small objects out of reach of children under age 3, and don't give them raw carrots, hot dogs, popcorn, peanuts, or hard candy. Examine toys carefully for small parts that could come loose; don't give plastic bags or balloons to small children.

Adults can also become choking victims, especially if they fail to chew food properly, eat hurriedly, or try to talk and eat at the same time. Many choking victims can be saved with abdominal thrusts, also called the Heimlich maneuver (see Figure A.1). Infants who are choking can be saved with blows to the upper back, followed by chest thrusts if necessary.

Incidents Involving Firearms

Firearms pose a significant threat of unintentional injury, especially to people between ages 5 and 29.

To prevent firearm injuries:

- Always treat a gun as though it were loaded, even if you know it isn't.
- Never point a gun—loaded or unloaded—at something you do not intend to shoot.
- Always unload a firearm before storing it. Store unloaded firearms under lock and key, away from ammunition.

- Inspect firearms carefully before handling them.
- If you own a gun, buy and use a gun lock designed specifically for that weapon.
- If you ever plan to handle a gun, take a firearms safety course first.

LEISURE INJURIES

Leisure injuries take place in public places but do not involve motor vehicles. Many injuries in this category involve such recreational activities as boating and swimming, playground activities, in-line skating, and sports.

Drowning and Boating Injuries

Although most drownings are reported in lakes, ponds, rivers, and oceans, more than half the drownings of young children take place in residential pools. Among adolescents and adults, alcohol plays a significant role in many boating injuries and drownings.

To prevent drowning and boating injuries:

- Develop adequate swimming skill and make sure children learn to swim.
- Make sure residential pools are fenced and that children are never allowed to swim without supervision.
- Don't swim alone or in unsupervised places.
- Use caution when swimming in unfamiliar surroundings or for an unusual length of time. To avoid being chilled, don't swim in water colder than 70°F.
- Don't swim or boat under the influence of alcohol or other drugs. Don't chew gum or eat while in the water.
- Check the depth of water before diving.
- When on a boat, use a life jacket (personal flotation device).

In-Line Skating and Scooter Injuries

Most in-line skating injuries occur because users are not familiar with the equipment and do not wear appropriate safety gear. Injuries to the wrist and head are the most common. To prevent injuries while skating, wear a helmet, elbow and knee pads, wrist guards, a long-sleeved shirt, and long pants.

Wearing a helmet and knee and elbow pads is also important for preventing scooter injuries. The rise in popularity of lightweight scooters has seen a corresponding increase in associated injuries. Scooters should not be viewed as toys, and young children should be closely supervised. Be sure that handlebars, steering column, and all nuts and bolts are securely fastened. Ride on smooth, paved surfaces away from motor vehicle traffic. Avoid streets and surfaces with water, sand, gravel, or dirt.

Sports Injuries

Since more people have begun exercising to improve their health, there has been an increase in sports-related injuries.

To prevent sports injuries:

- Develop the skills required for the activity. Recognize and guard against the hazards associated with it.
- Always warm up and cool down.
- Make sure facilities are safe.
- Follow the rules and practice good sportsmanship.

- Use proper safety equipment, including, where appropriate, helmets, eye protection, knee and elbow pads, and wrist guards. Wear correct footwear.
- When it is excessively hot and humid, avoid heat stress by following the guidelines given in Chapter 3.

WORK INJURIES

Many aspects of workplace safety are monitored by the Occupational Safety and Health Administration (OSHA), a federal agency. The Bureau of Labor Statistics estimates that more than 3 million Americans suffered injuries on the job in 2012. The highest rate of work-related injuries occurs among laborers, whose jobs usually involve extensive manual labor and lifting—two areas not addressed by OSHA safety standards. Back injuries are the most common work injury.

To protect your back when lifting:

- Don't try to lift beyond your strength. If you need it, get help.
- Get a firm footing, with your feet shoulder-width apart. Get a firm grip on the object.
- Keep your torso in a relatively upright position and crouch down, bending at the knees and hips. Avoid bending at the waist. To lift, stand up or push up with your leg muscles. Lift gradually, keeping your arms straight. Keep the object close to your body.
- Don't twist. If you have to turn with an object, change the position of your feet.
- Put the object down gently, reversing the rules for lifting.

Another type of work-related injury is damage to the musculoskeletal system from repeated strain on the hand, arm, wrist, or other part of the body. Such repetitive-strain injuries are proliferating due to increased use of computers. One type, carpal tunnel syndrome, is characterized by pain and swelling in the tendons of the wrists and sometimes numbness and weakness.

To prevent carpal tunnel syndrome:

- Maintain good posture at the computer. Use a chair that provides back support and place the feet flat on the floor or on a footrest.
- Position the screen at eye level and the keyboard so the hands and wrists are straight.
- Take breaks periodically to stretch and flex your wrists and hands to lessen the cumulative effects of stress.

VIOLENCE AND INTENTIONAL INJURIES

According to the Federal Bureau of Investigation (FBI), more than 1.2 million violent crimes occurred in the United States in 2012. Violence includes assault, sexual assault, homicide, domestic violence, suicide, and child abuse. Compared with rates of violence in other industrialized countries, U.S. rates are unusually high in two areas: homicide and firearm-related deaths.

Assault

Assault is the use of physical force to inflict injury or death on another person. Most assaults occur during arguments or in connection with another crime, such as robbery. Poverty, urban settings, and the use of alcohol and drugs are associated with higher rates of assault. Homicide victims are most likely to be male, between ages 19 and 24, and members of minority groups. Most homicides are committed with a firearm; the murderer and the victim usually know each other.

To protect yourself at home:

- Secure your home with good lighting and effective locks, preferably deadbolts. Make sure that all doors and windows are securely locked.
- Get a dog, or post "Beware of Dog" signs.
- Don't hide keys in obvious places, and don't give anyone the chance to duplicate your keys.
- Install a peephole in your front door. Don't open your door to people you don't know.
- If you or a family member owns a weapon, store it securely. Store guns and ammunition separately.
- If you are a woman living alone, use your initials rather than your full name on your door or buzzer. Don't use a greeting on your answering machine that implies you live alone or are not home.
- Teach everyone in the household how to get emergency assistance.
- Know your neighbors. Work out a system for alerting each other in case of an emergency.
- Establish a neighborhood watch program.

To protect yourself on the street:

- Avoid walking alone, especially at night. Stay where people can see and hear you.
- Walk on the outside of the sidewalk, facing traffic. Walk purposefully. Act alert and confident. If possible, keep at least two arm lengths between yourself and a stranger.
- Know where you are going. Appearing to be lost increases your vulnerability.
- Carry valuables in a fanny pack, pants pocket, or shoulder bag strapped diagonally across the chest.
- Always have your keys ready as you approach your vehicle or home.
- Carry a whistle to blow if you are attacked or harassed. If you feel threatened, run and/or yell. Go into a store or knock on the door of a home. If someone grabs you, yell for help.

To protect yourself in your car:

- Keep your car in good working condition, carry emergency supplies, and keep the gas tank at least half full.
- When driving, keep doors locked and windows rolled up at least three-quarters of the way.
- Park your car in well-lighted areas or parking garages, preferably those with an attendant or a security guard.
- Lock your car when you leave it, and check the interior before opening the door when you return.
- Don't pick up strangers. Don't stop for vehicles in distress; drive on and call for help.
- Note the location of emergency call boxes along highways and in public facilities. Carry a cell phone.

- If your car breaks down, raise the hood and tie a white cloth to the antenna or door handle. Wait in the car with the doors locked and windows rolled up. If someone approaches to offer help, open a window only a crack and ask the person to call the police or a towing service.
- When you stop at a light or stop sign, leave enough room to maneuver if you need an escape route.
- If you are involved in a minor automobile crash and you think you have been bumped intentionally, don't leave your car. Motion to the other driver to follow you to the nearest police station.
- If confronted by a person with a weapon, give up your car.

To protect yourself on public transportation:

- While waiting, stand in a populated, well-lighted area.
- Make sure that the bus, subway, or train is bound for your destination before you board it. Sit near the driver or conductor in a single seat or an outside seat.
- If you flag down a taxi, make sure it's from a legitimate service. When you reach your destination, ask the driver to wait until you are safely inside the building.

To protect yourself on campus:

- Make sure that door and window locks are secure and that halls and stairwells have adequate lighting.
- Don't give dorm or residence keys to anybody.
- Don't leave your door unlocked or allow strangers into your room.
- Avoid solitary late-night trips to the library or laundry room. Take advantage of on-campus escort services.
- Don't exercise outside alone at night. Don't take shortcuts across campus that are unfamiliar or seem unsafe.
- If security guards patrol the campus, know the areas they cover and stay where they can see or hear you.

Sexual Assault—Rape and Date Rape

The use of force and coercion in sexual relationships is one of the most serious problems in human interactions. The most extreme manifestation of sexual coercion—forcing a person to submit to another's sexual desires—is rape. Taking advantage of circumstances that render a person incapable of giving consent (such as when drunk) is also considered sexual assault or rape. Coerced sexual activity in which the victim knows or is dating the rapist is often referred to as date rape.

An estimated 700,000 females are raped annually in the United States, and some males—perhaps 10,000 annually—are raped each year by other males. Research shows that 1 in 5 women and 1 in 71 men have experienced an attempted or completed rape. A study of college students also found that between 1 in 4 and 1 in 5 women experience a completed or attempted rape during their college years. Rape victims suffer both physical and psychological injury. The psychological pain can be substantial and long-lasting.

To protect yourself against rape:

- Follow the guidelines listed earlier for protecting yourself against assault.
- Trust your gut feeling. If you feel you are in danger, don't hesitate to run and scream.

- Think out in advance what you would do if you were threatened with rape. However, no one knows what he or she will do when scared to death. Trust that you will make the best decision at the time—whether to scream, run, fight, or give in to avoid being injured or killed.

To protect yourself against date rape:

- Believe in your right to control what you do. Set limits and communicate them clearly, firmly, and early. Be assertive; men often interpret passivity as permission.
- If you are unsure of a new acquaintance, go on a group date or double date. If possible, provide your own transportation.
- Remember that some men think flirtatious behavior or sexy clothing indicates an interest in having sex.
- Remember that alcohol and drugs interfere with judgment, perception, and communication about sex. In a bar or at a party, don't leave your drink unattended, and don't accept opened beverages; watch your drinks being poured. At a party or club, check on friends and ask them to check on you.
- Use the statement that has proved most effective in stopping date rape: "This is rape and I'm calling the cops!"

If you are raped:

- Go to a safe place.
- Call the police. Tell them you were raped and give your location.
- Call someone you trust who can be with you and give support.
- Try to remember everything you can about your attacker and write it down.
- Don't wash or douche before the medical exam. Don't change your clothes, but bring a new set with you if you can.
- Be aware that at the hospital you will have a complete exam. Show the physician any bruises or scratches.
- Tell the police exactly what happened. Be honest and stick to your story.
- If you do not want to report the rape to the police, see a physician as soon as possible. Be sure you are checked for pregnancy and STDs.
- Contact an organization with skilled counselors so you can talk about the experience. Look in the telephone directory under "Rape" or "Rape Crisis Center" for a hotline number.

Guidelines for men (pursuing women, but the same guidelines apply to men pursuing men):

- Be aware of social pressure. It's OK not to score.
- Understand that "No" means "No." Stop making advances when your date says to stop. Remember that she has the right to refuse sex.
- Don't assume that flirtatious behavior or sexy clothing means a woman is interested in having sex, that previous permission for sex applies to the current situation, or that your date's relationships with other men constitute sexual permission for you.
- Remember that alcohol and drugs interfere with judgment, perception, and communication about sex.

Stalking and Cyberstalking

Stalking is characterized by harassing behaviors such as following or spying on a person and making verbal, written, or implied threats.

Cyberstalking, the use of electronic communications devices to stalk another person, is becoming more common. Although many cases are not reported, the U.S. Department of Justice estimates that about 900,000 people each year experience cyberstalking. Cyberstalkers may send harassing or threatening e-mails or chat room messages to the victim, or they may encourage others to harass the victim by posting inflammatory messages and personal information on bulletin boards or chat rooms.

To protect yourself online:

- Never use your real name as an e-mail user name or chat room nickname. Select an age- and gender-neutral identity.
- Avoid filling out profiles for accounts related to e-mail use or chat room activities with information that could be used to identify you.
- Do not share personal information in public spaces anywhere online or give it to strangers.
- Learn how to filter unwanted e-mail messages.
- If you experience harassment online, do not respond to the harasser. Log off or surf elsewhere. Save all communications for evidence. If harassment continues, report it to the harasser's Internet service provider, your Internet service provider, and the local police.
- Don't agree to meet someone you've met online face-to-face unless you feel completely comfortable about it. Schedule a series of phone conversations first. Meet initially in a very public place and bring along a friend to increase your safety.

Coping After Terrorism, Mass Violence, or Natural Disasters

Trauma from natural disasters—for example, hurricanes, tornadoes, floods, and earthquakes—can be similar to trauma experienced from violent attacks. Whether episodes of mass violence such as occurred in New York 2001 and Boston 2013 or the multiple shootings that happen around the country each year, some people suffer direct physical harm and loss of loved ones. Many others experience emotional distress and are robbed of their sense of security.

Each person reacts differently to traumatic disaster, and it is normal to experience a variety of responses. Reactions may include disbelief and shock, fear, anger and resentment, anxiety about the future, difficulty concentrating or making decisions, mood swings, irritability, sadness and depression, panic, guilt, apathy, feelings of isolation or powerlessness, and many of the behavioral signs such as headaches or insomnia that are associated with excess stress (see Chapter 10). Reactions may occur immediately or may be delayed until weeks or months after the event.

Taking positive steps can help you cope with powerful emotions. Consider the following strategies:

- Share your experiences and emotions with friends and family members. Be a supportive listener. Reassure children and encourage them to talk about what they are feeling.
- Take care of your mind and body. Choose a healthy diet, exercise regularly, get plenty of sleep, and practice relaxation techniques.

- Don't turn to unhealthy coping techniques such as using alcohol or other drugs.
- Take a break from media reports and images, and try not to develop nightmare scenarios for possible future events.
- Reestablish your routines at home, school, and work.
- Find ways to help others. Donating money, blood, food, clothes, or time can ease difficult emotions and give you a greater sense of control.

Everyone copes with tragedy in a different way and recovers at a different pace. If you feel overwhelmed by your emotions, seek professional help. Additional information about coping with terrorism and violence is available from the Federal Emergency Management Agency (www.fema.gov), the U.S. Department of Justice (www.usdoj.gov), and the National Mental Health Association (www.nmha.org).

Emergency Preparedness

Most prevention and coping activities related to terrorism, mass violence, and natural disasters occur at the federal, state, and community levels. However, one step you can take is to put together an emergency plan and kit for your family or household that can serve for any type of emergency or disaster.

Emergency Supplies   Your kit of emergency supplies should include everything you'll need to make it on your own for at least 3 days. You'll need nonperishable food, water, first-aid and sanitation supplies, a battery-powered radio, clothing, a flashlight, cash, keys, copies of important documents, and supplies for sleeping outdoors in any weather. Remember special-needs items for infants, seniors, and pets. Supplies for a basic emergency kit are listed in Figure A.2; add to your kit based on your family situation and the type of problems most likely to occur in your area.

You may want to create several kinds of emergency kits. The primary one would contain supplies for home use. Put together a smaller, lightweight version that you can take with you if you are forced to evacuate your residence. Smaller kits for your car and your workplace are also recommended.

A Family or Household Plan   You and your family or household members should have a plan about where to meet and how to communicate. Choose at least two potential meeting places—one in your neighborhood and one or more in other areas. Your community may also have set locations for community shelters. Where you go may depend on the circumstances of the emergency situation. Use your common sense, and listen to the radio or television for instructions from emergency officials about whether to evacuate or stay in place. In addition, know all the transportation options in the vicinity of your home, school, and workplace; roadways and public transit may be affected, so a sturdy pair of walking shoes is a good item to keep in your emergency kit.

Everyone in the family or household should also have the same emergency contact person to call, preferably someone who lives outside the immediate area and won't be affected by the same local disaster. Local phone service may be significantly disrupted, so long-distance

Basic emergency supplies

- Map of the area for locating evacuation routes or shelters
- Cash, coins, and credit cards
- Copies of important documents stored in watertight container
- Emergency contact list and phone numbers
- Extra sets of house and car keys
- Flashlights or lightsticks
- Battery- or solar-powered radio
- Battery-powered alarm clock
- Extra batteries and bulbs
- Cell phone

- Signal flares
- Fire extinguisher (small A-B-C type)
- Whistle
- Ladder
- Tube tent and rope
- Sleeping bags or warm blankets
- Foam pads, pillows, baby bed
- Complete change of warm clothing, footwear, outerware (jacket or coat, long pants, long-sleeved shirt, sturdy shoes, hat, gloves, raingear, extra socks and underwear, sunglasses)
- Work gloves

- Shutoff wrench for gas and water supplies
- Shovel, hammer, pliers, screwdriver, and other tools
- Compass
- Matches in a waterproof container
- Aluminum foil
- Plastic storage containers, bucket
- Duct tape, utility knife, and scissors
- Paper, pens, pencils
- Needles and thread

First aid kit

- First aid manual
- Thermometer
- Scissors
- Tweezers
- Safety pins, safety razor blades
- Needle
- Latex or other sterile gloves
- Sterile gauze pads
- Cleansing agents (soap, isopropyl alcohol, antiseptic towelettes)
- Sunscreen

- Insect repellent
- Antibiotic ointment
- Burn ointment
- Petroleum jelly or another lubricant
- Sterile adhesive bandages, several sizes
- Sterile rolled bandages and triangular bandages
- Cotton balls
- Eyewash solution
- Chemical heat and cold packs
- Aspirin or nonaspirin pain reliever

- Anti-diarrhea medication
- Laxative
- Antacid
- Activated charcoal (use if advised by Poison Control Center)
- Potassium iodide (use following radiation exposure if advised by local health authorities)
- Prescription medications and prescribed medical supplies
- List of medications, dosages, and any allergies
- Medicine dropper

Special needs items

- Infant care needs (formula, bottles, diapers, powdered milk, diaper rash ointment)
- Books or toys
- Extra eyeglasses, contact lenses and supplies

- Feminine hygiene supplies
- Denture needs
- Hearing aid or wheelchair batteries; other special equipment

- Pet care supplies, including leash, pet carrier, copy of vaccination history, and tie-out stakes
- Other (list)

Food and related supplies

- Manual (nonelectric) can opener
- Utility knife
- Paper towels

- Eating utensils: Mess kits, or paper cups and plates and utensils
- Plastic garbage bags and resealing bags

- Small cooking stove and cooking fuel (if food must be cooked)
- Water purification tablets

Water: Three-day-supply, at least 1 gallon of water per person per day, stored in plastic containers:

Number of people: _____ x 1 gallon x 3 days = _____ total minimum gallons of water

Store additional water if you live in a hot climate or if your household includes infants, pregnant women, or people with special health needs. Don't forget to store water for pets. Containers can be sterilized by rinsing them with a diluted bleach solution (one part bleach to ten parts water). Replace your water supply every six months.

Food: At least a three-day supply of nonperishable foods—those requiring no refrigeration, preparation, or cooking and little or no water. Choose foods from the following list and add foods that members of your household will eat. Replace items in your food supply every six months.

- Ready-to-eat canned meats, fruits, soups, and vegetables
- Protein or fruit bars
- Dry cereal or granola
- Peanut butter
- Sugar, salt, pepper

- Dried fruit
- Nuts
- Crackers
- Canned, powdered, or boxed juices
- Nonperishable pasteurized milk or powered milk
- Coffee, tea, sodas

- High-energy foods
- Comfort/stress foods
- MREs (military rations)
- Infant formula and baby foods
- Pet foods

Sanitation

- Plastic garbage bags (and ties)
- Toilet paper
- Moist towelettes or hand soap
- Washcloth and towel

- Personal hygiene items (toothbrush, shampoo, deodorant, comb, shaving cream, and so on)
- Plastic bucket with tight lid

- Household chlorine bleach, disinfectant
- Powdered lime
- Small shovel for digging latrine

For a clean air supply

Face masks or several layers of dense-weave cotton material (handkerchiefs, t-shirts, towels) that fit snugly over your nose and mouth.

Shelter-in-place supplies, to be used in an interior room to create a barrier between you and potentially contaminated air outside: Heavyweight plastic garbage bags or plastic sheeting; duct tape; scissors; and if possible, a portable air purifier with a HEPA filter.

Family emergency plan

Plan places where your family will meet; choose one location near your home and one outside your neighborhood.

Local _____ Outside neighborhood _____

Have one local and one out-of-state contact person for family members to call if separated during a disaster. (It may be easier to make long-distance calls than local calls.)

Local _____ Out-of state _____

FIGURE A.2 Sample emergency preparedness kit and plan.

calls may be more likely to go through. Everyone should carry the relevant phone numbers and addresses at all times.

It is also important to check into the emergency plans at any location where you or family members spend time, including schools and workplaces. For each location, know the safest place to be for different types of emergencies—for example, near load-bearing interior walls during an earthquake or in the basement during a tornado. Also know how to turn off water, gas, and electricity in case of damaged utility lines; keep the needed tools next to the shutoff valves.

Other steps you can take to help prepare for emergencies include taking a first-aid class and setting up an emergency response group in your neighborhood, residential building, or office. Talk with your neighbors: Who has specialized equipment (for example, a power generator) or expertise that might help in a crisis? Do older or disabled neighbors have someone to help them? More complete information about emergency preparedness is available from local government agencies and from the following:

American Academy of Pediatrics
   (www.aap.org)
American Red Cross
   (www.redcross.org)
Federal Emergency Management Agency
   (www.fema.gov)
U.S. Department of Homeland Security
   (www.ready.gov)

PROVIDING EMERGENCY CARE

You can improve someone else's chances of surviving if you are prepared to provide emergency help. A course in first aid offered by the American Red Cross and on many college campuses can teach you to respond appropriately when someone needs help. Emergency rescue techniques can save the lives of people who have stopped breathing, who are choking, or whose hearts have stopped beating. Pulmonary resuscitation (also known as rescue breathing, artificial respiration, or mouth-to-mouth resuscitation) is used when a person is not breathing (refer back to Figure A.1). Cardiopulmonary resuscitation (CPR) is used when a pulse can't be found. Training is required before a person can perform CPR. Significant changes were made to the guidelines for lay rescue CPR in 2005. Courses are offered by the American Red Cross and the American Heart Association.

When You Have to Provide Emergency Care Remain calm and act sensibly. The basic pattern for providing emergency care is *check-call-care*:

1. *Check the situation.* Make sure the scene is safe for both you and the injured person. Don't put yourself in danger; if you get hurt, too, you will be of little help to the injured person.
2. *Check the victim.* Conduct a quick head-to-toe examination. Assess the victim's signs and symptoms, such as level of responsiveness, pulse, and breathing rate. Look for bleeding and any indications of broken bones or paralysis.
3. *Call for help.* Call 9-1-1 or a local emergency number. Identify yourself and give as much information as you can about the condition of the victim and what happened.
4. *Care for the victim.* If the situation requires immediate action (no pulse, shock, etc.), provide first aid if you are trained to do so (refer back to Figure A.1).

Selected Bibliography

Bren, L. 2005. Prevent your child from choking. *FDA Consumer,* September/ October.

Centers for Disease Control and Prevention. 2014. Injury Prevention and Control: Key Data and Statistics. http://www.cdc.gov/injury/overview/data.html.

Central Intelligence Agency. 2011. *The World Factbook.* Washington, D.C.: Central Intelligence Agency.

Federal Bureau of Investigation. 2009. *Hate Crime Statistics,* 2008. Washington, D.C.: U.S. Department of Justice.

Federal Bureau of Investigation. 2010. *Crime in the United States:* 2009. Washington, D.C.: U.S. Department of Justice.

Insurance Information Institute. 2007. *Road Rage* (http://www.iii.org/individuals/auto /lifesaving/roadrage).

Iudice, A., et al. 2005. Effects of prolonged wakefulness combined with alcohol and hands-free cell phone divided attention tasks on simulated driving. *Human Psychopharmacology* 20(2): 125–132.

National Center for Health Statistics. 2012. Deaths: Preliminary data for 2010. *National Vital Statistics Reports* 64(4): 1–51.

National Safety Council. 2013. *Injury Facts 2013 Edition.* Itasca, IL: National Safety Council.

National Center for Health Statistics. 2013. Deaths: Final data for 2013. (http://www .cdc.gov/nchs/data/nvsr/nvsr64/nvsr64_02.pdf).

National Highway Traffic Safety Administration. *Safercar.gov.* Washington, D.C. (http://www.safercar.gov/Vehicle+Shoppers/Air+Bags/Side-Impact+Air+Bags).

Rape Treatment Center. Getting help: What to do if you are raped. (http://www.911rape .org/getting-help/what-to-do-if-you-are-raped).

U.S. Department of Homeland Security. 2014. *Ready America* (www.ready.gov).

EXERCISE GUIDELINES FOR PEOPLE WITH SPECIAL HEALTH CONCERNS

As explained in Chapters 2–7, regular, appropriate exercise is safe and beneficial for many people with chronic conditions or other special health concerns. In fact, for many people with special health concerns, the risks associated with not exercising are far greater than those associated with a moderate program of regular exercise.

The fitness recommendations made throughout this book are intended for the general population and can serve as basic guidelines for any exercise program. If you have a chronic health condition, however, you may need to modify your exercise program to accommodate your situation. This appendix presents precautions and specialized recommendations for people with a variety of special health concerns.

These recommendations, however, are not intended to replace a physician's advice. If you have a special health concern, talk to your physician before starting any exercise program.

ARTHRITIS

- Begin an exercise program as early as possible in the course of the disease.
- Warm up thoroughly before each workout to loosen stiff muscles and lower the risk of injury.
- For cardiorespiratory endurance exercise, avoid high-impact activities that may damage arthritic joints. Consider swimming, water walking, or another type of exercise that can be done in a warm pool.
- Strength train the whole body. Pay special attention to muscles that support and protect affected joints. For example, build the quadriceps, hamstrings, and calf muscles to support and protect arthritic knees. Start with small amounts of weight and gradually increase the intensity of your workouts.
- Perform flexibility exercises daily to maintain joint mobility.

ASTHMA

- Exercise regularly. Acute attacks are more likely to occur if you exercise only occasionally.
- Carry medication during workouts and avoid exercising alone. Use your inhaler as recommended by your physician.
- Warm up and cool down slowly to reduce the risk of acute attacks.
- When starting an exercise program, choose self-paced endurance activities, especially those involving interval training (short bouts of exercise followed by a rest period). Gradually increase the intensity of your cardiorespiratory endurance workouts.
- Educate yourself about situations that can trigger an asthma attack and act accordingly when exercising. For example, cold, dry air can trigger or worsen an attack. Pollen, dust, and polluted air can also trigger an attack. To avoid attacks in dry air, drink water before, during, and after a workout to moisten your airways. In cold weather, cover your mouth with a mask or scarf to warm and humidify the air you breathe. Also, avoid outdoor activities during pollen season or when the air is polluted or dusty.

DIABETES

- Don't begin an exercise program unless your diabetes is under control and you have discussed exercise safety with your physician. Because people with diabetes have an increased risk for heart disease, an exercise stress test may be recommended.
- Don't exercise alone. Wear a bracelet that identifies you as someone with diabetes.
- If you take insulin or another medication, adjust the timing and amount of each dose as needed. Work with your physician and check your blood sugar level regularly so you can learn to balance your energy intake and output and your medication dosage.
- To prevent abnormally rapid absorption of injected insulin, inject it over a muscle that will not be exercised, and wait at least an hour before exercising.
- Check your blood sugar before, during, and after exercise. Adjust your diet and insulin dosage as needed. Keep high-carbohydrate foods on hand during a workout. Avoid exercise if your blood sugar level is above 250 mg/dl; if your blood sugar level is below 100 mg/dl, eat some carbohydrate-rich food before exercising.
- If you have poor circulation or numbness in your extremities, check your skin regularly for blisters and abrasions, especially on your feet. Avoid high-impact activities and wear comfortable shoes.
- For maximum benefit and minimum risk, choose moderate-intensity activities.

HEART DISEASE AND HYPERTENSION

- Check with your physician about exercise safety before increasing your activity level. Your doctor may recommend that you take an exercise stress test before starting your program.
- Exercise at moderate intensity rather than high intensity. Keep your heart rate below the level at which abnormalities appear on an exercise stress test.
- Warm up and cool down gradually. Every warm-up and cool-down session should last at least 10 minutes.

- Monitor your heart rate during exercise, and stop if you experience dizziness or chest pain.
- If your physician prescribes nitroglycerin, carry it with you during exercise. If you take a beta-blocker to manage hypertension, use RPE rather than heart rate to monitor your exercise intensity (beta-blockers reduce heart rate). Exercise at an RPE level of "fairly light" to "somewhat hard." Your breathing should be unlabored, and you should be able to talk during exercise.
- Don't hold your breath when exercising. Doing so can cause sudden, steep increases in blood pressure. Take special care during weight training and do not lift heavy loads. Exhale during the exertion phase of each lift.
- Increase exercise frequency, intensity, and time very gradually.

OBESITY

- For maximum benefit and minimum risk, begin by choosing low- to moderate-intensity activities. Increase intensity slowly as your fitness improves. Studies of overweight people show that exercising at moderate to high intensities causes more fat loss than training at low intensities.
- People who want to lose weight or maintain weight loss should exercise moderately for 60 minutes or more every day. To get the benefit of 60 minutes of exercise, you can exercise all at once or divide your total activity time into sessions of 10, 20, or 30 minutes.
- Choose non- or low-weight-bearing activities such as swimming, water exercises, cycling, or walking. Low-impact activities are less likely to cause joint problems or injuries.

- Stay alert for symptoms of heat-related problems during exercise (as described in Chapter 3). Obese people are vulnerable to heat intolerance.
- Ease into your exercise program and increase overload gradually. Increase time and frequency of exercise before increasing intensity.
- Include strength training in your fitness program to build or maintain muscle mass.
- Try to include as much lifestyle physical activity in your daily routine as possible.

OSTEOPOROSIS

- For cardiorespiratory endurance activities, exercise at the maximum intensity that causes no significant discomfort. If possible, choose low-impact, weight-bearing exercises to help safely maintain bone density. (See Chapter 8 for strategies for building and maintaining bone density.)
- To prevent fractures, avoid any activity or movement that stresses the back or carries a risk of falling.
- Include weight training in your exercise program to improve strength and balance and to reduce the risk of falls and fractures. Always use proper exercise technique and avoid lifting heavy loads.
- Include muscle-strengthening exercises three days per week.
- Include bone-strengthening exercises, such as jumping, at least three days per week, if they are safe for you. If you already have bone loss, avoid high-impact activities.

MONITORING YOUR PROGRESS

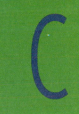

NAME _____ **SECTION** _____ **DATE** _____

As you completed the labs listed below, you entered the results in the Preprogram Assessment column of this appendix. Now that you have been involved in a fitness and wellness program for some time, do the labs again and enter your new results in the Postprogram Assessment column. You will probably notice improvement in several areas. Congratulations! If you are not satisfied with your progress thus far, refer to the tips for successful behavior change in Chapter 1 and throughout this book. Remember fitness and wellness are forever. The time you invest now in developing a comprehensive, individualized program will pay off in a richer, more vital life in the years to come.

	Preprogram Assessment	Postprogram Assessment
LAB 2.3 Pedometer	Daily steps: _____	Daily steps: _____
LAB 3.1 Cardiorespiratory Endurance		
1-mile walk test	$\dot{V}O_{2max}$: _____ Rating: _____	$\dot{V}O_{2max}$: _____ Rating: _____
3-minute step test	$\dot{V}O_{2max}$: _____ Rating: _____	$\dot{V}O_{2max}$: _____ Rating: _____
1.5-mile run-walk test	$\dot{V}O_{2max}$: _____ Rating: _____	$\dot{V}O_{2max}$: _____ Rating: _____
Beep test	$\dot{V}O_{2max}$: _____ Rating: _____	$\dot{V}O_{2max}$: _____ Rating: _____
12-minute swim test	Rating: _____	Rating: _____
LAB 4.1 Muscular Strength		
Maximum bench press test	Weight: _____ lb Rating: _____	Weight: _____ lb Rating: _____
LAB 4.2 Muscular Endurance		
Curl-up test	Number: _____ Rating: _____	Number: _____ Rating: _____
Push-up test	Number: _____ Rating: _____	Number: _____ Rating: _____
Squat endurance test	Number: _____ Rating: _____	Number: _____ Rating: _____
LAB 5.1 Flexibility		
Sit-and-reach test	Score: _____ cm Rating: _____	Score: _____ cm Rating: _____
LAB 5.3 Low-Back Muscular Endurance		
Side bridge endurance test	Right: _____ sec. Rating: _____	Right: _____ sec. Rating: _____
	Left: _____ sec. Rating: _____	Left: _____ sec. Rating: _____
Trunk flexors endurance test	Trunk flexors: _____ sec. Rating: _____	Trunk flexors: _____ sec. Rating: _____
Back extensors endurance test	Back extensors: _____ sec. Rating: _____	Back extensors: _____ sec. Rating: _____

	Preprogram Assessment	**Postprogram Assessment**
LAB 6.1 Body Composition Body mass index Skinfold measurements (or other methods for determining percent body fat) Waist circumference Waist-to-hip ratio	BMI: _____ kg/m² Rating: _____ Sum of 3 skinfolds: _____ mm % body fat: _____% Rating: _____ Circumf.: _____ Rating: Ratio: _____ Rating: _____	BMI: _____ kg/m² Rating: _____ Sum of 3 skinfolds: _____ mm % body fat: _____% Rating: _____ Circumf.: _____ Rating: _____ Ratio: _____ Rating: _____
LAB 8.1 Daily Diet Number of oz-eq Number of cups Number of cups Number of cups Number of oz-eq Number of tsp Number of g Number of g or tsp	Grains: _____ Vegetables: _____ Fruits: _____ Milk: _____ Meat or beans: _____ Oils: _____ Solid fats: _____ Added sugars: _____	Grains: _____ Vegetables: _____ Fruits: _____ Milk: _____ Meat or beans: _____ Oils: _____ Solid fats: _____ Added sugars: _____
LAB 8.2 Dietary Analysis Percentage of calories Percentage of calories Percentage of calories Percentage of calories	From protein: _____ % From fat: _____ % From saturated fat: _____ % From carbohydrate: _____ %	From protein: _____ % From fat: _____ % From saturated fat: _____ % From carbohydrate: _____ %
LAB 9.1 Daily Energy Needs	Daily energy needs: _____ cal/day	Daily energy needs: _____ cal/day
LAB 10.1 Identifying Stressors	Average weekly stress score: _____	Average weekly stress score: _____
LAB 11.1 Cardiovascular Health CVD risk assessment Hostility assessment	Score: _____ Estimated risk: _____ Score: _____ Rating: _____	Score: _____ Estimated risk: _____ Score: _____ Rating: _____
LAB 12.1 Cancer Prevention Diet: Number of servings Skin cancer	Fruits/vegetables: _____ Score: _____ Risk: _____	Fruits/vegetables: _____ Score: _____ Risk: _____

CREDITS

Design Elements

Wellness in Digital Age(smart watch): © Hong Li/ Getty RF; Evidence for Exercise(sneakers & stethoscope): © VstockLLC/Getty Images RF; Critical Consumer(scale): © pagadesign/Getty RF; Take Charge(women red shirt): © VisualsCommuncaitions/ Getty RF; Diversity Matters(large group): © Tetra Images/ Getty RF; Fitness Tips(dumbbells): © Image Source; Hands-on lab activities(smart phone): © McGraw-Hill Education/Mark Dierker; Exercise photos and online videos(squat): © Taylor Robertson Photography

Front Matter

p. i: © Yuri_Arcurs/Getty Images RF; p. xi: © McGraw-Hill Education. Mark Dierker, photographer

Chapter 1

Opener: © Image Source/Getty Images RF; p. 4: © Jonathan Goldberg/Alamy; p. 5: © Robin Lund/ Alamy RF; p. 7: © Cultura Creative/Alamy RF; p. 11: © yellowdog/Getty Images RF; p. 12: Tetra Images/ Getty Images RF; p. 14: © Tony Tallec/Alamy RF; 1.6(bike): © Adam Brown/Getty Images RF; (desk): Ray Kachatorian/Getty Images; p. 18: © Tony Tallec/ Alamy RF.

Chapter 2

Opener: © Lane Oatey/Blue Jean Images/Getty Images RF; p. 32: © moodboard/Alamy RF; p. 33: © John P Kelly/Getty Images; p. 35: © Getty Images; p. 36: © Harold Cunningham/Getty Images; p. 37: © Hero Images/Getty Images RF; 2.3(sedentary): © Stockbyte/ PunchStock RF; (Strength): © Ryan McVay/Getty Images RF; (Flexibility): Courtesy Shirlee Stevens; (Cardiorespiratory): © Joaquin Palting/Getty Images RF; (Moderate-Intensity): © Doug Menuez/Getty Images RF; (raking leaves): © UpperCut Images/Alamy RF; 2.4(physical): © RubberBall Productions RF; (moderate); © Royalty Free/Corbis; (vigorous): © Thinkstock Images/ Jupiterimages RF; p. 41: © JoseGirarte/Getty RF; p. 44: © IT Stock/PunchStock RF.

Chapter 3

Opener: © Michael Heffernan/Getty Images; p. 65: © Paul Burns/Digital Vision/Getty Images RF; 3.4(both): Courtesy Robin Mouat; p. 68: © Stephen Barnes/Northern Ireland/Alamy; p. 69: © Blend Images/Alamy; p. 73: © keepics/Alamy; p. 74: © Cultura RM/Edwin Jimenez/Getty Images; p. 75: © Tetra Images/Alamy RF; p. 80(shoe): © Siede Preis/ PhotoDisc/Getty Images RF.

Chapter 4

Opener: © Juriah Mosin/Alamy RF; p. 100: © JGI/ Tom Grill/Getty Images RF; 4.2a: © grant pritchard/ Alamy RF; 4.2b,c: Courtesy Neil A. Tanner; p. 103(left): © McGraw-Hill Education/David Scott; (middle): © Assembly/Getty Images RF; (right): © Taylor Robertson Photography; p. 107: Courtesy Neil A. Tanner; p. 110(all): © Taylor Robertson Photography; p. 111(Ex 3a–c): © Taylor Robertson Photography; (Ex 4a,b): Courtesy Neil A. Tanner; p. 112(Ex 5a,b): © Wayne Glusker; (Ex 6): Courtesy Joseph Quever; p. 113(all): © Taylor Robertson Photography; p. 114(Ex 10): © Taylor Robertson Photography; (Ex 1a,b): © Wayne Glusker; p. 115(Ex 2a–c): © Taylor Robertson Photography; (Ex 3a,b): Courtesy Joseph Quever; (Ex 4a,b): © Wayne Glusker; p. 116(Ex 5a,b): Courtesy Joseph Quever; (Ex 6a,b): Courtesy Neil A. Tanner; (Ex 7a,b): © Taylor Robertson Photography; p. 117 (Ex 8a,b): Courtesy Shirlee Stevens; (Ex 9a–10b); © Taylor Robertson Photography; p. 118(Ex 11–1b): © Taylor Robertson Photography; (Ex 2a,b): Courtesy Neil A. Tanner; p. 119 (Ex 3a,b): © Wayne Glusker; (Ex 4a–5b): Courtesy Joseph Quever; p. 120(Ex 6a,b): Courtesy Neil A. Tanner; (Ex 7a–8b): Courtesy Joseph Quever; p. 121(Ex 9a,b): © Taylor Robertson Photography; (Ex 10a,b): © Wayne Glusker; (Ex 11a,b): Courtesy Joseph Quever; p. 122(Ex 12a,b): © Wayne Glusker; (Ex 13a,b): Courtesy Joseph Quever; p. 127: © Wayne Glusker; p. 129(all): Courtesy Tom Fahey; p. 130–131: © Wayne Glusker; p. 133–134: Courtesy Neil A. Tanner; p. 135: © Wayne Glusker.

Chapter 5

Opener: © Andres Rodriguez/Alamy RF; p. 142: © Dougal Waters/Getty Images RF; p. 143: © Image Source/Alamy RF; p. 145(both): Courtesy Shirlee Stevens; p. 147(Ex 1): © Taylor Robertson Photography; (Ex 2–3b): © Wayne Glusker; p. 148(Ex 4&5): © Taylor Robertson Photography; (Ex 6): Courtesy Neil A. Tanner; p. 149(Ex 7); (Ex 8): © Taylor Robertson Photography); (Ex 9&10): © Wayne Glusker; p. 150(Ex 11a–c): Courtesy Shirlee Stevens; (Ex 12a,b): Courtesy Neil A. Tanner; (Ex 13): © Taylor Robertson Photography; p. 155: © Wavebreakmedia Ltd/Getty Images RF; p. 156(Ex 1a,b): © Wayne Glusker; (Ex 4): © Taylor Robertson Photography; p. 157(Ex 8): Courtesy Neil A. Tanner; p. 158(Ex 9–11): © Taylor Robertson Photography; p. 163: Courtesy Shirlee Stevens; p. 164: © Wayne Glusker; p. 171(top, middle): © Taylor Robertson Photography; (bottom): © Wayne Glusker; p. 172(top): Courtesy Joseph Quever; (bottom): © Taylor Robertson Photography.

Chapter 6

Opener: © Cultura Creative/Alamy RF; p. 177: © imtmphoto/Alamy RF; p. 180: © Fertnig/Getty Images RF; p. 181(jogging): © EyeWire Collection/ Getty Images RF; p. 185(top): BOD POD® Body Composition Tracking System photo provided courtesy of COSMED USA, Inc.; (bottom): © Julie Brown/ Custom Medical Stock Photo; p. 186(handheld BIA): © Lebazele/Getty Images RF; (varying body shapes): © FredFroese/Getty Images RF; p. 192(all): Courtesy Shirlee Stevens.

Chapter 7

Opener: © Getty Images/iStockphoto RF; p. 202: yellowdog/Getty Images RF; p. 206: © Vadym Drobot/ Alamy RF; p. 208: © mezzotint-alamy/Alamy RF; p. 209: © Zia Soleil/Iconica/Getty Images.

Chapter 8

Opener: © Fotokia/Getty Images; p. 230: © Diana Haronis/Getty Images; 8.2: © Brand X Pictures/ PunchStock RF; p. 232: © Smneedham/Getty Images p. 233: © Richard Levine/Alamy; p. 239: © Getty Images; p. 242: © Blend Images/SuperStock RF; p. 244: © Marc Romanelli/Getty Images; p. 246: © Nicolas McComber/Getty Images RF; p. 249: © Patrick Murphy-Racey/Sports Illustrated/Getty Images; p. 254: © Joe Madeira/Getty Images RF.

INDEX

Page numbers followed by b indicate boxes; f, figures; (lab), laboratory activities; t, tables. **Boldface** page numbers indicate where terms are defined. Page numbers preceded by capitalized A, B, or C indicate Appendixes.

C